Practical Intracardiac
Echocardiography in
Electrophysiology

This book is dedicated to my wife, Helen, our daughter, Kenna, and her children, Jonathan and Jeremy [Jian-Fang Ren]

Practical Intracardiac Echocardiography in Electrophysiology

Jian-Fang Ren, MD
Senior Research Investigator
Clinical and Experimental Electrophysiology Laboratories
University of Pennsylvania School of Medicine
Philadelphia, PA, USA

Francis E. Marchlinski, MD
Professor of Medicine and Director of Electrophysiology
University of Pennsylvania Health System
Philadelphia, PA, USA

David J. Callans, MD
Professor of Medicine and
Director of the Cardiac Electrophysiology Laboratory
Hospital of the University of Pennsylvania
Philadelphia, PA, USA

David Schwartzman, MD
Associate Professor of Medicine
University of Pittsburgh
Pittsburgh, PA, USA

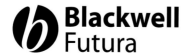

© 2006 Jian-Fang Ren, Francis E. Marchlinski, David J. Callans, and David Schwartzman
Published by Blackwell Publishing
Blackwell Futura is an imprint of Blackwell Publishing

Blackwell Publishing, Inc., 350 Main Street, Malden, Massachusetts 02148-5020, USA
Blackwell Publishing Ltd, 9600 Garsington Road, Oxford OX4 2DQ, UK
Blackwell Science Asia Pty Ltd, 550 Swanston Street, Carlton, Victoria 3053, Australia

ISBN-13: 978-1-4051-3500-9
ISBN-10: 1-4051-3500-X

Library of Congress Cataloging-in-Publication Data

Ren, Jian-Fang.
    Practical intracardiac Echocardiography in electrophysiology/author and co-authors,
    Jian-Fang Ren . . . [et al.].
        p.; cm.
    1. Echocardiography. 2. Cardiac catheterization. I. Title.
    [DNLM: 1. Echocardiography–methods. 2. Electrophysiologic
    Techniques, Caridiac–methods. 3. Heart Catheterization.
    4. Ultrasonography, Interventional–methods. WG 141.5.E2 R393 2005]
    RC683.5.U5R46 2005
    616.1'207543–dc22   2005010455

A catalogue record for this title is available from the British Library

Commissioning Editor: Gina Almond
Development Editor: Vicki Donald
Set in 9/12 pt Minion by Newgen Imaging Systems (P) Ltd., Chennai, India
Printed and bound by Replika Press, PVT Ltd., Haryana, India

For further information on Blackwell Publishing, visit our website:
www.blackwellcardiology.com

The publisher's policy is to use permanent paper from mills that operate a sustainable
forestry policy, and which has been manufactured from pulp processed using acid-free and
elementary chlorine-free practices. Furthermore, the publisher ensures that the text paper
and cover board used have met acceptable environmental accreditation standards.

Notice: The indications and dosages of all drugs in this book have been recommended in the
medical literature and conform to the practices of the general community. The medications
described do not necessarily have specific approval by the Food and Drug Administration for
use in the diseases and dosages for which they are recommended. The package insert for
each drug should be consulted for use and dosage as approved by the FDA. Because standards
for usage change, it is advisable to keep abreast of revised recommendations, particularly those
concerning new drugs.

Contents

Contributors

David J. Callans, MD
Professor of Medicine and
Director of the Cardiac Electrophysiology Laboratory
Hospital of the University of Pennsylvania
Philadelphia, PA, USA

Francis E. Marchlinski, MD
Professor of Medicine and Director of Electrophysiology
University of Pennsylvania Health System
Philadelphia, PA, USA

Jian-Fang Ren, MD
Senior Research Investigator
Clinical and Experimental Electrophysiology Laboratories
University of Pennsylvania School of Medicine
Philadelphia, PA, USA

David Schwartzman, MD
Associate Professor of Medicine
University of Pittsburgh
Pittsburgh, PA, USA

Jeffrey P. Weiss, MD
Associate Professor of Radiology
Temple University
Philadelphia, PA, USA

Preface

Tremendous advances in intracardiac echocardiography (ICE) have coincided with the evolution of interventional electrophysiology. The development of the latter has created a pressing need to directly image cardiac anatomy during catheter manipulation and ablative therapy. The lower frequency (12.5–9 MHz) mechanical ultrasound catheter and, more recently, the electronic phased-array diagnostic ultrasound catheter with Doppler color flow imaging have facilitated the use of an intravascular approach to image cardiac and adjacent non cardiac structures accurately, assess function and monitor closely for complications. *Practical Intracardiac Echocardiography in Electrophysiology* is designed to provide the electrophysiologist and echocardiographer with an in-depth view of the role and value of ICE during electrophysiologic procedures. A guide to techniques used for optimal ICE imaging in cardiac electrophysiology is provided. In addition, new and less well-recognized uses of ICE in electrophysiological procedures are described and their clinical applications are presented. This book can also be used as a practical atlas as it has over 500 illustrations, many of which are in color. Readers need not be experts in the field of echocardiography to benefit from this practical approach to intracardiac imaging in electrophysiology.

Organized into 12 chapters, this text begins with Chapter 1 describing the basic concepts of ICE imaging. Chapter 2 deals with imaging equipment, ultrasound catheters, technical controls, and right heart catheterization techniques. Information regarding optimal image acquisition and Doppler recording is presented and identification of acoustic artifacts on ICE image is described. Chapter 3 is devoted to ICE imaging techniques. Major emphasis has been placed on optimizing transducer positioning and imaging specific cardiac structures especially as they relate to electrophysiological arrhythmia substrate.

Chapter 4 describes commonly encountered cardiac anatomic and functional abnormalities. The next six chapters cover current clinical applications of ICE that include guiding and monitoring of transseptal catheterization (Chapter 5) as well as mapping/ablating of inappropriate sinus tachycardia/atrial tachycardias, atrial fibrillation, ventricular tachycardia, and Wolff–Parkinson–White syndrome (Chapters 6–10). One of the more powerful applications of ICE imaging lies in its ability to efficiently identify procedural complications before they become life threatening. Chapter 11 provides a detailed description of these complications in addition to those described throughout the text. The final chapter describes experimental applications of ICE in swine.

This book would not have been possible without the effort and dedication of its numerous contributors and for this, I owe them my highest regard. I am also honored to have had the privilege of working with Drs Francis E. Marchlinski, David J. Callans, and David Schwartzman, to whom I owe the success of my career. I am also grateful for the support of Acuson-Siemens Medical Solutions USA, Inc. especially in sponsoring the AcuNav peer training courses in which I had the pleasure to participate. These sessions provided me the opportunity to meet so many enthusiastic echocardiographers and electrophysiologists eager to learn about this new technology and imaging application and sharpened my focus on what information needed to be conveyed about this exciting new field. In addition, this book is a tribute to the magnificent work of all the personnel at Blackwell Publishing Ltd. Last, I would like to take this opportunity to express my appreciation of all the cardiologists, trainees, and staff who have worked tireless with me over the years in the University of Pennsylvania Health System.

Jian-Fang Ren

CHAPTER 1

Intracardiac Echocardiography: Basic Concepts

Jian-Fang Ren, MD*, & Francis E. Marchlinski,* MD

Introduction

Intracardiac echocardiography (ICE), also termed intracardiac ultrasound catheter imaging, allows visualization of the heart from within the cardiac chambers or from within the great vessels. Catheter-based ICE has advanced from devices bearing single-element transducers and M-mode transducers [1,2] to the current technology, which allows for higher resolution two-dimensional imaging with pulsed/continuous-wave Doppler and color flow evaluation of blood vessels and intracardiac structures.

Historical developments

Over the past 15 years, transducer miniaturization and advances in microelectric and piezoelectric crystal technology have allowed ICE to become an invaluable tool for cardiac assessment. No other technology allows for such superb temporal and spatial resolution through opaque blood [3–7]. In the late 1970s and early 1980s, real-time M-mode echocardiography was tested for intracardiac imaging [8,9]. In the 1990s, modified transesophageal transducers with low frequency (5 or 7 MHz) were used as ultrasound catheters for intracardiac imaging research in animal models but were not in clinical use due to the large size (24–30 Fr) of the transducer [5,6,10,11]. A higher frequency (20 MHz) intravascular ultrasound catheter was available for intracardiac imaging in 1990 [12] but was suboptimal for imaging of cardiac structures due to its diminished tissue penetration. One of the initial limitations of this growing technology was the large size of the lower frequency ICE catheters. Clinical usage of these devices was limited until a 12.5 MHz (6 Fr, mechanical system, Boston Scientific Co., Watertown, MA) and a 10 MHz (10 Fr, mechanical system, Cardiovascular Imaging System, Sunnyvale, CA) ultrasound catheter were developed in the early 1990s. Clinical acceptance of these lower frequency ultrasound catheter transducers was rapid in that detailed cardiac anatomy and function could be easily defined [13–15]. The clinical efficacy and safety of ICE for diagnosis of cardiac structure and function, for guidance of radiofrequency catheter ablation, and for transseptal catheterization have been extensively described [13–20]. With further lowering of ultrasound frequency, ICE with 9 MHz mechanical ultrasound catheter (9 Fr, Boston Scientific, Co., Watertown, MA) showed enhanced imaging capability with greater depth of imaging field compared with the 12.5 and 10 MHz catheters [21,22], but they still did not allow satisfactory imaging of the left heart from the right atrium or the right ventricle in adults or an enlarged heart. Recently, a new 5.5–10 MHz, 10 Fr, electronic phased-array ultrasound catheter with pulsed/continuous-wave Doppler and color flow imaging has been developed (AcuNav, Siemens Medical Solutions USA, Inc., Mountain View, CA). This device can be used for imaging of left heart structures, for visualization of mapping/ablation catheters, and for evaluation of pulmonary vein flow [23–25]. This ultrasound catheter has a flexible tip that provides for higher resolution and deeper penetration of the left side of the heart from the right atrium during interventional cardiac electrophysiologic procedures [24,26–27].

ICE in electrophysiology

During the past 20 years, interventional cardiac electrophysiology procedures have been performed almost exclusively under fluoroscopic guidance. Although this two-dimensional "silhouette" imaging provides a general representation of cardiac anatomy, it requires substantial experience to position the intracardiac catheter at a specific intracardiac target. However, with the increasing complexity of interventional electrophysiologic procedures, accurate imaging of intracardiac anatomic structures and interventional catheter devices has been required. So transesophageal echocardiography has been used as a major complement to fluoroscopy for imaging of intracardiac structures for guidance of interventional procedures, such as radiofrequency ablation and transseptal catheterization [28–32], and for assessing/monitoring the placement of transcatheter devices [33,34]. However, several disadvantages have limited its routine use during interventional procedures, including prolonged placement of the transesophageal transducer requiring heavy sedation and/or general anesthesia [30,35], the risk of vagal nerve stimulation that can be a potentially serious complication, and problems with inadequate orientation of transesophageal imaging planes for visualization of specific cardiac structures [10]. The new catheter-based ICE with mechanical radial imaging (9 MHz, 9 Fr) has demonstrated its utility for the safe and efficient guidance of transseptal catheterization [22]. For anatomically based ablation procedures in the right heart, this device can provide real-time guidance and monitoring of catheter location, its tissue contact and stability, and assessment of the targeted lesion, such as in sinus node ablation [36]. Electronically phased-array ICE can provide cardiac structural and functional imaging in more detail, especially for the left heart, which is comparable with transesophageal echocardiography, but without manipulation in a limited esophageal space. In contrast to the mechanical radial imaging catheter with a fixed ultrasound frequency and rigid tip, the electronic phased-array ICE catheter has variable ultrasonic frequency from 5.5 to 10 MHz and a deflectable tip, which provides greater detail and increased imaging depth, even in patients with cardiomegaly [24]. It also provides hemodynamic evaluation with Doppler and color flow imaging for the atria, ventricles, and the great vessels. An additional benefit of this newer technology is that the imaging catheter can remain in the right heart safely during the entire procedure with excellent patient tolerance [24]. The role of ICE during electrophysiologic procedures

has been further demonstrated not only in guiding transseptal catheterization and assistance in catheter placement in the right heart, but also with assistance in placement of mapping/ablation catheters in the left heart, for instance in the pulmonary vein ostia or at the aortic valve cusps [37–39]. Rapid assessment of the pulmonary vein flow velocity and identification of hemodynamically significant stenosis can be made during pulmonary vein ablation procedures [25]. Instant detection of procedural complications, such as left atrial thrombus formation [40] and pericardial effusion, has allowed for early management strategies that limit adverse outcome [24]. More recently, ICE has been used to prevent esophageal damage during radiofrequency catheter ablation at the posterior left atrial wall adjacent to the esophagus by online assessment of lesion development [41,42]. Additionally, appropriate utilization of these powerful imaging tools has been accompanied by a reduction of fluoroscopic exposure time for both the patient and the physician which has been another benefit of ICE guidance [16,20,22].

Future directions

ICE heralds a novel era of catheter-based intracardiac ultrasound imaging technology. Additional improvement can be expected in the near future allowing multiplane and computer-reconstructed three-dimensional imaging [43,44], which will provide more rapid and efficient diagnosis, guidance, and monitoring. Although there are no reported complications directly related to the use of the ultrasound catheter, further refinement and miniaturization will expand its clinical applications and ease of use of ICE imaging in diagnostic and therapeutic interventional electrophysiologic procedures, especially for ventricular tachyarrhythmia ablation directed at the ventricular endo- and/or epicardium.

References

1 Cieszynski T. Intracardiac method for the investigation of structure of the heart with the aid of ultrasonics. *Arch Immun Ter Dosw* 1960; **8**: 551–553.
2 Kossof G. Diagnostic applications of ultrasound in cardiology. *Australas Radiol* 1996; **10**: 101–106.
3 Seward JB, Khandheria BK, Oh JK, *et al.* Transesophageal echocardiography: technique, anatomic correlations,

implementation, and clinical applications. *Mayo Clin Proc* 1988; **63**: 649–680.

4 Bom N, ten Hoff H, Lancee CT, Gussenhoven WJ, Bosch JG. Early and recent intraluminal ultrasound devices. *Int J Card Imaging* 1989; **4**: 79–88.

5 Schwartz SL, Pandian NG, Kusay BS, *et al.* Real-time intracardiac two-dimensional echocardiography: an experimental study of in vivo feasibility, imaging planes, and echocardiographic anatomy. *Echocardiography* 1990; **7**: 443–456.

6 Seward JB, Khandheria BK, McGregor CGA, Locke TJ, Tajik AJ. Transvascular and intracardiac two-dimensional echocardiography. *Echocardiography* 1990; **7**: 457–464.

7 Seward JB, Packer DL, Chan RC, Curley M, Tajik AJ. Ultrasound cardioscopy: embarking on a new journey. *Mayo Clin Proc* 1996; **71**: 629–635.

8 Conetta DA, Christie LG, Pepine CJ, Nichols WW, Conti CR. Intracardiac M-mode echocardiography for continuous left ventricular monitoring: methods and potential application. *Cathet Cardiovasc Diagn* 1979; **5**: 135–143.

9 Glassman E, Kronzon I. Transvenous intracardiac echocardiography. *Am J Cardiol* 1981; **47**; 1255–1259.

10 Valdes-Cruz LM, Sideris E, Sahn DJ, *et al.* Transvascular intracardiac applications of a miniaturized phase-array ultrasonic endoscope: initial experience with intracardiac imaging in piglets. *Circulation* 1991; **83**: 1023–1027.

11 Ren JF, Schwartzman D, Michele JJ, *et al.* Lower frequency (5 MHz) intracardiac echocardiography in a large swine model: imaging views and research applications. *Ultrasound in Med & Biol* 1997; **23**: 871–877.

12 Weintraub AR, Schwartz SL, Smith J, Hsu TL, Pandian NG. Intracardiac two-dimensional echocardiography in patients with pericardial effusion and cardiac temponade. *J Am Soc Echocardiogr* 1991; **4**: 571–576.

13 Pandian NG, Kumar R, Katz SE, *et al.* Real-time intracardiac two-dimensional echocardiography: enhanced depth-of-field with a low frequency (12.5 MHz) ultrasound catheter. *Echocardiography* 1991; **8**: 407–422.

14 Schwartz SL, Gillam LD, Weintraub AR, *et al.* Intracardiac echocardiography in humans using a small sized (6 French), low frequency (12.5 MHz) ultrasound catheter: methods, imaging planes, and clinical experience. *J Am Coll Cardiol* 1993; **21**: 189–198.

15 Schwartz SL, Pandian NG, Hsu T-L, Weintraub A, Cao Q-L. Intracardiac echocardiographic imaging of cardiac abnormalities, ischemic myocardial dysfunction, and myocardial perfusion: studies with a 10 MHz ultrasound catheter. *J Am Soc Echocardiogr* 1993; **6**: 345–355.

16 Chu E, Kalman JM, Kwasman MA, *et al.* Intracardiac echocardiography during radiofrequency catheter ablation of cardiac arrhythmias in humans. *J Am Coll Cardiol* 1994; **24**: 1351–1357.

17 Mitchel JF, Gillam LD, Sanzobrino BW, Hirst JA, McKay RG. Intracardiac ultrasound imaging during transseptal catheterization. *Chest* 1995; **108**: 104–108.

18 Hung J-S, Fu M, Yeh K-H, Wu C-J, Wong P. Usefulness of intracardiac echocardiography in complex transseptal catheterization during percutaneous transvenous mitral commissurotomy. *Mayo Clin Proc* 1996; **71**: 134–140.

19 Ren JF, Schwartzman D, Lighty GW, *et al.* Multiplane transesophageal and intracardiac echocardiography in large swine: imaging technique, normal values and research applications. *Echocardiography* 1997; **14**: 135–147.

20 Kalman JM, Olgin JE, Karch MR, Lesh MD. Use of intracardiac echocardiography in interventional electrophysiology. *PACE* 1997; **20**[Pt.1]: 2248–2262.

21 Ren JF, Schwartzman D, Callans D, Marchlinski FE, Gottlieb CD, Chaudhry FA. Imaging technique and clinical utility for electrophysiologic procedures of lower frequency (9 MHz) intracardiac echocardiography. *Am J Cardiol* 1998; **82**: 1557–1560.

22 Ren JF, Schwartzman D, Callans DJ, Brode SE, Gottlieb CD, Marchlinski FE. Intracardiac echocardiography (9 MHz) in humans: methods, imaging views and clinical utility. *Ultrasound in Med & Biol* 1999; **25**: 1077–1086.

23 Packer DL, Stevens CL, Curley MG, *et al.* Intracardiac phased-array imaging: methods and initial clinical experience with high resolution, under blood visualization – initial experience with intracardiac phased-array ultrasound. *J Am Coll Cardiol* 2002; **39**: 509–516.

24 Ren JF, Marchlinski FE, Callans DJ, Herrmann HC. Clinical use of AcuNav diagnostic Ultrasound catheter imaging during left heart radiofrequency ablation and transcatheter closure procedures. *J Am Soc Echocardiogr* 2002; **15**: 1301–1308.

25 Ren JF, Marchlinski FE, Callans DJ, Zado ES. Intracardiac Doppler echocardiographic quantification of pulmonary vein flow velocity: an effective technique for monitoring pulmonary vein ostia narrowing during focal atrial fibrillation ablation. *J Cardiovasc Electrophysiol* 2002; **13**: 1076–1081.

26 Cooper JM, Epstein LM. Use of intracardiac echocardiography to guide ablation of atrial fibrillation. *Circulation* 2001; **104**: 3010–3013.

27 Marrouche NF, Martin DO, Wazni O, *et al.* Phased-array intracardiac echocardiography monitoring during pulmonary vein isolation in patients with atrial fibrillation: impact on outcome and complications. *Circulation* 2003; **107**: 2710–2716.

28 Goldman AP, Irwin JM, Glover MU, Mick W. Transesophageal echocardiography to improve positioning of radiofrequency ablation catheters in left-sided Wolff–Parkinson–White syndrome. *Pacing Clin Electrophysiol* 1991; **14**: 1245–1250.

29 Lai WW, al-Khatib Y, Klitzner TS, *et al.* Biplanar transesophageal echocardiographic direction of radiofrequency catheter ablation in children and adolescents with the Wolff–Parkinson–White syndrome. *Am J Cardiol* 1993; **71**: 872–874.

30 Saxon LA, Stevenson WG, Fonarow GC, *et al.* Transesophageal echocardiography during radiofrequency catheter ablation of ventricular tachycardia. *Am J Cardiol* 1993; **72**: 658–661.

31 Drant SE, Klitzner TS, Shannon KM, Wetzel GT, Williams RG. Guidance of radiofrequency catheter ablation by transesophageal echocardiography in children with palliated single ventricle. *Am J Cardiol* 1995; **76**: 1311–1312.

32 Tucker KJ, Curtis AB, Murphy J, *et al.* Transesophageal echocardiographic guidance of transseptal left heart catheterization during radiofrequency ablation of left-sided accessory pathways in humans. *Pacing Clin Electrophysiol* 1996; **19**: 1702–1703.

33 Ge S, Shiota T, Rice MJ, Hellenbrand WM, Sahn DJ. Images in cardiovascular medicine: transesophageal ultrasound imaging during stent implantation to relieve superior vena cava to intra-atrial baffle obstruction after mustard repair of transposition of the great arteries. *Circulation* 1995; **91**: 2679–2680.

34 Fenske W, Pfeiffer D, Babic U, Luderitz B. Images in cardiovascular medicine: multiplane transesophageal imaging during transcatheter closure of an atrial septal defect. *Circulation* 1997; **96**: 1702–1703.

35 Jaarsma W, Visseer CA, Suttorp MJ, Haagen FDH, Ernst SMPG. Transesophageal echocardiography during percutaneous balloon mitral valvuloplasty. *J Am Soc Echocardiogr* 1990; **3**: 384–391.

36 Ren JF, Marchlinski FE, Callans DJ, Zado ES. Echocardiographic lesion characteristics associated with successful ablation of inappropriate sinus tachycardia. *J Cardiovasc Electrophysiol* 2001; **12**: 814–818.

37 Lamberti F, Calo L, Pandozi C, *et al.* Radiofrequency catheter ablation of idiopathic left ventricular outflow tract tachycardia: utility of intracardiac echocardiography. *J Cardiovasc Electrophysiol* 2001; **12**: 529–535.

38 Marchlinski FE, Lin D, Dixit S, *et al.* Ventricular tachycardia from the aortic cusps: localization and ablation. In: Raviele A, ed. *Cardiac Arrhythmias.* Springer-Verlag Italia, Milan, 2003: 357–370.

39 Callans DJ, Ren J-F. Ablation of ventricular tachycardia: can the current results be improved using intracardiac echocardiography? In: Raviele A, ed. *Cardiac Arrhythmias.* Springer-Verlag Italia, Milan, 2003: 451–462.

40 Ren JF, Marchlinski FE, Callans DJ. Left atrial thrombus associated with ablation for atrial fibrillation: identification with intracardiac echocardiography. *J Am Coll Cardiol* 2004; **43**: 1861–1867.

41 Ren JF, Marchlinski FE, Callans DJ. Esophageal imaging characteristics and structural measurement during left atrial ablation for atrial fibrillation: an intracardiac echocardiographic study (abstr). *J Am Coll Cardiol* 2005; **45**: 114A.

42 Ren JF, Callans DJ, Marchlinski FE, Nayak H, Lin D, Gerstenfeld EP. Avoiding esophageal injury with power titrating during left atrial ablation for atrial fibrillation: an intracardiac echocardiographic study (abstr). *J Am Coll Cardiol* 2005; 45: 114A.

43 Okumura Y, Watanabe I, Yamada T, *et al.* Comparison of coronary sinus morphology in patients with and without atrioventricular nodal reentrant tachycardia by intracardiac echocardiography. *J Cardiovasc Electrophysiol* 2004; **15**: 269–273.

44 Ren JF, Marchlinski FE. Intracardiac ultrasound catheter imaging for electrophysiologic substrate of AV nodal reentrant tachycardia: anatomic versus electrophysiologic evidence (editorial comment). *J Cardiovasc Electrophysiol* 2004; **15**: 274–275.

2

CHAPTER 2

Imaging Equipment and Right Heart Catheterization Technique

Jian-Fang Ren, MD, *& Jeffrey P. Weiss,* MD

Imaging equipment and ultrasound catheter technology

Two types of real-time ultrasound catheter imaging systems are currently available.

The electronic phased-array ultrasound catheter (AcuNav) sector imaging system

Intracardiac echocardiography (ICE) imaging can be performed using a Sequoia ultrasound system (Acuson Corporation, Siemens Medical Solutions USA, Inc.) (Figure 2.1) with an AcuNav diagnostic ultrasound catheter (Figure 2.2). The tip of this 10 Fr catheter contains a forward facing 64-element vector phased-array transducer scanning in the longitudinal plane. Both 90° sector two-dimensional (Figure 2.3) and M-mode (Figure 2.4) imaging technology is available with tissue penetration up to 16 cm. This catheter includes variable ultrasound frequency (5.5, 7.5, 8.5, and 10 MHz), and has a four-way steerable tip (160° anteroposterior or left–right deflections), with color flow (Figure 2.5) and pulsed-/continuous-wave Doppler imaging capability (Figure 2.6). Due to the depth of our experience using this system, it will be emphasized in the remainder of this chapter.

The mechanical ultrasound catheter radial imaging system

ICE imaging can also be performed using a Hewlett-Packard Sonos intravascular imaging system with a 9 MHz catheter-based ultrasound transducer (EP Technologies™, Boston Scientific Co., San Jose, California, USA). The transducer is contained within

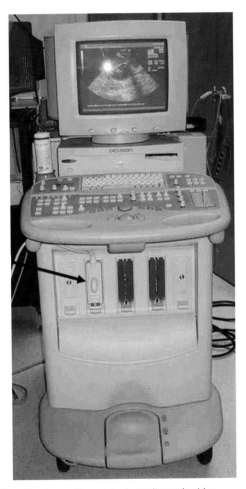

Figure 2.1 Acuson (Sequoia) echocardiograph with a keyboard of major controls below the monitor. The system is connected with an AcuNav diagnostic ultrasound catheter through the Swiftlink catheter connector (arrow).

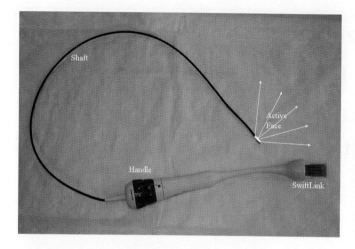

Figure 2.2 An AcuNav diagnostic ultrasound catheter with its steerable tip (active face), base of SwiftLink, and handle controls including steerable anteroposterior and left–right tip controls as well as tension control knobs.

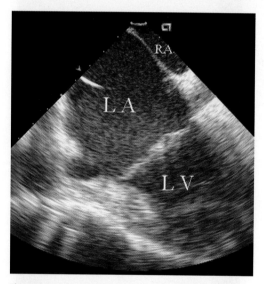

Figure 2.3 ICE image with the transducer placed near the atrial septum in the high right atrium (RA), showing a 90° sector two-dimensional image of the left atrium (LA) and left ventricle (LV).

a 9 Fr (110-cm length) polyethylene catheter shaft and has a small ultrasound element implanted in the catheter tip rotated by an external motor at 600 rpm. The ultrasound beam is emitted from a 10° forward-angled tip of the single crystal focused element (Figure 2.7). The transducer produces circular real-time images with the catheter located centrally (Figure 2.8). A frame rate of up to 30/s is available with approximately 6–8 cm of radial imaging depth. The best axial resolution is specified

to be 0.2–0.3 mm. This technology has application in transseptal catheterization and is of particular value in certain electrophysiologic procedures such as radiofrequency ablation of supraventricular tachyarrhythmias. Major limitations of this technology include lack of Doppler capability and catheter nondeflectability (see Chapter 3).

Technical controls related to basic diagnostic ultrasound physical principles

Imaging controls

Several controls are available for ICE imaging quality modification, especially for the AcuNav ultrasound catheter. These controls alter transducer frequency, imaging depth and "time-gain-compensation" (depth compensation) [1] and are important for two-dimensional imaging of specific targeted cardiac structures. However, their misuse can rapidly degrade image quality. Therefore, a thorough knowledge of their function is essential. First, one has to select a proper ultrasound frequency based on targeted imaging depth. The frequency of the ultrasonic beam is one of the more important determinants of axial resolution, which represents the ability to distinguish structures located along the axial ultrasound beam propagation. Increasing ultrasound frequency improves axial image resolution. However, tissue penetration decreases, resulting in decreased imaging depth. The 7.5 MHz for AcuNav catheter is useful for imaging of most cardiac structures.

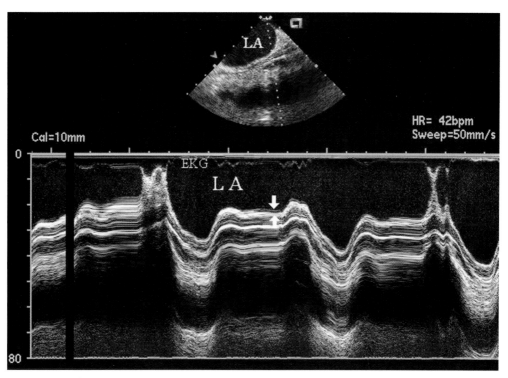

Figure 2.4 ICE image of an M-mode recording with the transducer in the right atrium, showing left atrial (LA) wall thickness (2.5 mm in diastole, between arrows) and motion during the cardiac cycle.

Figure 2.9 demonstrates how changing ultrasound frequency alters imaging quality and depth. Based on this one can then select a higher frequency (such as 8.5 or 10 MHz) for imaging of structures in the near field (lesser depth) or a lower frequency (5.5 MHz) for those in the far field (greater depth). The ultrasonic beam width or the interrogating ultrasonic pulse width is one of the important determinants in lateral resolution, which represents the ability to distinguish structures located perpendicularly to the axis of ultrasound beam propagation. Using a minimum amount of gain or focusing the ultrasonic beam can enhance lateral resolution [2].

The Acuson imaging system has a variable depth-compensation control that consists of a series of levers that alter the relative gain throughout the entire depth (Figure 2.10, arrow). The depth-compensation control can be confusing and is often difficult for the clinical electrophysiologist to employ. If one understands that this control can be used to compensate for ultrasonic attenuation as the beam passes through

cardiac structures, then one can better understand how the control should be used. For example, when the ICE transducer is placed along the aortic root or a thickened right atrial septum, one should increase the gain in order to optimize imaging of near-field structures, such as the aortic valves or the right pulmonary vein ostia. However, when performing transthoracic echocardiography, gain should be adjusted in order to suppress echoes in the near field and enhance it in the far field. In addition, when operating the depth-compensation or any other control for mechanical radial ICE imaging, it is important that the catheter tip be unsheathed especially when a long-length sheath is used. Otherwise, images will be severely degraded by the overlying sheath. Lastly, the orientation of a circular image can be controlled by adjusting the image rotation button.

Doppler controls

Several controls are specifically used for the pulsed- or continuous-wave and color flow Doppler imaging on the AcuNav ultrasound catheter imaging

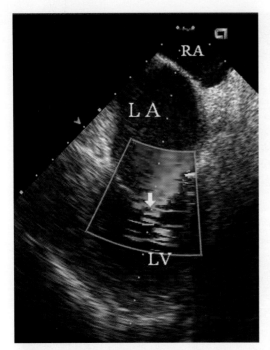

Figure 2.5 ICE Doppler color flow image of the left ventricular (LV) inflow with the transducer placed in the right atrium (RA), showing blood flow (blue color, arrow) filling from left atrium (LA) into the LV.

system. Doppler spectral and color flow imaging is used for blood flow and hemodynamic assessment. The information obtained with Doppler echocardiography includes presence or absence of flow, its direction, velocity, and flow characteristics (laminar or turbulent). This Doppler capability has unsurpassed utility in the identification of flow disturbances and changes in flow velocity especially in venous structures and across cardiac valves during radiofrequency catheter ablation procedures in these regions.

Ultrasound frequency reflected from a moving target is different from that transmitted by the ultrasound transducer. This effect is called the Doppler shift. For example, reflected (backscattered) ultrasound from a moving target has a frequency (f_r) that is higher than the transmitted frequency (f_t) when the target is moving toward the transducer, whereas it is lower when the target moves away from the transducer. The Doppler frequency shift (f_d) is the difference between the transmitted (from the transducer) and reflected (from a moving target, such as blood cells) frequencies. The Doppler equation expresses the mathematical relationship between the velocity of the moving target (v) and the Doppler frequency (f_d) as follows [2]:

$$f_d = f_r - f_t$$

$$f_d = 2f_t \cdot v \cdot \cos\theta / c$$

$$v = f_d \cdot c / 2f_t(\cos\theta)$$

where c is the velocity of sound and θ is the angle between the direction of the moving target and the path of the ultrasonic beam.

As noted in the Doppler equations, the velocity is a function of the Doppler frequency and the angle since the velocity of sound in the medium being examined (blood or cardiac tissues) is reasonably constant and the transmitted frequency is known. Importantly, the equation shows that the relationship between the Doppler frequency and the velocity is a function of the cosine of the angle. The angle becomes critical if the velocity is calculated from the Doppler frequency. For example, if the angle is $\leq 20°$, the percentage of underestimation of flow velocity is $\leq 6\%$ [3], which can almost be ignored. However, as the angle increases, the maximum underestimation of the flow velocity is increased (Figure 2.11). When it reaches $90°$, $\cos\theta$ is zero and no Doppler velocity is detected. Therefore, the most accurate Doppler velocity is obtained when the ultrasonic beam is parallel (if the angle is zero then $\cos\theta$ is one) to the moving target (blood flow) (Figure 2.11). With pulsed Doppler, one needs to use a track ball to position the sampling volume in the desired location, keeping the ultrasonic beam as parallel as possible to the targeted blood flow to accurately measure the flow velocity from a specific depth or area. The maximal velocity detected with pulsed Doppler is limited by the pulsed repetition frequency (PRF) and transducer frequency (maximum $v = \text{PRF} \cdot c/4f_t\cos\theta$) [4], which in turn depends on the maximum depth of measurement. When flow velocities exceed maximal measurable velocity (the Nyquist limit = PRF/2 for Doppler shift frequency), aliasing occurs and velocities above this limit "wrap around" to the maximum value of the opposite scale, and the actual value of maximal velocity cannot be determined. However, aliasing can be reduced by transmitting a lower frequency (f_t) or by increasing the angle θ. One can also

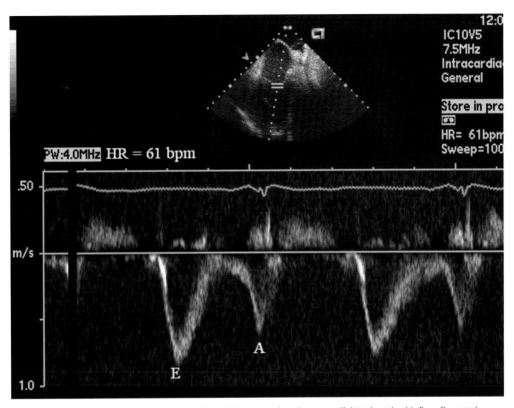

Figure 2.6 Pulsed-wave Doppler spectral recording with the sample volume parallel to the mitral inflow flow at the orifice of the mitral valve (see Figure 2.5), showing characteristic mitral flow velocity including an early diastolic filling (E peak) velocity and late diastolic (A peak) velocity following atrial contraction.

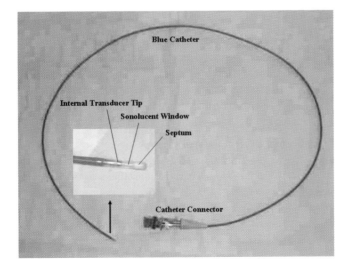

Figure 2.7 A mechanical ultrasound blue catheter is constructed with a rotational internal catheter shaft and transducer tip, and a proximal connector (to be attached to the motor drive unit). Before using this imaging catheter, its lumen needs to be filled with sterile water (about 5 cc) following insertion of a 26-gauge needle through the distal catheter tip, carefully just across the white self sealing septum, avoiding contact with the internal transducer tip. A continuous bubble-free column of water should be visible. If persistent bubbles remain in the sonolucent window area, remove the needle, hold the catheter about 30–50 cm from the tip and swirl fast the distal catheter section around. This should force the water column to the tip displacing the remaining air bubbles away from the tip.

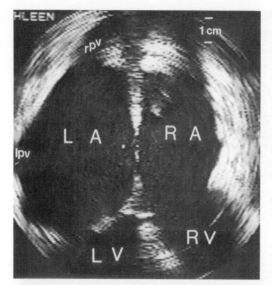

Figure 2.8 Mechanical radial ICE image with the transducer placed at the fossa ovalis of the interatrial septum in the right atrium (RA), showing a four-chamber view including the left atrium (LA) with the upper left (lpv) and right pulmonary vein (rpv) ostia, RA, and truncated left (LV) and right ventricle (RV).

increase the maximal velocity detected by sampling more superficially or by shifting the spectral baseline to remove aliasing with greater velocity excursion in one direction. High pulse repetition frequency (HPRF) ultrasound allows more efficient velocity determination and localization of blood flow at increased depth and it can be used to detect higher Doppler velocities than pulsed-wave Doppler can provide (press the "scale" button up to enter HPRF mode on Sequoia 512 system). Continuous-wave Doppler ultrasound does not allow detection of blood flow at a specific depth. However, it does allow the measurement of blood flow in all paths intercepted by the ultrasonic beam. Continuous-wave Doppler is more suitable for measuring high blood flow velocities, such as those encountered with jets.

Color flow Doppler imaging is a form of pulsed Doppler that trades off detailed velocity information for increased spatial information. Here velocity data are transformed into a color spectrum, which is superimposed on the two-dimensional image in real time. The color flow gain setting of the ultrasound system controls the sensitivity of this technology. An optimal gain setting can be obtained first by increasing the gain gradually until noise just begins to appear

around the flow of interest, then by slightly decreasing the gain until the noise disappears. The area of a color flow of interest can be adjusted from a wide sector down to less than a few centimeters. With such small areas of interrogation, the sensitivity and real-time nature of color approaches that of spectral Doppler. Thus, decreasing the size of the region of interest increases the sensitivity of color flow Doppler imaging. The ability to change the size of the region of interest combined with a pre-processing control allows one to optimize one of three parameters, which are line density (affecting the spatial resolution of the color), number of samples per line or packet size (affecting the accuracy of the derived color), and frame rate (affecting the real-time nature of the display) [5]. As a result, a wide range of flow velocity information can be displayed simultaneously with accurate anatomic and functional real-time ultrasound imaging.

Artifact
Side lobes
Side lobes are represented by a weakened duplicate of the original image that is superimposed adjacent to it. They are produced by a beam (or beams) of ultrasound generated from individual transducer elements that is returned at a slight angle to that of the main ultrasonic beam. This artifact occurs with greater frequency when using phased-array transducers. A large, relatively echo-free cavity, such as an enlarged left atrium, provides an opportunity for side lobes to be displayed within the left atrium (Figure 2.12). Echoes that originate from a strong reflecting surface increase the risk of this artifact [2]. Lesser degrees of side lobe artifact can merely increase the general noise level of the system and thus decrease the dynamic range. They may be eliminated or reduced by gently changing the transducer angle, by increasing the reject level, or by decreasing the gain.

Reverberations
Reverberations occur when a portion of the returning echo encounters and bounces off a reflective surface traveling in the same direction as the original ultrasonic beam. This echo then encounters the original reflective surface and returns to the transducer, resulting in a time delay, which is interpreted as a deeper surface. Multiple reflections and re-reflections may

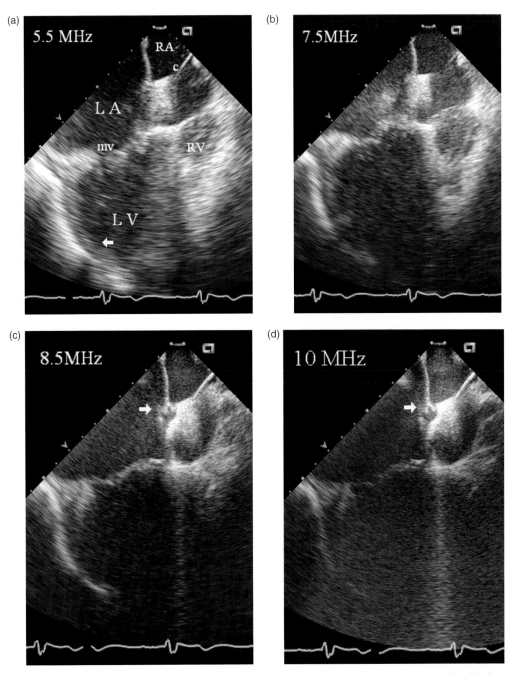

Figure 2.9 Serial four-chamber view ICE images using different ultrasonic frequencies with the transducer placed in the right atrium (RA), showing the effect of ultrasound frequencies on imaging quality and depth: (a) at 5.5 MHz, imaging depth reaches left ventricular apex (maximum 16 cm) with fair imaging quality of all cardiac structures including Left atrium (LA), mitral valve (mv), right ventricle (RV) and left ventricular (LV) wall near the apex (arrow); (b) at 7.5 MHz, imaging depth reaches almost all the cardiac structures except the LV apex area with good imaging resolution; (c) at 8.5 MHz, imaging depth is further reduced with increased imaging resolution of the mitral valve and inferior limbus of the interatrial septum (arrow) in the near and middle field, but the RV and LV wall are not visualized in the far field; (d) at 10 MHz, imaging depth is further decreased and the highest imaging resolution is obtained in the near field (inferior limbus, arrow). C: coronary sinus catheter.

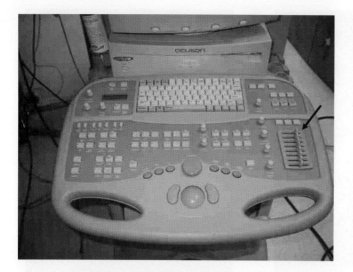

Figure 2.10 The controls on the keyboard are grouped by function allowing efficient imaging and Doppler processing. Depth compensation control (arrow) allows gain control at any depth within the imaging range. The standard position of each lever is demonstrated.

(a)

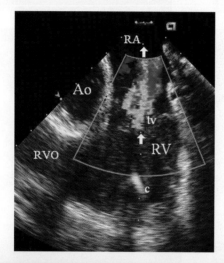

(b)

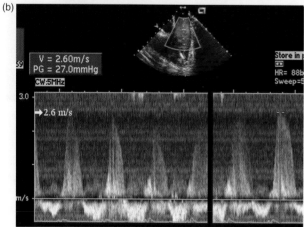

Figure 2.11 ICE Doppler color flow and continuous-wave spectral images: (a) recorded with the transducer placed in the right atrium (RA), with the ultrasonic sampling beam parallel to the tricuspid regurgitant flow (arrows, red color, flow toward the RA during systole); (b) a maximum velocity of 2.6 m/s is recorded without underestimation; (c) when the sampling beam angle θ is 25°; (d) a maximum velocity of 2.2 m/s recorded with significant underestimation. Ao: aortic root; c: catheter; RV and RVO: right ventricle and RV outflow tract; tv: tricuspid valve.

(c)

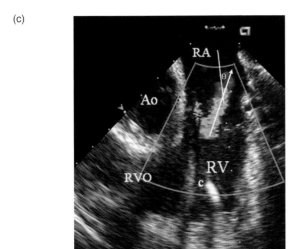

(d)

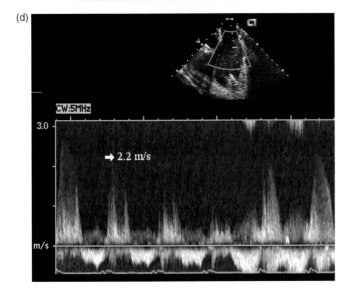

Figure 2.11 Continued.

occur resulting in multiple spurious parallel surfaces and weak images. Images from reverberation artifact may be intra-cardiac or extra-cardiac (Figure 2.13). Intra-cardiac reverberation artifact may not have an obvious origin [6] and can therefore be particularly troublesome [2]. By readjusting the angle, depth, or frequency of the transducer, these artifacts can be identified, reduced, or eliminated.

Acoustic shadowing

Acoustic shadowing artifact can be induced by structures with high density, such as calcium, prosthetic valves, central venous catheters, or pacemaker leads. Virtually 100% of the ultrasonic beam encountering these surfaces is reflected preventing visualization of deeper structures. The artifact can be easily recognized (Figure 2.14) but is troublesome when trying to visualize anatomy beyond this strong reflective surface. Another similar artifact can occur when the ultrasonic beam encounters the sharp edge of certain anatomic structures, which may act as a strong edge reflector even though the tissue is of low density (Figure 2.15). Acoustic shadowing can be avoided by moving the transducer and changing the angle of insonation so

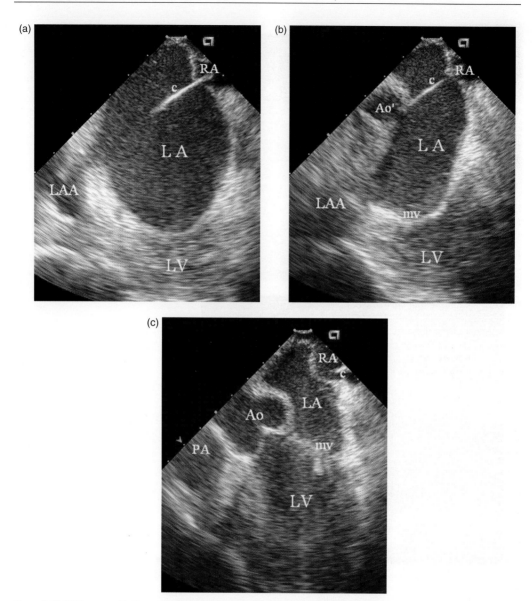

Figure 2.12 ICE images with the transducer placed in the right atrium (RA) showing: (a) an enlarged left atrium (LA); (b) side lobe artifact originating from the aortic root (Ao') seen in the left atrium (LA) during a cardiac cycle; (c) with slight counterclockwise rotation of the transducer, the aortic root (Ao) adjacent to LA is visualized. C: catheter; LAA: LA appendage; LV: left ventricle; mv: mitral valve; PA: pulmonary artery.

that it no longer encounters the offending reflective surface.

Right heart catheterization

The AcuNav diagnostic ultrasound imaging catheter, as well as the mechanical radial imaging catheter, is intended for use in the right side of the heart only. The percutaneous left femoral vein approach [7,8] is used in almost all ICE imaging procedures. After palpation of the femoral arterial pulse within the inguinal skin crease, a local anesthetic is introduced into an area 3–4 cm in diameter, 1–2 cm below the inguinal crease, medial to the femoral pulse. A small incision (about 0.5 cm long) is made over the vessels to be used for the imaging

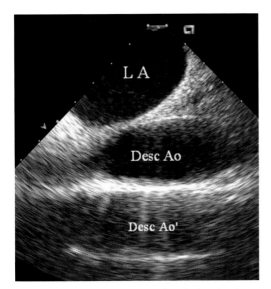

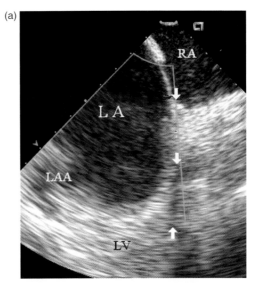
(a)

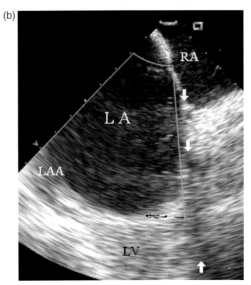
(b)

Figure 2.13 ICE image with the transducer placed in the right atrium, showing the part of the left atrium (LA) and the descending aorta (Desc Ao). Below the border of the posterior wall of the Desc Ao, an artifact is visualized (Desc Ao') which represents reverberations from echoes originating in the Desc Ao wall.

Figure 2.15 ICE images of left atrium (LA) and ventricle (LV) with the transducer placed in the right atrium (RA), showing: (a and b) a linear imaging drop-out shadowing artifact (upward arrow) seen behind strong edged cardiac structures (between two downward arrows). This artifact should not be mistaken for pericardial effusion since this finding changes location relative to the ultrasonic beam during a cardiac cycle. LAA: LA appendage.

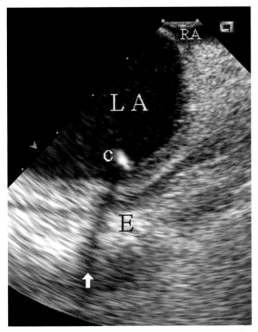

Figure 2.14 ICE image of an ablation catheter electrode (c) attached at the left atrial (LA) posterior wall with the transducer placed in the right atrium (RA), showing the shadowing artifact behind it (arrow). E: esophagus.

catheter introduction and passage, after which a "tunnel" is constructed with a straight hemostat from the skin incision directed toward the femoral vein. An 18-gauge thin-walled Seldinger needle is introduced through the skin incision and tunneled at a 30–45° angle into the lumen of the femoral vein.

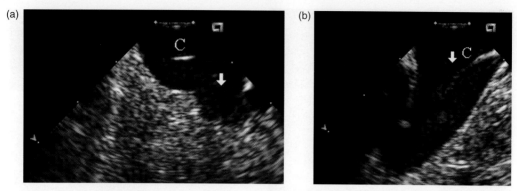

Figure 2.16 ICE images showing: (a) ICE catheter encountering resistance as it is advanced toward a venous bifurcation; (b) it is corrected by withdrawal and anterior tip deflection toward the larger venous branch (arrow). This maneuver also allows redirection of a second catheter "c" facilitating transfemoral right heart catheterization.

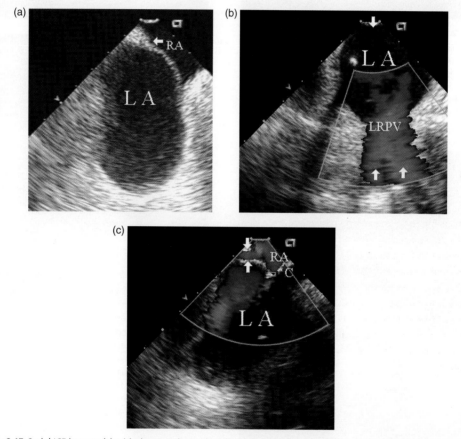

Figure 2.17 Serial ICE images: (a) with the transducer placed in the high right atrium (RA) showing the limbus at the superior portion of the foramen ovale (arrow) without any echo-free space indicating that the foramen ovale is not "patent"; (b) with imaging catheter forced into the left atrium (LA) (downward arrow) through the superior limbus, showing the lower right pulmonary vein (LRPV) with a red color flow jet entering the LA from its two branches (upward arrows); (c) following imaging catheter withdrawal from the limbus, posterior tip deflection and advancement more superiorly in the RA, a red color flow jet (new left to right shunt) is visualized originating from the superior limbus of the now "patent" foramen ovale (between arrows). C: catheter.

The needle is slowly pulled back while gently applying negative pressure using a syringe. Once blood is aspirated, a guide wire is advanced into the lumen of the punctured vein. The wire is held firmly in place as the needle is removed. With the wire in the femoral vein, a 10–11 Fr introducer sheath is threaded over it and into the vein lumen, and the wire is removed [7,8]. The imaging catheter is then inserted into the femoral vein through the introducer sheath. Under fluoroscopic or ultrasound imaging guidance the catheter is advanced into the right atrium, superior vena cava or right ventricle. The desired diagnostic and/or therapeutic procedures can then begin.

If resistance is encountered when advancing the imaging catheter, it should never be overcome by force. A small luminal echo-free space (such as the lumbar branch) around the catheter tip may be revealed; the catheter can be drawn back under imaging guidance until a large lumen (or bifurcation) is observed (Figure 2.16). The catheter tip can then be redirected and advanced using slight anterior deflection. Resistance can also be encountered while advancing the catheter from the right atrium into the superior vena cava when it encounters the superior limbus of the interatrial septum. This is especially problematic in patients with lipomatous hypertrophy of the interatrial septum. Then the catheter can be pulled back and redirected with slight posterior deflection and then advanced.

Advancing the catheter when encountering resistance in this scenario can result in an iatrogenic patent foramen ovale (Figure 2.17).

Following catheterization by this approach, the catheter and sheath are removed, and hemostasis is achieved by manual compression over the puncture site until bleeding stops; this usually occurs after 5 min, longer if the patient is heparinized. Subsequently, the patient must remain in bed with the involved leg immobilized for 6–12 h.

Right heart catheterization is usually contraindicated in the presence of conditions that create unacceptable risk, such as sepsis, major coagulation abnormalities, class IV angina, heart failure, right heart thrombus, deep vein thrombosis, or significant peripheral vascular disease. Lack of femoral venous access due to chronic venous occlusion or any other reason presents additional contraindication to this approach. The catheters described in this text are not for use in coronary vessels, for insertion into the arterial system, or for fetal use.

References

1 Pye SD, Wild SR, McDicken WN. Adaptive time gain compensation for ultrasonic imaging. *Ultrasound in Med & Biol* 1992; **18**: 205–212.

2 Feigenbaum H. *Echocardiography*, 5th edn. Lea & Febiger, Philadelphia, 1994: 19–47.

3 Hatle L, Angelsen B. *Doppler Ultrasound in Cardiology*, Lea & Febiger, Philadelphia, 1985: 104–108.

4 Sehgal CM. Principles of ultrasonic imaging and Doppler ultrasound. In: St. John Sutton MG, Oldershaw PJ, Kotler MN, eds. *Textbook of Echocardiography and Doppler in Adults and Children*, 2nd edn. Blackwell Science, Inc., Cambridge, 1996: 26–27.

5 Durell M, Mandel L. Instrumentation for Doppler echocardiography. In: Nanda NC, ed. *Doppler Echocardiography*, 2nd edn. Lea & Febiger, Philadelphia, 1993: 51–53.

6 Yeh EL. Reverberations in echocardiograms. *J Clin Ultrasound* 1977; **5**: 84–86.

7 Hills LD, Lange RA, Cigarroa RG. Cardiac Catheterization. In: Kloner RA, ed. *The Guide to Cardiology*, 2nd edn. Le Jacq Communications, New York, 1990: 113–114.

8 Baim DS. Percutaneous approach, including transseptal and apical puncture. In: Baim DS, Grossman W, eds. *Grossman's Cardiac Catheterization, Angiography, and Intervention*, 6th edn. Lippincott Williams & Wilkins, Philadelphia, 2000: 69–80.

3 CHAPTER 3

Imaging Technique and Cardiac Structures

Jian-Fang Ren, MD, *& Jeffrey P. Weiss*, MD

Sector electronic phased-array ultrasound catheter intracardiac echocardiographic imaging

Image orientation and transducer control

Understanding the relationship between the sector ultrasound catheter face and the anatomic structures being imaged is critical for proper catheter manipulation. Intracardiac echocardiography (ICE) two-dimensional 90° sector scanning demonstrates a cross-sectional anatomic view oriented from the tip to the shaft of the imaging catheter's active face (see Figure 2.2). The left/right (L/R) orientation marker indicates the catheter's shaft side. For example, when the L/R orientation marker is set to the operator's right (Figure 3.1a) and the catheter is advanced from the inferior vena cava into the right atrium, the cranial-caudal axis projects from image left to right and the posterior to anterior axis projects from image top to bottom. This occurs only when the catheter's face is oriented anteriorly. Changing the L/R marker to the left side (Figure 3.1b), inverts the image but does not change top to bottom image orientation. Traditionally, the "L/R" orientation marker is set to the operator's right [1] and the anatomic views obtained are consistent with those previously published in ICE images [2].

Using the above described relationships, the operator may adjust imaging orientation by simple catheter advancement or withdrawal, by tip deflection in four directions (anterior/posterior and left/right), or by catheter rotation thus using image guidance to reach and visualize targeted structures. For example, using an imaging catheter with the tip undeflected placed just above the inferior vena cava in the right atrium, the right ventricular inflow and outflow tract can be viewed (Figure 3.1a). To image more superior/anterior structures, such as the pulmonary artery, the catheter transducer should be advanced superiorly (Figure 3.1c). Similarly, deflecting the catheter tip posteriorly increases the distance between the transducer and the atrial septum allowing more effective monitoring and guiding of catheters along the right atrial side of the interatrial septum during transseptal catheterization (Figure 3.2a,b). Figure 3.3a–f illustrates how to view cardiac anatomy using catheter rotation, and Figure 3.4a,b shows how to use anterior tip deflection and catheter advancement into the right ventricle.

Transducer location and normal cardiac imaging views

From the right atrium

With the catheter transducer placed in the right atrium just above the inferior vena cava orifice and oriented anteriorly and to the left, the right atrium and ventricle are viewed (Figure 3.1). With rotation of the catheter transducer anterolaterally (counterclockwise), the right atrial appendage is imaged. The superior crista terminalis is identified when the catheter is advanced forward to the junction of the right atrium and superior vena cava (Figure 3.5). When the catheter transducer is placed near the fossa ovalis and interatrial septum and oriented anteriorly and to the left, the left ventricular outflow tract (Figure 3.6) and left atrial appendage and truncated left ventricle are imaged (Figure 3.7). With clockwise rotation and slight adjustment of the transducer level, the left ventricular inflow

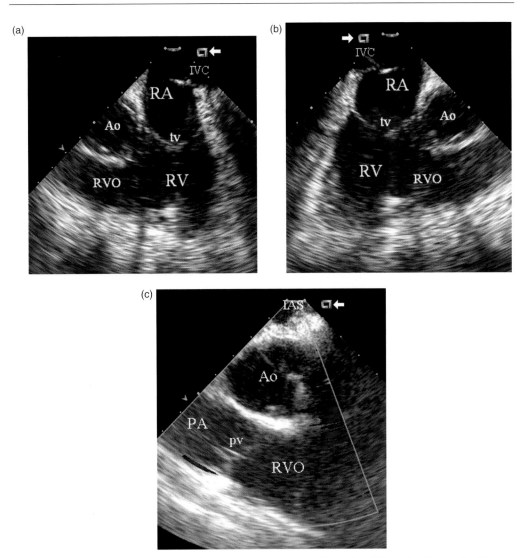

Figure 3.1 ICE images with the transducer facing anteriorly, placed in the right atrium (RA) passing through the inferior vena cava (IVC) orifice, demonstrate: (a) anatomic structures with the L/R orientation marker (arrow) on the right side indicating the shaft side of the imaging catheter's active face. The anatomic structures in this view are oriented with superior structures on the left and inferior structures on the right. Posterior to anterior structures descend from the top to bottom of the image. The aortic root (Ao) and right ventricular (RV) outflow tract (RVO) are located on the left side, near the bottom of the image are located superiorly and anteriorly when compared to the IVC which is located on the right side and top of the image (i.e., inferior and posterior structure); (b) the same view when displayed with the L/R orientation marker (arrow) changed to the left side, the image becomes inverted, reversing structures on the right and left, but not the posterior and anterior orientation; (c) with the transducer advanced superiorly and anteriorly toward the interatrial septum (IAS) in the RA, the pulmonic valve (pv) and pulmonary artery (PA) come into view. tv: tricuspid valve.

(mitral valve) and apex can be viewed (Figure 3.8). Continued clockwise rotation of the transducer allows visualization of the lower and upper left pulmonary veins (Figure 3.9a,b). When the catheter transducer is advanced toward the superior vena cava – right atrial junction and rotated posteriorly (clockwise) – the lower and upper (or shared middle) right pulmonary veins are imaged (Figure 3.10). When the transducer is deflected slightly to the right, the upper and middle right pulmonary veins and their

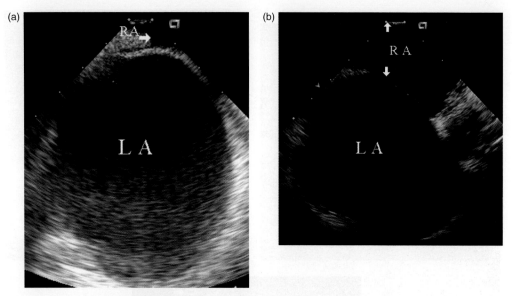

Figure 3.2 ICE images with the transducer placed in the right atrium (RA), demonstrate: (a) limited space between the transducer and interatrial septum (arrow); (b) as the imaging catheter is withdrawn and deflected posteriorly, the space on the RA side between the transducer and interatrial septum increases (arrows) allowing more effective monitoring and guidance of RA catheters along the septum during transseptal catheterization. LA: left atrium.

proximal lumens are imaged (Figure 3.11a–c). With the pulmonary vein ostia in view, each of their ostial flow velocities can be sampled and determined using the Doppler technology described in Chapter 2 (Figure 3.12a,b) [3]. When the transducer is placed in the mid-right atrium with an appropriate deflection to right, a short-axis view of the aortic root and aortic valve cusps are visualized anteriorly (Figure 3.13).

From the tricuspid valve annulus and right ventricle

Catheterization of the right ventricle from the right atrium can be performed while simultaneously deflecting the catheter tip anteriorly and advancing it forward, toward the tricuspid valve annulus or across it. Images of the left ventricle can then be obtained in short-axis (Figure 3.14) or long-axis views (Figure 3.15).

Radial mechanical ultrasound catheter ICE imaging

Image orientation and transducer manipulation

Radial ICE imaging is performed with the ultrasound catheter transducer located in one of the four specific regions of the right heart and left atrium. As with the sector electronic phased-array imaging catheter, this device is typically advanced into the right atrium via femoral vein access (Chapter 2). The preferred orientation of the circular image generated when using this technology displays right sided structures to the operator's right [2,4]. Cephalic and posterior structures are typically displayed at the top of the image, while caudal and anterior structures are typically displayed at the image bottom. When the transducer is advanced into the right atrium via the superior vena cava, the orientation of the image then changes with the right-sided heart structures to the viewer's left. At present, available radial catheters using this technology are not deflectable. Therefore, change in image orientation or location can only be made by catheter advancement and withdrawal. The lack of catheter tip deflectability can be overcome by using pre-shaped angled sheaths available with $15°, 30°, 60°$, or $120°$ angles. For example, a $15°$ sheath can be used for guiding transseptal catheterization and a sheath with a $120°$ deflection can be used for imaging the tricuspid valvular annulus or isthmus region. However, using these sheaths can be cumbersome, especially if numerous sheath angles (and therefore sheath exchanges) are required.

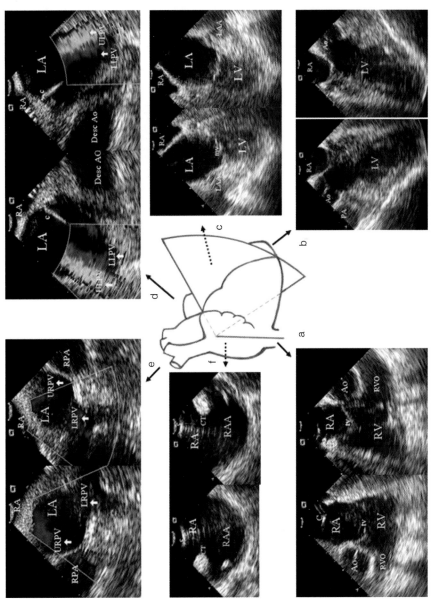

Figure 3.3 ICE serial images with the transducer placed in the middle or high right atrium (RA), demonstrate serial changes in tomographic imaging views following clockwise rotation of the transducer. Each view displays both "L/R" orientation options: (a) the vertical plane of the transducer projecting anteriorly toward the right ventricular (RV) inflow and outflow (RVO); (b) following clockwise rotation toward the left ventricular (LV) outflow tract; (c) the LV inflow; (d) the lower (LLPV) and upper (ULPV) left pulmonary vein ostia with color flow imaging; (e) the lower (LRPV) and upper (URPV) right pulmonary vein with color flow imaging on the opposite side of the anterior RV; (f) the right atrial appendage (RAA). Ao: aortic root; c: catheter; CT: crista terminalis; Desc Ao: descending aorta; LA and LAA: left atrium and LA appendage; RPA: right pulmonary artery.

(a)

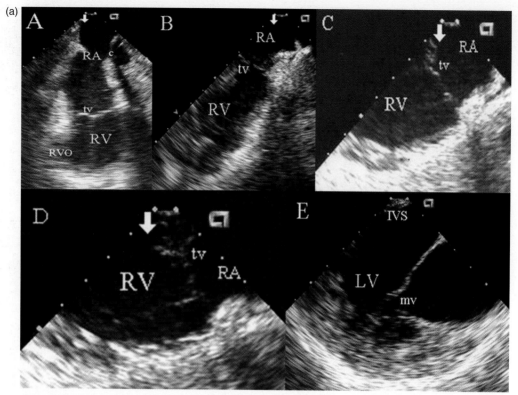

Figure 3.4 ICE serial images showing imaging guidance of an imaging catheter transducer tip (arrow) into the right ventricle (RV) from right atrium (RA) through the tricuspid valve (tv) orifice. In panel A, the imaging catheter tip (arrow) requires withdrawal as no chamber space exists in front of the catheter tip. The imaging catheter is then advanced into the RV with anterior tip deflection (panel B through D). With proper rotation of the transducer in the RV, a truncated long-axis view of the left ventricle (LV) is obtained (panel E). c: catheter; IVS: interventricular septum; mv: mitral valve; RVO: RV outflow. (b) ICE serial images recorded with reverse L/R orientation showing imaging guidance of an imaging catheter tip (arrow) entering the right ventricle (RV) from right atrium (RA) through the tricuspid valve (tv) orifice with anterior tip deflection (panel A through D). With proper rotation of the transducer in the RV, a truncated long-axis view of the left ventricle (LV) is obtained (panel E). pm: papillary muscle; RVO: RV outflow tract.

Transducer location and normal cardiac imaging views

From the right atrium

With the transducer placed at the junction of the inferior vena cava and right atrium (Figure 3.16), then advanced into the lower (Figure 3.17) and middle right atrium (Figure 3.18), the eustachian valve and the lateral crista terminalis at different levels are visualized. With the transducer placed at the limbus fossa ovalis or at the anterosuperior part of the limbus, the left atrium, the left pulmonary vein orifice and aortic root are imaged (Figure 3.19). With manipulation of the transducer near the medial aspect of the atrioventricular junction, a truncated five-chamber view is obtained (Figure 3.20).

From the superior vena cava

When the transducer is advanced from the superior vena cava – right atrium junction (Figure 3.21) into the superior vena cava (Figure 3.22), the ascending aorta, the pulmonary artery bifurcation and, occasionally, the right pulmonary vein are viewed. With the transducer advanced further cephalad, the azygos vein orifice is imaged (Figure 3.23).

From the right ventricle and its outflow tract

With the transducer placed in the right ventricle through the tricuspid valvular orifice (Figure 3.24), and further advanced into the right ventricular outflow tract (Figure 3.25), both ventricles and the pulmonary artery are imaged.

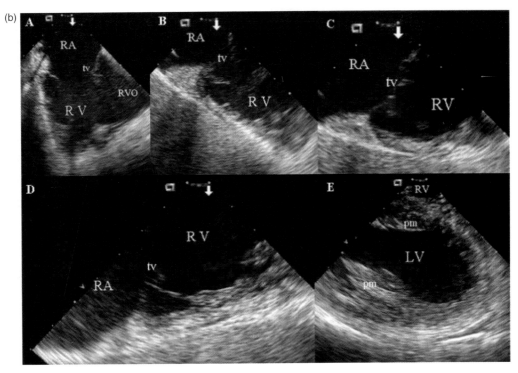

Figure 3.4 Continued.

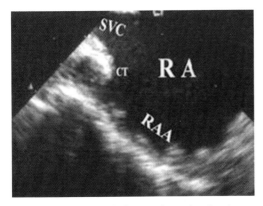

Figure 3.5 ICE image with the transducer placed at the junction of the right atrium (RA) and superior vena cava (SVC), showing the superior crista terminalis (CT) and RA appendage (RAA). Reproduced with permission [1].

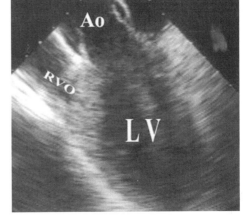

Figure 3.6 ICE image with the transducer placed in the right atrium, showing the left ventricle (LV) with its outflow. Ao: aorta; RVO: right ventricular outflow. Reproduced with permission [1].

From the interatrial septal limbus or left atrium

The 9 MHz mechanical radial imaging ultrasound catheter is limited when imaging the left atrium during pulmonary vein ostial ablation for atrial fibrillation due to its limited penetration depth. Visualization of pulmonary vein ostia, especially left-sided ones, is facilitated by placing the transducer in the interatrial septal limbus (Figure 3.26) or directly into

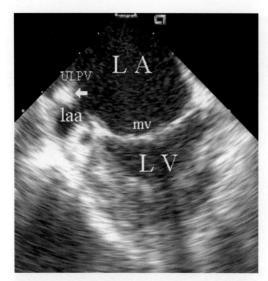

Figure 3.7 ICE image with the transducer placed near the fossa ovalis in the right atrium, showing the left ventricular (LV) inflow and left atrial appendage (laa). The Marshall ligament (arrow) appears as an echogenic mass between laa and upper left pulmonary vein ostium (ULPV). mv: mitral valve. Reproduced with permission [1].

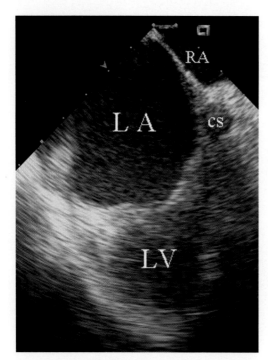

Figure 3.8 ICE image with the transducer placed in the right atrium (RA), showing the left ventricular (LV) inflow with mitral valve. CS: coronary sinus; LA: left atrium.

(a)

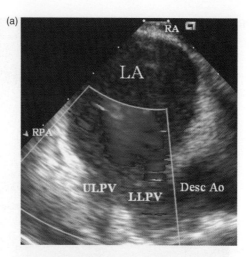

(b)

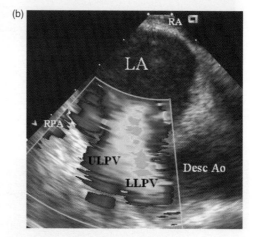

Figure 3.9 (a,b) ICE images demonstrating the ostia of the upper (ULPV) and lower left pulmonary veins (LLPV) and color flow imaging (panel A). Ostial flow (red color) demonstrates flow directed from the ostia toward the left atrium (LA) (panel B). Desc Ao: descending aorta; RA: right atrium; RPA: right pulmonary artery.

the pulmonary vein following transseptal catheterization (see Chapter 8). The pulmonary venous ostia and wall structures are imaged in detail in Figure 3.27.

Intracardiac anatomic landmarks

There are many important intracardiac structures which can be used as anatomic landmarks during interventional electrophysiologic procedures. Imaging technique of important cardiac anatomy, including normal variants, is described as follows.

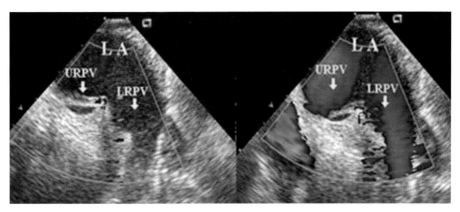

Figure 3.10 ICE images demonstrating the ostia (arrows) of the upper (URPV) and lower right pulmonary veins (LRPV). The LRPV ostium is shared with a superior branch of LRPV as seen with color flow. LA: left atrium. Reproduced with permission [3].

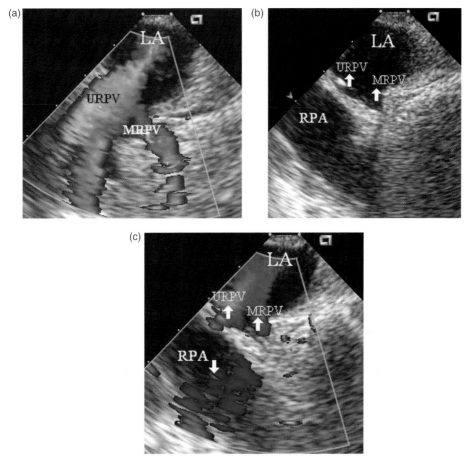

Figure 3.11 ICE Doppler color flow images with the transducer placed at the junction of the right atrium and superior vena cava showing: (a) the upper (URPV) and middle (MRPV) right pulmonary vein with red color flow toward the left atrium (LA); (b) During a cardiac cycle, the right pulmonary artery (RPA) comes into view; (c) with blood flowing away from the transducer (blue color).

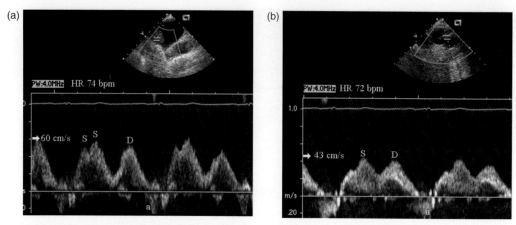

Figure 3.12 ICE Doppler spectra: with sampling volume recorded from: (a) the upper left; (b) and lower right pulmonary vein ostia, showing the maximal peak flow velocities with two systolic components (S), as well as early diastolic (D) and late reversal (a) waves.

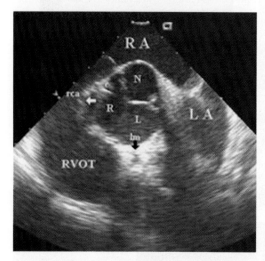

Figure 3.13 Short-axis view of the aortic root recorded with the transducer tip deflected to the right within the anterior right atrium (RA), showing the three cusps of the aortic valve during diastole; the noncoronary cusp (N) is most posterior. It is proximal to the interatrial septum and, of the three cusps, is closest to the posteriorly located transducer. The right cusp (R) is anterior, and contains the right coronary ostium (rca, white arrow). The left cusp (L) is identified by the left main coronary ostium (lm, black arrow). c: catheter; LA: left atrium; RVOT: right ventricular outflow tract.

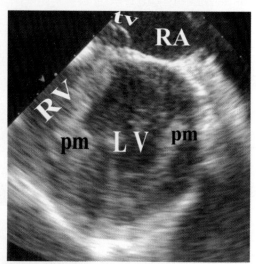

Figure 3.14 ICE image with the transducer placed just above the tricuspid valve (tv) in the right atrium (RA), showing the left ventricle (LV) with its papillary muscles (pm) in short-axis. RV: right ventricle. Reproduced with permission [1].

Right atrium

Eustachian valve

The anterior aspect of the inferior vena caval orifice is bordered by the eustachian valve [5]. The eustachian valve is a common ICE finding that is visualized as an echogenic rim of tissue at the junction of the inferior vena cava and right atrium when the ICE transducer is placed in the right atrium just at or above the orifice of the inferior vena cava (Figures 3.16 and 3.28).

Coronary sinus and its orifice

The coronary sinus runs along the posterior atrio-ventricular groove toward the septal surface and

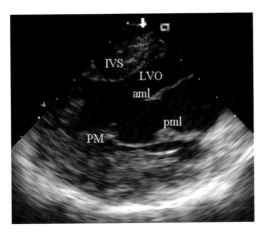

Figure 3.15 ICE image with the transducer placed at the right atrio-ventricular junction (arrow), showing the left ventricular inflow and outflow (LVO) tracts. A papillary muscle (PM) is visualized in truncated long-axis. aml and pml: anterior and posterior mitral leaflets; IVS: interventricular septum.

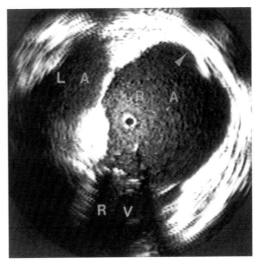

Figure 3.17 Mechanical radial ICE image recorded with the transducer in the lower right atrium (RA), showing the interatrial septum (fossa ovalis) between the RA and left atrium (LA), the lateral crista terminalis (arrowhead) and tricuspid valve. RV: right ventricle. Reproduced with permission [4].

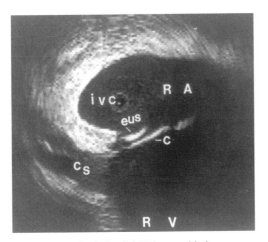

Figure 3.16 Mechanical radial ICE image with the transducer placed at the junction of inferior vena cava (ivc) and the right atrium (RA), showing the eustachian valve (eus), ivc and coronary sinus (CS) orifice. C: catheter; RV: right ventricle. Reproduced with permission [4].

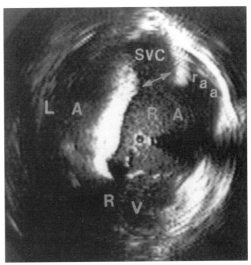

empties into the right atrium close to the inferior vena cava, just anterior to the medial aspect of the eustachian valve. Its orifice may be guarded by the thebesian valve (Figure 3.29). The long and short axis of the coronary sinus as well as the coronary sinus orifice (Figure 3.30a,b) can be visualized from the right atrium using the AcuNav imaging catheter following clockwise rotation from the tricuspid orifice

Figure 3.18 Mechanical radial ICE image recorded with the transducer in the right atrium (RA), showing the superior portion (lateral and medial) of crista terminalis (bilateral arrow) at the junction of the superior vena cava (SVC) and RA appendage (raa). LA: left atrium; RV: right ventricle. Reproduced with permission [4].

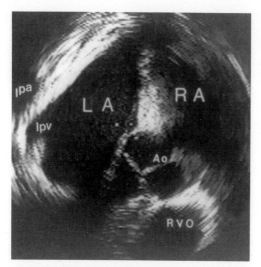

Figure 3.19 Mechanical radial ICE image recorded with the transducer in the anterosuperior part of the interatrial septal limbus, showing the left atrium (LA) with left pulmonary vein (lpv) orifice, aortic root (Ao) and aortic valve cusps. lpa: left pulmonary artery; RA: right atrium; RVO: right ventricular outflow. Reproduced with permission [4].

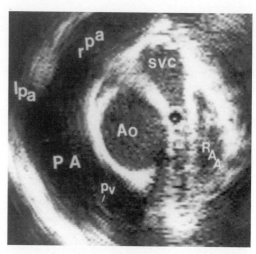

Figure 3.21 Mechanical radial ICE image recorded with the transducer at the junction of superior vena cava (SVC) and right atrial appendage (RAA), showing ascending aorta (Ao), pulmonary artery (PA) and its bifurcation, right (rpa) and left pulmonary (lpa) arteries. pv: pulmonic valve. Reproduced with permission [4].

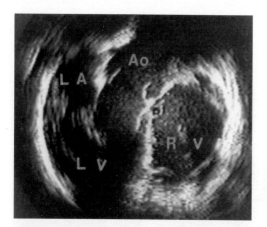

Figure 3.20 Mechanical radial ICE image with the transducer at the right cardiac crux, showing the aortic root (Ao) with right and noncoronary cusps, left atrium (LA) and ventricle (LV) and mitral valve, right ventricle (RV) with a truncated right atrium. Reproduced with permission [4].

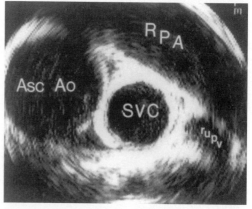

Figure 3.22 Mechanical radial ICE image recorded with the transducer in the superior vena cava (SVC), showing the ascending aorta (Asc Ao), right pulmonary artery (RPA) and right upper pulmonary vein (rupv). Reproduced with permission [4].

and posterior deflection toward the atrio-ventricular septal junction and left atrium.

Right atrial appendage

The right atrial appendage is located anterior to the ascending aorta and is lined by easily visualized pectinate muscles. This structure is visualized using the AcuNav imaging catheter following counter-clockwise rotation from the tricuspid orifice view (Figure 3.31). The pectinate muscles may be prominent and appear as a mass within the right atrial appendage (Figure 3.32) [6].

Crista terminalis

The crista terminalis is a ridge of muscle which separates the smooth-walled and trabeculated parts of the right atrium. This ridge is most prominent superiorly, next to the superior vena cava orifice;

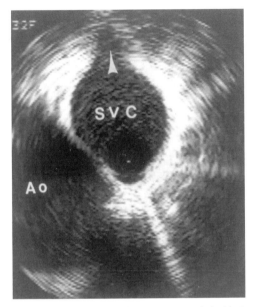

Figure 3.23 Mechanical radial ICE image recorded with the transducer in the superior vena cava (SVC) at the level of the azygos vein, showing the azygos vein orifice (arrowhead) and ascending aorta (Ao). Reproduced with permission [4].

it fades out to the right of the inferior vena cava ostium [5]. The superolateral crista terminalis is the largest part of this structure and is visualized at the level of the superior vena cava–right atrial appendage junction. The sinus node is located in this region [7]. The superolateral crista terminalis can be visualized during sinus node ablation with either the AcuNav (Figure 3.5) or the mechanical radial (Figure 3.18) imaging catheter placed in the right atrium or at the junction of the superior vena cava and right atrium.

Interatrial septum

The interatrial septum forms the posteromedial wall of the right atrium. The ovoid, central portion of this structure represents the fossa ovalis which is easily identified as it is thin and fibrous. The remainder of the septum is muscular. The limbus fossa ovalis is a muscular ridge around the fossa ovalis. The fossa ovalis and limbus may be visualized with AcuNav imaging catheter placed in the middle/lower right atrium facing the interatrial septum and left atrium (Figure 3.33). The interatrial septum, fossa ovalis, and limbus may be imaged using the mechanical radial ICE transducer from the right atrium (Figure 3.17).

Isthmus region

The "posterior" or inferior isthmus border includes the area between the eustachian valve or ridge posteriorly, and the hinge of the tricuspid valve anteriorly. The

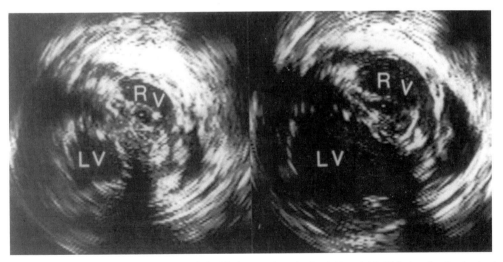

Figure 3.24 Mechanical radial ICE images recorded with the transducer in the right ventricle (RV), showing the short-axis view of the left ventricle (LV) and RV (crescent shape). The LV and RV chamber size and wall thickening can be evaluated at end-systole (left panel) and end-diastole (right panel). Reproduced with permission [4].

septal (superior) isthmus border includes the smooth vestibule of the tricuspid valve between the margin of the coronary sinus and the hinge of the septal leaflet of the tricuspid valve [8,9]. The "central" (inferior) isthmus (Figure 3.34a) and septal isthmus (Figure 3.34b) can be visualized using the AcuNav catheter placed in

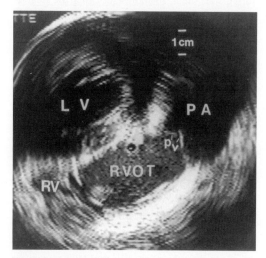

Figure 3.25 Mechanical radial ICE image recorded with the transducer in the right ventricular outflow tract (RVOT), showing the pulmonary artery (PA) and pulmonic valve (pv). LV: left ventricle; RV: right ventricle. Reproduced with permission [2].

the middle or lower right atrium facing slightly posterior to the interventricular septum and the insertion of the tricuspid septal leaflet. Slight anterior deflection of the catheter tip may be needed for imaging of the septal isthmus. The isthmus has a thicker muscular wall between the orifice of the inferior vena cava and the hinge of the tricuspid valve. This subeustachian region has been recognized as a potential zone of slow conduction with resultant atrial flutter and is therefore a common target for radiofrequency ablation when treating this condition [10,11].

Right ventricle
Tricuspid valve and tricuspid annulus
The tricuspid valve is situated in the fibromuscular annulus of the right heart between the right atrium and right ventricle. It is the posteroinferior inflow portion of the right ventricular cavity and it consists of three leaflets (anterior, posterior, and septal) of unequal size with subvalvular components, including chordae tendineae attached to papillary muscles. The anterior leaflet (infundibular cusp) is the largest and is attached to the anterior annular ring from the region of the infundibulum to the inferolateral right ventricular wall. The posterior leaflet is typically the smallest and is

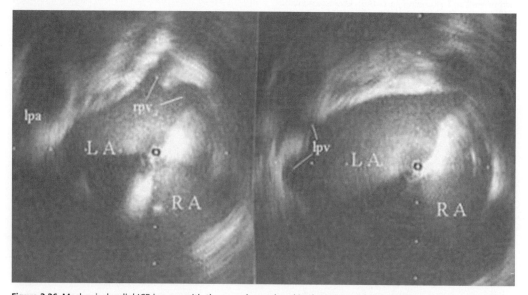

Figure 3.26 Mechanical radial ICE images with the transducer placed in the interatrial septal limbus, showing the right pulmonary vein (rpv) (left panel) and left pulmonary veins (lpv). LA: left atrium; lpa: left pulmonary artery; RA: right atrium.

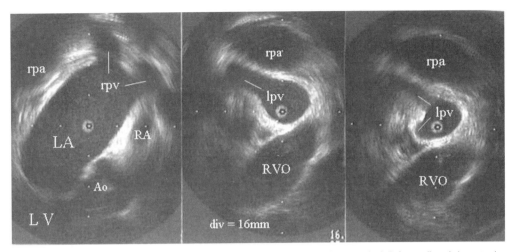

Figure 3.27 Mechanical radial ICE images with the transducer placed in the left atrium (LA) (left panel) and closer to the left pulmonary vein (lpv) ostia (the middle and right panels) through a transseptal sheath, showing the right pulmonary veins (rpv) and lpv with their ostia and luminal wall structures. Ao: aortic root; LV: left ventricle; RA: right atrium; rpa: right pulmonary artery; RVO: right ventricular outflow tract.

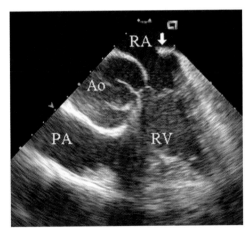

Figure 3.28 ICE image with the transducer placed in the right atrium (RA), showing a prominent eustachian valve (arrow), right ventricular (RV) inflow and outflow. Ao: aortic root; PA: pulmonary artery.

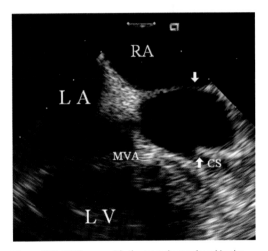

Figure 3.29 ICE image with the transducer placed in the right atrium (RA), showing the thebesian valve (upward arrow) guarding the coronary sinus (CS) orifice, and a variant Eustachian valve (downward arrow) connecting from the inferior vena cava orifice to the lower interatrial septum. LA: left atrium; LV: left ventricle; MVA: mitral annulus.

attached to the posterior annulus from the inferolateral to the septal wall. The septal (medial) leaflet is attached to the septal annular ring in the region of ventricular septum between the anterior and posterior leaflets. The tricuspid annular septal insertion is inferior to the mitral septal annular insertion [12]. The right ventricular inflow and tricuspid valve can be visualized with AcuNav transducer placed in the middle/lower right atrium facing anteriorly and inferiorly (Figure 3.35). Tricuspid regurgitation jets are often directed toward the transducer even without tip deflection, allowing excellent continuous-wave Doppler interrogation for estimation of right ventricular systolic pressure. ICE imaging of different regions along the annulus may provide anatomic guidance for catheter ablation of accessory atrioventricular pathways in patients with supraventricular tachycardia [13].

(a)

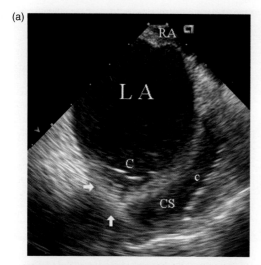

(b)

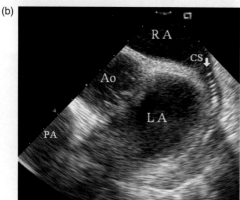

Figure 3.30 (a) ICE image with the transducer placed in the high right atrium (RA), showing a long-axis view of the coronary sinus (CS) containing a CS catheter (c). A Lasso catheter (C) is placed in the common left pulmonary vein ostium in the left atrium (LA). The region of the oblique vein of Marshall and ligament of Marshall is located between the distal CS and the upper left pulmonary vein ostium (arrows). (b) ICE image with the transducer placed in the lower right atrium (RA) deflected to the left, showing the long-axis view of the coronary sinus (CS) with a CS catheter seen inside (arrow). Ao: aortic root; LA: left atrium; PA: pulmonary artery.

Papillary muscles and moderator band

There are multiple separate papillary muscles connected to the free edges of the tricuspid leaflets through the chordae tendineae. Of these, the anterior papillary muscle is easy to distinguish as it arises from the moderator band and the anterior septal right ventricular wall. The posterior and septal papillary muscles originate from the posterior and septal

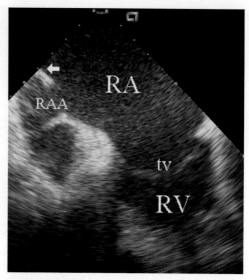

Figure 3.31 ICE image with the transducer placed at the junction of superior vena cava and right atrium (RA) and deflected posteriorly, showing RA appendage (RAA) with pectinate muscles, the superior crista terminalis (arrow) and right ventricle (RV). tv: tricuspid valve.

wall of the right ventricle, respectively. The posterior papillary muscle usually has multiple heads. There may also be multiple smaller papillary muscles in addition to those described earlier. The papillary muscles and moderator band can be visualized with the AcuNav transducer placed in the atrium near the atrioventricular junction (Figure 3.36) or with the mechanical radial ICE transducer placed in the right ventricle (Figure 3.37a) or right ventricular outflow tract (Figure 3.37b).

Right ventricular outflow tract and pulmonic valve

The right ventricular outflow tract is the anterosuperior outflow portion of the right ventricle, from which the pulmonary artery originates. The infundibulum (right ventricular outflow tract) and pulmonic valve can be visualized with the AcuNav transducer placed in the right atrium, facing anterosuperiorly and scanning from the right ventricle inflow to the right ventricular outflow (Figure 3.38a,b). These structures can also be visualized with mechanical radial ICE transducer in the right ventricular outflow tract (Figure 3.37c).

Pulmonary artery and right pulmonary artery

The pulmonary artery arises superiorly from the right ventricle, passes backward and slightly upward and

(a)

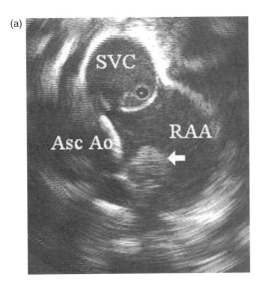

(b)

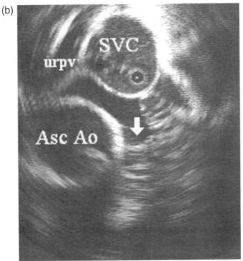

Figure 3.32 Mechanical radial ICE images of the right atrial appendage (RAA) with the transducer placed in the superior vena cava (SVC), showing: (a) a mass (arrow); (b) representing a partial cross-section view through pectinate muscles (arrow) within the RAA. The radius of the image = 60 mm. Asc Ao: ascending aorta; urpv: upper right pulmonary vein.

bifurcates into the right and left pulmonary arteries. The main and right pulmonary artery can be imaged with the AcuNav transducer in the right atrium while scanning upward from the pulmonic valve (Figure 3.38b). Rotating the transducer clockwise with slight anterior deflection allows additional views of the main pulmonary artery and its bifurcation (Figure 3.38c). In addition, when the transducer

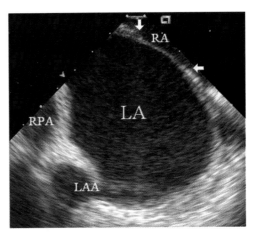

Figure 3.33 ICE image with the transducer placed in the right atrium (RA), showing the interatrial septum. The central portion is the fossa ovalis and the limbus (arrows) is a muscular ridge around it. LA and LAA: left atrium and LA appendage; RPA: right pulmonary artery.

is advanced superiorly, slight posterior tip deflection allows visualization of the right pulmonary artery in its long-axis as it passes alongside an upper or middle right pulmonary vein (Figure 3.39). The main pulmonary artery and its bifurcation can also be visualized with the mechanical radial ICE transducer placed at the junction of superior vena cava and right atrial appendage (Figure 3.21).

Left atrium

Left and right pulmonary veins and ostia

The left atrium consists mainly of a smooth-walled sac, the transverse axis of which is somewhat larger than the vertical and sagittal axes [5]. When the left atrium is enlarged it becomes more spherical. Two pulmonary veins enter the left atrium from the left. Occasionally they share a common trunk. On the right, there are two or, occasionally, three pulmonary veins. All these veins and their ostia are easily visualized using the AcuNav transducer (Figures 3.9a,b and 3.10) or the mechanical radial ICE transducer (Figure 3.26) from the right atrium. ICE is an extremely valuable imaging technique for guiding mapping and ablation catheters at pulmonary vein ostia, and for monitoring ostial flow velocity during radiofrequency pulmonary vein ostial ablation procedures [3].

Left atrial appendage

The left atrial appendage originates from the superior aspect of the left atrium on the left, anteriorly.

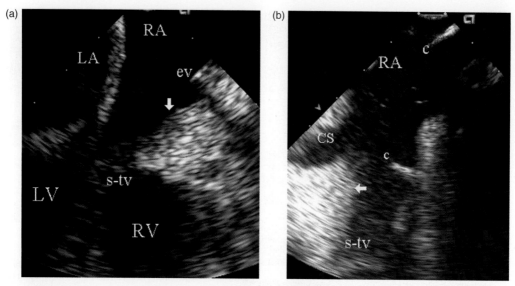

Figure 3.34 (a) ICE images with the transducer placed in the lower right artrium (RA), showing the inferior vena cava-tricuspid valve (tv) isthmus region. The "central" (inferior) isthmus is visualized with the transducer oriented inferiorly and posteriorly. This area (arrow) is located between the Eustachian valve (ev) posteriorly and the insertion of septal leaflet of the tv (s-tv) anteriorly. (b) A magnified view of the septal isthmus (arrow) is also demonstrated. This septal isthmus is located between the coronary sinus (CS) ostium and the insertion of the s-tv. The anterior section close to the hinge of the s-tv consists of myocardium formed by the full thickness of the atrial wall and demonstrates increased echogenicity. c: catheter; LV and RV: left and right ventricle.

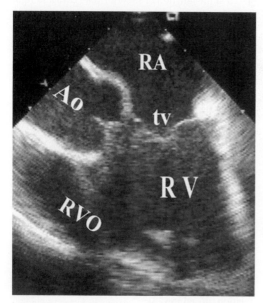

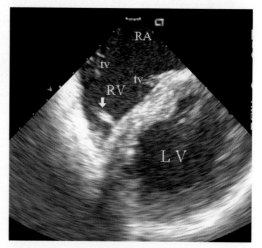

Figure 3.36 ICE image with the transducer placed near the atrioventricular junction in the right atrium (RA), showing the moderator band (arrow) between the anterior and septal right ventricular (RV) wall. LV: left ventricle; tv: anterior or septal leaflet of the tricuspid valve.

Figure 3.35 ICE image with the transducer placed in the mid-right atrium (RA), showing the right ventricular (RV) inflow with tricuspid valve (tv, anterior and posterior leaflets). Ao: aorta; RVO: RV outflow tract. Reproduced with permission [1].

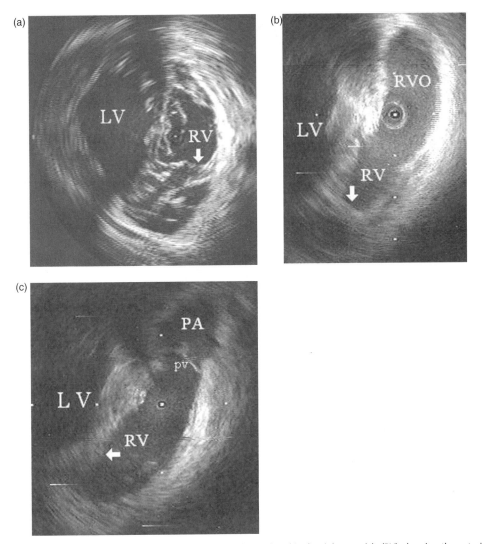

Figure 3.37 Mechanical radial ICE images: (a) with the transducer placed in the right ventricle (RV), showing the anterior papillary muscle arising from the moderator band (arrow) and the anterior septal RV wall (radius = 60 mm); (b) with the transducer placed in the RV outflow tract (RVO), showing the moderator band (arrow) attached to the anterior papillary muscle (each scale = 16 mm); (c) with transducer advanced further in the RVO, showing the pulmonic valve (pv) and pulmonary artery (PA), and initial septal band (arrow) (each scale = 32 mm). LV: left ventricle.

Its lumen contains small pectinate muscles proximally with a distinct waistlike narrowing. Catheterization of this structure must be performed with caution as its walls are thin, especially between the pectinate muscles where it can be easily perforated. Visualization from the right atrium using the AcuNav catheter is straightforward (Figure 3.7), and is of particular importance in monitoring upper left pulmonary vein catheterization especially in patients with an enlarged left atrial appendage (see Figure 11.4) or a transverse heart where accidental catheterization of this structure is more common.

Ligament of Marshall

The ligament of Marshall is a fold of the left superior vena cava [5] running downward to the oblique (Marshall) vein of the left atrium (Figure 3.40). During heart development at 10 weeks the distal part of the left sinus horn develops into the oblique vein of Marshall, while the proximal portion of the horn and

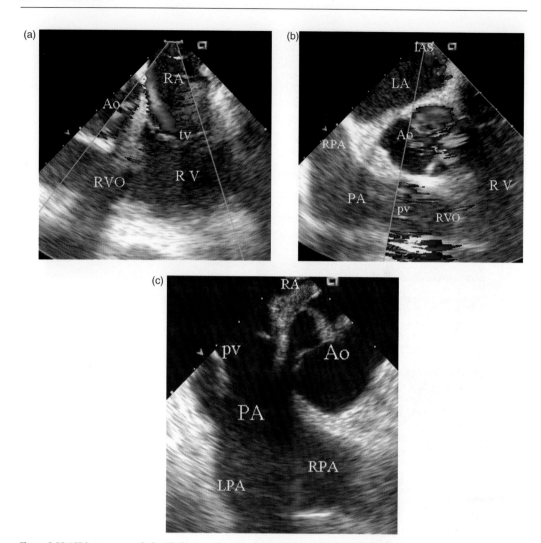

Figure 3.38 ICE images recorded with the transducer in the right atrium (RA): (a) demonstrates the right ventricular (RV) inflow and outflow tract (RVO) with mixed color flow in the RA at end-systole; (b) with the transducer advanced superiorly and anteriorly up to the interatrial septum (IAS), demonstrates the pulmonic valve (pv), the pulmonary artery (PA), the right pulmonary artery (RPA) and the aortic root (Ao), and shows mixed color flow in the Ao at early systole; (c) with the transducer rotated clockwise and deflected anteriorly, demonstrates the proximal left pulmonary artery (LPA) at the bifurcation of the PA. LA: left atrium; tv: tricuspid valve.

the transverse portion of the sinus become the coronary sinus [14]. From the right atrium, the ligament of Marshall may be visualized with the AcuNav transducer in two cross-sectional views: a short-axis view of the ligament of Marshall between the left upper pulmonary vein ostium and the left atrial appendage (Figure 3.41), and a longitudinal cross-sectional view of it (Figure 3.42) between the distal coronary sinus and the left pulmonary vein ostia adjacent to the left wall of the descending aorta anteriorly [15]. It has a

distinctly echogenic appearance compared to adjacent tissue and is therefore easily visualized [15]. This structure contains important neuromuscular bundle where autonomic activity can be a frequent source of paroxysmal atrial fibrillation, and this structure is commonly ablated in this setting [16].

Left ventricle

The left ventricle is shaped like an egg with its base located superiorly and posteriorly. The inferior mitral

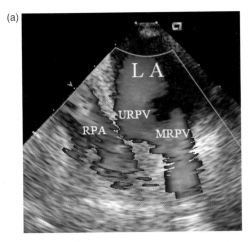

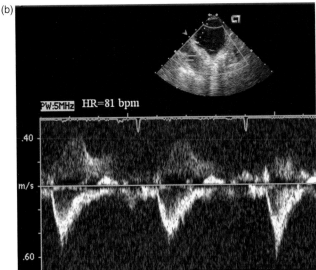

Figure 3.39 ICE images with the transducer placed in the high right atrium, showing: (a) the right pulmonary artery (RPA) with its blue color flow directed away from the transducer. This vessel passes alongside the upper (URPV) and middle right pulmonary vein (MRPV) with their red color flow directed toward the transducer, entering the left atrium (LA); (b) pulsed-wave Doppler spectrum recorded peak flow velocity from RPA during systole.

and the superior aortic valves are located adjacent to each other along the posterior wall. Both valves are separated by a fibrous band from which the anterior mitral leaflet and the adjacent portions of the left and posterior (noncoronary) aortic-valve cusps originate [5].

Mitral valve and mitral annulus

The mitral valve is situated in the fibromuscular annulus of the left heart between the left atrium and the left ventricle. It resides in the posteroinferior inflow portion of the left ventricular cavity and consists of an anterior (septal) and a posterior (lateral) leaflet with their basal portions attached to the mitral annulus. The free edges of the leaflets are connected to

the papillary muscles through chordae tendineae. The mitral annulus is formed from two strong fibrous trigones, one on the right and one on the left. The right fibrous trigone is situated between the tricuspid, aortic and mitral valves, comprising the largest portion of the cardiac skeleton. The left fibrous trigone separates the anterior mitral leaflet and the adjacent portions of the left and posterior (noncoronary) aortic-valve cusps [5].

Papillary muscles

Two stout papillary muscles originate from anteriolateral and posteromedial free wall at the level of the middle third and posterior aspect of the left ventricle. Each of them receives chordae tendineae from

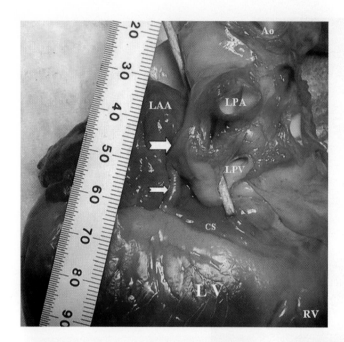

Figure 3.40 Gross anatomic specimen of the heart (swine), demonstrating the ligament of Marshall (large arrow) located between the oblique (Marshall) vein of left atrium (small arrow) and the left pulmonary artery (LPA). Ao: aorta; CS: coronary sinus; LAA: left atrial appendage; LPV: left pulmonary vein; LV: left ventricle; RV: right ventricle.

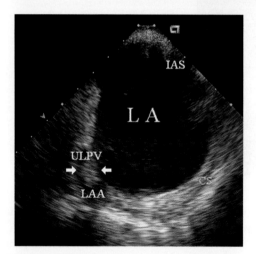

Figure 3.41 ICE image with the transducer placed in the high right atrium, showing a cross-sectional view of the ligament of Marshall (arrows) between the upper left pulmonary vein (ULPV) and left atrial (LA) appendage (LAA). CS: coronary sinus; IAS: interatrial septum.

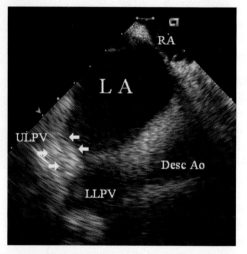

Figure 3.42 ICE image with the transducer placed in the high right atrium (RA), showing a long-axis view of the ligament of Marshall (arrows) between the upper (ULPV) and lower left pulmonary vein (LLPV) ostia and distal coronary sinus, adjacent to the left front wall of the descending aorta (Desc Ao). LA: left atrium.

both the major mitral valvular leaflets. Occasionally, a third small papillary muscle is present laterally (Figure 3.43).

Interventricular septum

Most of the interventricular septum is muscular except the membranous portion. Normally it bulges into the right ventricle so that in transverse section, the left ventricle is almost circular (Figure 3.24). Its muscular portion has approximately the same thickness as the left ventricular free wall and consists of two layers, a thin one on the right ventricular side and a thicker one on the left ventricular side.

(a)
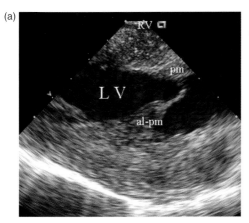

(b)
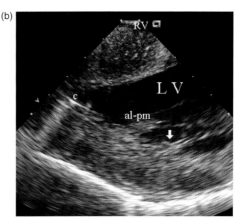

Figure 3.43 ICE images with the transducer placed in the right ventricle (RV), showing: (a) the anterolateral (al-pm) and posteromedial (pm) papillary muscles and (b) a third small papillary muscle (arrow) visualized laterally in a long-axis view of a hypertrophic left ventricle (LV). c: catheter.

The mitral valve, papillary muscles and left ventricular wall can be visualized using the AcuNav imaging catheter from the right atrium near the atrioventricular junction (Figures 3.14 and 3.15) or from the right ventricle (Figure 3.43). Accurate and efficient imaging of these structures is extremely important for guiding left ventricular mapping and ablation procedures.

Aortic valve and sinuses of Valsalva

The aortic valve consists of the three semilunar cusps (left, right, and noncoronary), which arise from the left ventricular outflow tract. Unlike the mitral valve, the aortic valve is not anchored by a distinct fibrous ring; rather, the aortic wall expands into three dilated pouches – the sinuses of Valsalva [5] whose walls are much thinner than that of the aorta. The origin of the valve cusps is, therefore, not straight but scalloped. The three aortic cusps are easily visualized in the short-axis view of the aortic valve using the AcuNav transducer from the right atrium near the posterior wall of the aortic root (Figure 3.13). ICE imaging provides important anatomic identification during mapping and radiofrequency ablation of the aortic-valve cusp especially for treatment of ventricular tachycardia where it plays a critical role in preventing damage to the coronary artery ostia [17].

References

1 Ren JF, Marchlinski FE, Callans DJ, Herrmann HC. Clinical use of AcuNav diagnostic ultrasound catheter imaging during left heart radiofrequency ablation and transcatheter closure procedures. *J Am Soc Echocardiogr* 2002; **15**: 1301–1308.

2 Ren JF, Schwartzman D, Callans D, Marchlinski FE, Gottlieb CD, Chaudhry FA. Imaging technique and clinical utility for electrophysiologic procedures of lower frequency (9 MHz) intracardiac echocardiography. *Am J Cardiol* 1998; **82**: 1557–1560.

3 Ren JF, Marchlinski FE, Callans DJ, Zado ES. Intracardiac Doppler echocardiographic quantification of pulmonary vein flow velocity: an effective technique for monitoring pulmonary vein ostia narrowing during focal atrial fibrillation ablation. *J Cardiovasc Electrophysiol* 2002; **13**: 1076–1081.

4 Ren JF, Schwartzman D, Callans DJ, Brode SE, Gottlieb CD, Marchlinski FE. Intracardiac echocardiography (9 MHz) in humans: methods, imaging views and clinical utility. *Ultrasound in Med & Biol* 1999; **25**: 1077–1086.

5 Netter FH, Yonkman FF. The CIBA Collection of Medical Illustrations, Volume 5. *A compilation of paintings on the normal and pathologic anatomy and physiology, embryology, and diseases of the heart.* Summit: CIBA, 1974: 8–12.

6 Ren JF, Schwartzman D, Chaudhry FA. Intracardiac echocardiographic imaging of right atrial appendage: mass vs. pectinate muscle. *J Interventional Cardiac Electrophysiol* 1998; **2**: 247–248.

7 Ren JF, Marchlinski FE, Callans DJ, Zado ES. Echocardiographic lesion characteristics associated with successful ablation of inappropriate sinus tachycardia. *J Cardiovasc Electrophysiol* 2001; **12**: 814–818.

8 Cabrera JA, Sanchez-Quintana D, Ho SY, Medina A, Anderson RH. The architecture of the atrial musculature

between the orifice of the inferior caval vein and the tricuspid valve: the anatomy of the isthmus. *J Cardiovasc Electrophysiol* 1998; **9**: 1186–1195.

9 Cabrera JA, Sanchez-Quintana D, Ho SY, *et al.* Angiographic anatomy of the inferior right atrial isthmus in patients with and without history of common atrial flutter. *Circulation* 1999; **99**: 3017–3023.

10 Cosio FG, Arribas F, Barbero JM, Kallmeyer C, Goicolea A. Validation of double spike electrograms as markers of conduction delay or block in atrial flutter. *Am J Cardiol* 1998; **61**: 775–780.

11 Nakagawa H, Lazzara R, Khastgir T, *et al.* Role of the tricuspid annulus and Eustachian valve/ridge on atrial flutter: relevance to catheter ablation of the septal isthmus and a new technique for rapid identification of ablation success. *Circulation* 1996; **94**: 407–424.

12 Silver MD, Lam JHC, Ranganathan N, Wigle ED. Morphology of the human tricuspid valve. *Circulation* 1971; **43**: 333–348.

13 Ren JF, Schwartzman D, Callans DJ, Marchlinski FE, Zhang LP, Chaudhry FA. Intracardiac echocardiographic imaging in guiding and monitoring radiofrequency catheter ablation at the tricuspid annulus. *Echocardiography* 1998; **15**: 661–664.

14 Sadler TW. *Langman's Medical Embryology.* Lippincott Williams & Wilkins, Philadelphia, 2000: 217–220.

15 Ren JF, Lin D, Gerstenfeld EP, Lewkowiez L, Callans DJ. Ligament of Marshall tissue related to pulmonary vein ostial ablation: an intracardiac echocardiographic imaging study (abstr). *Circulation* 2003; **108**: IV-646.

16 Katritsis D, Ioannidis JPA, Anagnostopoulos CE, *et al.* Identification and catheter ablation of extracardiac and intracardiac components of ligament of Marshall tissue for treatment of paroxysmal atrial fibrillation. *J Cardiovasc Electrophysiol* 2001; **12**: 750–758.

17 Marchlinski FE, Lin D, Dixit S, *et al.* Ventricular tachycardia from the aortic cusps: localization and ablation. In: Raviele A, ed. *Cardiac Arrhythmias.* Springer-Verlag, Italia, Milan, 2003: 357–370.

CHAPTER 4

Cardiac Anatomic and Functional Abnormalities Commonly Diagnosed in Patients Undergoing Electrophysiological Procedures

Jian-Fang Ren, MD, *& David J. Callans,* MD

Variant eustachian valve and Chiari network

Congenital remnants of the sinus venosus may appear as residual tissue echodensities within the right atrium. These include the eustachian valve and Chiari network. A prominent eustachian valve may commonly be seen at the junction of the inferior vena cava and the right atrium (see Chapter 3, Figures 3.15 and 3.27). The Chiari network, which is due to incomplete resorption of the right valve of the sinus venosus, is less frequently seen. The Chiari network represents persistence of fibrous strands attached to the edges of the eustachian valve and/or the coronary sinus (thebesian) valve and/or crista terminalis [1–3]. The Chiari network is a thin, fenestrated, web-like membrane that appears with ICE imaging as a highly reflective freely mobile, filamentous echodensity within the right atrium. The network generally originates at the junction of the inferior vena cava and right atrium, extends across the right atrium toward the tricuspid valve ring, and inserts into the atrial septum or right atrial wall (Figure 4.1). It is important to search and visualize this structure fully with the transducer placed in the middle of right atrium, rotating clockwise from imaging of the junction of the inferior vena cava and the right atrium, and tricuspid valve annulus, interatrial septum, then to imaging of the right atrium wall or crista terminalis (Figure 4.2).

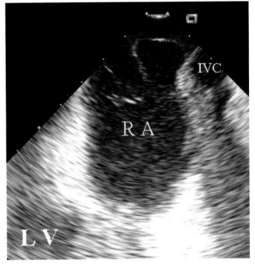

Figure 4.1 ICE image with the transducer placed in the right atrium (RA) above the orifice of inferior vena cava (IVC), showing the Chiari network as a freely mobile, filamentous echodensity originating at the junction of IVC and RA, across the RA chamber, and inserting into the interatrial septum. LV: left ventricle.

Lipomatous hypertrophy of the interatrial septum

Lipomatous hypertrophy of the atrial septum is characterized by excessive accumulation of adipose tissue

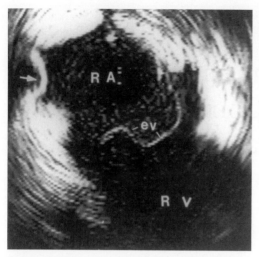

Figure 4.2 Mechanical radial ICE image with the transducer placed in the right atrium (RA), showing a delicate lace-like structure attached to the lateral crista terminalis, known as a variant eustachian valve (ev) or the network of Chiari, and an interatrial septal aneurysm (arrow) bulging toward the RA in diastole. RV: right ventricle.

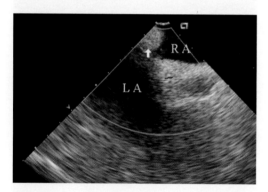

Figure 4.3 ICE image with the transducer placed in the right atrium (RA), showing lipomatous hypertrophy of interatrial septum (IAS) (17 mm, arrow). LA: left atrium.

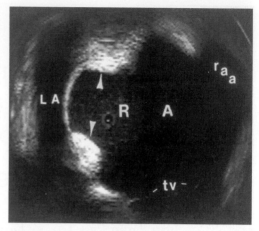

Figure 4.4 Mechanical radial ICE image with transducer placed in the right atrium (RA), showing a dumbbell-shaped lipomatous hypertrophy of the interatrial septum (arrowheads). LA: left atrium; raa: right atrial appendage; tv: tricuspid valve.

in the septum that produces globular thickening of the septum (≥ 15 mm).

The central membrane of the fossa ovalis is always spared; thus the mass may have a characteristic "dumbbell" appearance [4–7]. Some reports have suggested that supraventricular arrhythmias of atrial origin and abnormal P waves on the electrocardiogram may be a consequence of this fatty deposition in the atrial septum, especially seen among older (mean age 70 years) or obese patients [5–7]. Interatrial septum with differing degrees of thickening or the characteristic "dumbbell" appearance (Figures 4.3 and 4.4)

can be easily identified with ICE before transseptal catheterization. As transseptal puncture may be more difficult in this setting, ICE imaging guidance to ensure puncture at the fossa ovalis proper may be helpful.

Atrial septal aneurysm

The interatrial septal aneurysm is recognized as a bulging of the thin, billowing septal tissue typically involving the region of the fossa ovalis. The redundant aneurysmal septum may bulge back and forth between the right and the left atrium within the cardiac cycle (Figure 4.5). The diagnosis of the aneurysm can be made qualitatively, but a displacement ≥ 15 mm beyond the plane of the interatrial septum is also applied [8]. The septal aneurysm is not an uncommon abnormality, and in many cases may be an incidental finding. Although an atrial septal aneurysm is generally considered to be benign, it has been associated with atrial septal defects, atrial arrhythmias, atrioventricular valvular prolapse, and embolic events [8–10].

Patent foramen ovale

A patent foramen ovale is a channel through or interruption of the superior portion of the fossa ovalis membrane and the atrial septum [11]. This channel may be just a barely detectable slit or may be

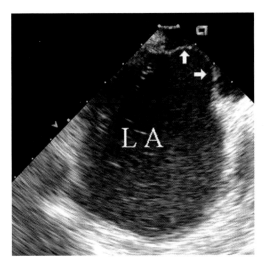

Figure 4.5 ICE image with the transducer placed in the right atrium, showing interatrial septal (IAS) aneurysm bulging into the right atrium (arrows). LA: left atrium.

large enough to allow intermittent or persistent left-to-right shunting although usually without hemodynamic consequences. With ICE color Doppler imaging, the patent foramen ovale can be easily detected (Figure 4.6a,b) and its size often varies throughout the respiratory cycle. Both the size of the defect and the degree of right-to-left shunting may increase with increased right atrial blood flow during inspiration, especially with the Valsalva maneuver. The significance of finding a patent foramen ovale and attributing an ischemic event to paradoxical embolism remains controversial [12]. A higher prevalence of a patent foramen ovalis has been demonstrated in patients with unexplained cerebral ischemia and embolic events [13]. However, no difference in the prevalence of patent foramen ovale was reported in patients with cerebral ischemia compared to matched patients without unexplained cerebral ischemia [14]. With recent advances in the percutaneous transcatheter closure technique, many investigators argue about closure of the anatomic defect in patients with presumed or high risk of paradoxical embolism [15–17].

Atrial septal defect

Four types of atrial septal defects are conventionally described: secundum, sinus venosus, coronary sinus,

and ostium primum. Of these, only the secundum defect represents a true deficiency of the atrial septum since the atrial septum is defined as that part of the wall separating the two atrial cavities which is thus confined to the floor of the fossa ovalis and its immediate surroundings [18]. It is also the most common atrial septal defect that appears as a deficiency in the midportion of the septum with a T-shaped sign at its margin (Figure 4.7). ICE with Doppler color flow imaging may provide transatrial flow shunting and hemodynamic features (Figure 4.8). The other three types of the atrial septal defects are rarely diagnosed during electrophysiologic procedures. The sinus venosus defect occurs when the superior or inferior vena cava is anomalously connected to both atria. The rarer coronary sinus defect is also an anomalous communication between the roof of the coronary sinus and the left atrium. The ostium primum atrial septal defect is an interatrial communication through a deficiency at the site of the atrioventricular septum, that is, absence of tissue in the most inferior portion of the atrial septum (at the level of insertion of the septal leaflets of the atrioventricular valves). Thus, an ostium primum defect may occur alone (partial atrioventricular canal) or in association with defect in the inlet ventricular septum (complete atrioventricular canal or endocardial cushion defect) [19]. Although these defects are not typically diagnosed during electrophysiological procedures, ICE does provide detailed anatomic or Doppler color flow imaging to better define sinus venous (Figure 4.9), coronary sinus (Figure 4.10) or ostium primum defects (Figure 4.11).

Ventricular septal defect

The interventricular septum is composed of membranous and muscular portions. Ventricular septal defects are rarely limited to the membranous septum, but more often extend into the muscular (inlet, trabecular or outlet) region ("perimembranous") [19]. Perimembranous defects are the most common ventricular septal defect (Figure 4.12). Ventricular septal defect may be a small or large defect, or may occur as part of complex cardiovascular malformations such as in Fallot's tetralogy. These defects and malformations are usually not diagnosed incidentally, but may be seen after surgical repair during electrophysiologic procedures.

(a)

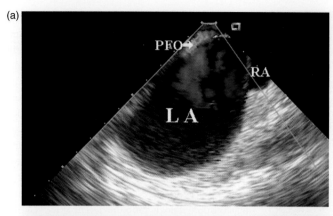

(b)

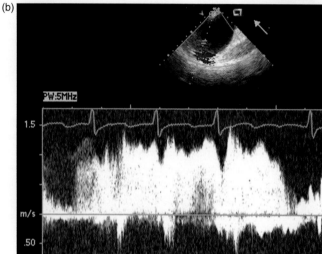

Figure 4.6 (a) ICE image with the transducer placed in the right atrium (RA), showing septal aneurysm bulging into the RA and a patent foramen ovale (PFO) as indicated by color flow imaging with the red turbulent flow across the superior limbus (arrow) in a left to right direction. (b) High pulsed repetition frequency pulsed Doppler echocardiogram with the sample volume at the PFO from the RA side. Flow above the baseline indicates left to right shunting through the PFO. Turbulent flow persists throughout the cardiac cycle and reaches a maximal velocity of approximately 1.5 m/sec.

Ebstein's anomaly

Ebstein's anomaly is characterized by a downward displacement of the tricuspid valve into the right ventricle due to anomalous attachment of the tricuspid leaflets [20,21]. The pathologic anatomy of the tricuspid valve is better demonstrated with these newer echocardiographic techniques (Figure 4.13a,b) than with angiography [22]. The clinical presentation and prognosis are related to the degree of atrialization of the right ventricle, the severity of tricuspid regurgitation, the presence of significant arrhythmias and the coexistence of other congenital malformations [22,23].

Left ventricular hypertrophy

Left ventricular hypertrophy is commonly seen in aged patients with arrhythmias, arterial hypertension, or calcified aortic valves (Figure 4.14a). It (Figure 4.14b) can be simply indicated by ICE imaging showing a thickened ventricular wall (>11 mm during diastole). A more detailed evaluation of left ventricular hypertrophy is performed by measuring left ventricular mass using the biplane area-length formula for volumetric determinations ($v = 8A_1 \times A_2/3\pi L$, where A_1 and A_2 represent the enclosed area of a chamber of two orthogonal views, respectively, and L is the common axis shared). The left ventricular mass is determined as follows: (Epicardial enclosed volume − Endocardial enclosed volume) × 1.05, where 1.05 is the specific gravity of the myocardium [24].

Valvular regurgitation

Cardiac functional and organic valvular regurgitation may be qualitatively and quantitatively evaluated by

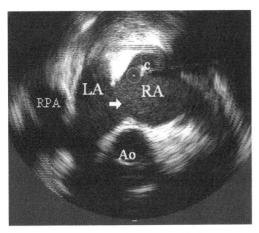

Figure 4.7 Mechanical radial ICE image with the transducer placed near the septum in the right atrium (RA), showing a secundum atrial septal defect (arrow) with a 16 mm diameter. A T-sign (thickened) is seen at the superior edge of the defect. Ao: aorta; C: catheter; LA: left atrium; RPA: right pulmonary artery.

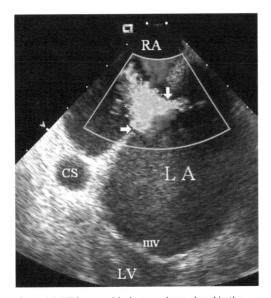

Figure 4.8 ICE image with the transducer placed in the high right atrium (RA), showing color flow imaging of a secundum atrial septum defect (17 mm diameter) with left to right shunt (red mosaic color). CS: coronary sinus; LA: left atrium; LV: left ventricle; mv: mitral valve.

ICE with pulsed, continuous wave and color flow Doppler imaging.

Tricuspid regurgitation

The severity of tricuspid regurgitation may be evaluated primarily by the size of the regurgitant jet on the

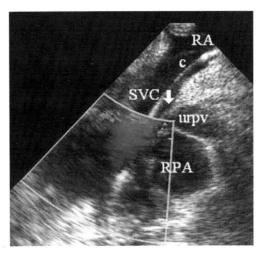

Figure 4.9 ICE of image with the transducer placed in the junction of the right atrium (RA) and superior vena cava (SVC) and its tip slightly anteriorly deflected, showing an anatomic region of the high septum near the junction of the SVC and the RA (arrow) and color flow imaging of SVC flow toward RA (red color). If the upper right pulmonary vein (urpv) drains anomalously into that site, a sinus venosus defect can be detected by color flow imaging of an abnomal flow communication. C: catheter; RPA: right pulmonary artery.

color flow image. Continuous wave Doppler recording of tricuspid regurgitation is used to calculate the right atrial–right ventricular systolic pressure difference from the modified Bernoulli equation ($P_1 - P_2 = 4V^2$), using the peak velocity of the regurgitant jet [25–27]. Pulmonary artery systolic pressure can be estimated by adding 10–14 mmHg which represents an empiric value of right atrial systolic pressure, provided no pulmonic valve stenosis is present (Figure 4.15).

Mitral regurgitation

ICE may be used for diagnosis of mitral regurgitation with the same high degree of accuracy as transesophageal echocardiography [28]. With ICE imaging, semiquantitation of mitral regurgitation from a mitral valve prostheses can be made without interference from prosthetic acoustic shadow. For imaging of an entire left atrium, ICE may have real advantage (Figure 4.16a,b) over transesophageal echocardiography because of the limitation in space within the esophagus to manipulate the transducer and the difficulty in imaging the entire left atrium because the probe is placed in close apposition. ICE may

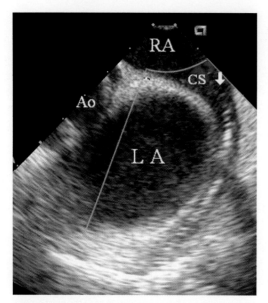

Figure 4.10 ICE of image with the transducer placed in the lower right atrium (RA) and its tip deflected slightly leftward, showing the long-axis view of the coronary sinus (CS) with a CS catheter from its orifice (arrow) to distal lumen, and color flow imaging of CS ostial flow toward RA (red color). If an anomalous communication exists through the defect of the roof of the CS wall, a CS defect can be detected by color flow imaging of an abnormal flow communication between CS and LA. Ao: aorta.

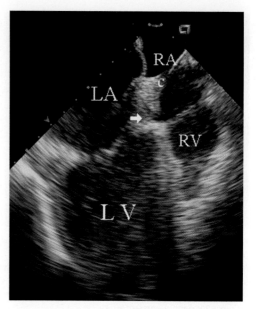

Figure 4.11 ICE of image with the transducer placed in the high right atrium (RA), showing a four-chamber view including the crux at the site of the ostium primum (arrow). If an interatrial communication exists through a deficiency at the site of the most inferior portion of the atrial septum, an ostium primum defect can be detected by color flow imaging of flow shunting and tissue dropout at the lower end of the atrial septum. Mitral regurgitation can be detected if an accompanied cleft in the mitral valve is present. c: catheter; LA and LV: left atrium and ventricle.

provide the ratio of maximal regurgitant area to left atrial area for semiquantitative evaluation of the mitral regurgitation (Figure 4.17a,b and c) [29]. Left atrial emptying volume may be measured and used for quantifying the degree of nonrheumatic mitral regurgitation [30]. ICE can be of great assistance in clarifying the cause of regurgitation (endocarditis, flail leaflets, or valve chordal ruptures) and identify associated complications (such as valve perforation, intracardiac fistulas) during electrophysiologic procedures.

Aortic insufficiency

The severity of aortic insufficiency can be semi-quantitatively evaluated using ICE Doppler color flow imaging based on mapping the length of the diastolic regurgitant turbulent color-flow jet of the left ventricle [31]. Mild (1+) aortic regurgitation is defined by a diastolic regurgitant flow jet reaching subjacent to the aortic valve; moderate (2+) aortic regurgitation is regurgitant flow jet reaching the left ventricular

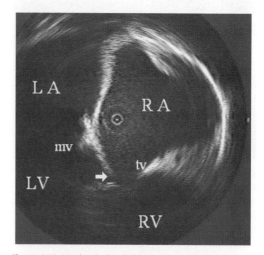

Figure 4.12 Mechanical radial ICE image with the transducer placed near the crux of the heart in the right atrium (RA), showing the anatomic tricuspid annulus and apical displacement of the insertion of the tricuspid septal leaflet (tv). A perimembranous ventricular septal defect (arrow, 6 mm diameter) is imaged. LA and LV: left atrium and ventricle; mv: mitral valve; RV: right ventricle.

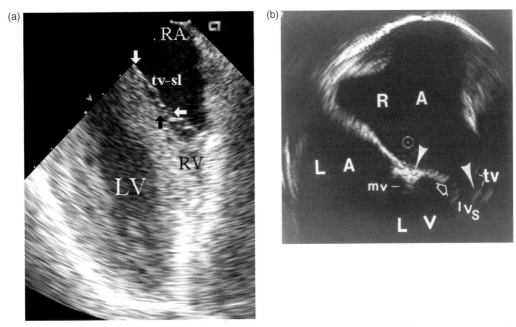

Figure 4.13 (a) ICE image of Ebstein's anomaly with the transducer placed in the right atrium (RA), showing the anatomic tricuspid annulus and apical displacement (between the two white arrows) of the insertion of the tricuspid septal leaflet (tv-sl) with tethering to the septum (upward arrow). (b) Mechanical radial ICE image with the transducer placed near the crux of the heart in the right atrium (RA), showing the anatomic tricuspid annulus and apical displacement of the insertion of the tricuspid septal leaflet (tv, two arrowheads = 3.9 cm). A perimembranous ventricular septal defect (arrow) is imaged (6 mm in diameter). The crista terminalis seen as a prominent ridge extended from the RA posterior wall (oriented at 11 o'clock). IVS: interventricular septum; LA: left atrium; LV: left ventricle; RV: right ventricle.

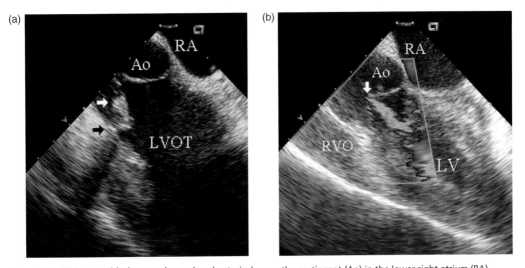

Figure 4.14 ICE image with the transducer placed anteriorly near the aortic root (Ao) in the lower right atrium (RA), showing: (a) calcified/thickened aortic valve cusp (white arrow) and annulus (black arrow) with distal acoustic shadowing; (b) color flow imaging of aortic regurgitant flow (arrow) toward apex (blue mosaic color) indicating a moderate to severe aortic insufficiency, and thickened left ventricular (LV) wall (14 mm) during diastole. LVOT: LV outflow tract; RVO: RV outflow tract.

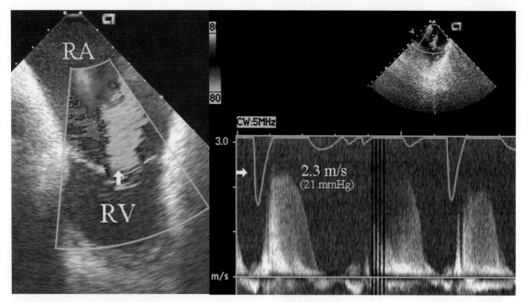

Figure 4.15 ICE image with the transducer placed in the right atrium (RA), showing right ventricular (RV) inflow with tricuspid regurgitant color-flow jet (red mosaic color) during systole (the left panel), and a 2.3 m/s (estimated the systolic pressure gradient = 21 mmHg between the RV and RA) of the regurgitant peak flow velocity recorded with continuous-wave Doppler spectrum (the right panel). The pulmonary atery systolic pressure was estimated as 31 mmHg by adding 10 mmHg for the RA systolic pressure.

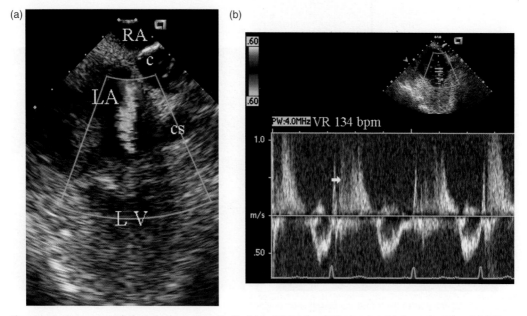

Figure 4.16 ICE images with the transducer placed in the high right atrium (RA), showing: (a) the entire left atrial (LA) area and color flow imaging of maximal mitral regurgitant flow area during systole; (b) pulsed wave Doppler spectra of mitral regurgitation (arrow) recorded with sampling volume placed on the LA side of the mitral valvular orifice during atrial fibrillation. C: catheter; CS: coronary sinus; LV: left ventricle; VR: ventricular rate.

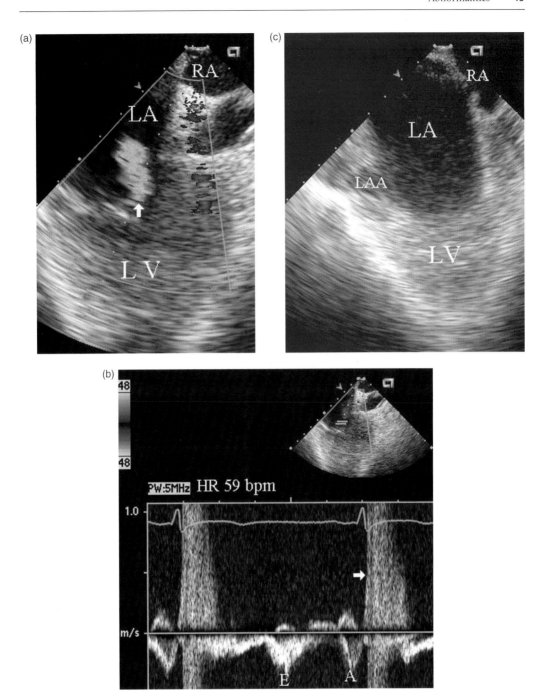

Figure 4.17 ICE images with the transducer placed in the right atrium (RA), showing: (a) color flow imaging of maximal mitral regurgitant flow area (arrow, red mosaic color) during systole; (b) pulsed wave Doppler spectra of mitral regurgitation (arrow) recorded with the sampling volume placed on the left atrial (LA) side of the mitral valvular orifice; (c) with the transducer placed in the high RA an entire LA area is imaged for calculation of the ratio of the color regurgitant flow area to the entire atrial area. LAA: LA appendage; LV: left ventricle.

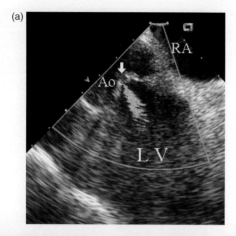

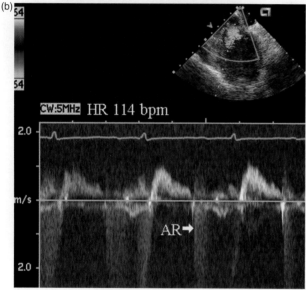

Figure 4.18 ICE images with the transducer placed in the right atrium (RA), showing: (a) color flow imaging of aortic regurgitant (AR) flow toward left ventricular (LV) outflow tract (arrow, blue mosaic color) during diastole; (b) continuous wave Doppler spectra of AR recorded with the sampling beam placed in the LV outflow tract.

outflow tract (Figure 4.18a,b); moderate to severe (3+) aortic regurgitation (Figure 4.14b) is regurgitant flow jet reaching to the papillary muscles, and severe (4+) aortic regurgitation is regurgitant jet flow visible in the left ventricular apex. Instrumental and physiologic (not directly related to the severity of regurgitation) factors potentially affecting the spatial extent of the color-flow jet include transducer frequency, gain setting, pulse repetition frequency, and the driving diastolic pressure of the aorta, compliance of the left ventricle, duration of diastole and left ventricular end-diastolic pressure [32,33]. These factors have to be considered in quantification of aortic regurgitation.

Pulmonary regurgitation

The severity of pulmonary regurgitation can be semi-quantitatively evaluated using ICE Doppler color flow imaging. With proper imaging of the pulmonic valve, the severity of pulmonary regurgitation may be assessed by mapping the regurgitant turbulent flow jet of the right ventricle (Figure 4.19). Moderate to severe pulmonary regurgitation is frequently a sign of pulmonary hypertension. In pulmonary hypertension, the gradient between the pulmonary artery and the right ventricle remains high throughout diastole [31]. The intensity of the regurgitant signal may vary with respiration. The peak velocity recorded at end-diastole may be used to calculate pulmonary arterial

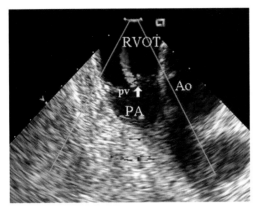

Figure 4.19 ICE image with the transducer placed in the right ventricle, showing the right ventricular outflow tract (RVOT) and pulmonary artery (PA), and color flow imaging of a mildly pulmonary regurgitant flow jet (red color) through the pulmonic valve (pv) during diastole. Ao: aorta.

end-diastolic pressure using the modified Bernoulli equation.

However, if the right ventricle is relatively noncompliant, the added volume with atrial contraction into the ventricle may substantially raise the right ventricular pressure and as a result decrease the diastolic gradient driving the pulmonary regurgitation.

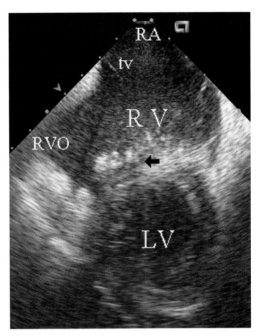

Figure 4.20 ICE image with the transducer placed in the right atrium (RA), showing dilated RA and right ventricle (RV) as compared to the left ventricular (LV) diameter. Because of dilatation, the RV is no longer triangle shaped (arrow). tv: tricuspid valve; RVO: RV outflow tract.

Dilated atria and ventricles

Dilated atrial and ventricular volumes caused by valvular regurgitation, intracardiac septal defect, arrhythmia-induced cardiomyopathy, and other cardiac diseases may be accurately assessed by ICE imaging. Volumetric overload alters both the ventricular size and the shape. For the largest short-axis diameter of normal adults, the left atrium (end-systole) is 4.1 ± 0.7 cm; the left ventricle (end-diastole) 4.7 ± 0.4 cm; the right atrium (end-systole) 3.7 ± 0.4 cm; the right ventricle 3.1 ± 0.4 cm [34]. During chamber enlargement, the shape of the left atrium, left ventricle or right atrium becomes less elliptical and more global and the shape of the right ventricle becomes less triangular and more elliptical (Figure 4.20).

Left ventricular global systolic dysfunction

The common measurement for left ventricular global function is ejection fraction. It represents the

percentage or fraction of left ventricular diastolic volume that is ejected in systole. Ejection fraction is made by calculation of ICE-determined left ventricular volumes as follows: Left ventricular ejection fraction = End-diastolic volume − End-systolic volume/End-diastolic volume = Stroke volume/End-diastolic volume. Left ventricular diastolic and systolic volumes (Figure 4.21a,b) can be determined by digitized area measurements using the single-plane ellipsoid area–length formula: $v = 8A^2/3\pi L$, where A is the area and L is the length, or the biplane area–length formula: $v = 8A_1 \times A_2/3\pi L$, where A_1 and A_2 represent the enclosed area of a chamber of two orthogonal views, respectively, and L is the common axis shared [35,36]. An abnormal left ventricular ejection fraction is <0.51 [37].

Left ventricular regional wall motion abnormalities

ICE may provide tomographic views of different regions of the left ventricle with the ICE transducer

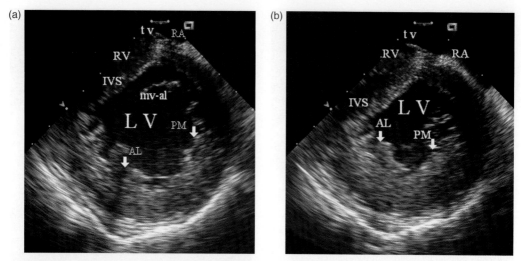

Figure 4.21 ICE images with the transducer placed near the ventricular septum at the right atrioventricular junction, showing: (a) short-axis views of the left ventricle (LV) at end-diastole; and (b) at end-systole. LV volumes and LV ejection fraction can be calculated based on digitized area border and measurements of these areas. AL and PM: anterolateral and posteromedial papillary muscles; IVS: interventricular septum; mv-al: anterior leaflet of mitral valve; RA and RV: right atrium and ventricle; tv: tricuspid valve.

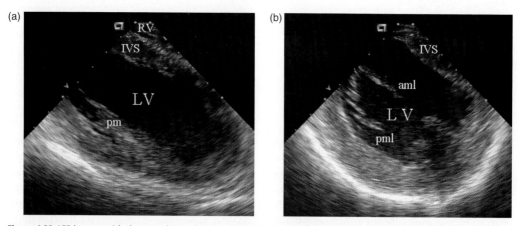

Figure 4.22 ICE images with the transducer placed near the tricuspid valvular orifice in the right ventricle (RV), showing: (a) interventricular septum (IVS) and left ventricular (LV) wall to be evaluated for wall segmental function in the LV long-axis view; and (b) short-axis view. aml and pml: anterior and posterior leaflet of mitral valve; pm: papillary muscle.

placed in the right atrium or near the atrioventricular annulus; more detailed left ventricle imaging is obtained with the transducer advanced into the right ventricle (Figure 4.22a,b). The simplest and most common technique is to qualitatively analyze wall motion in real time and to indicate which segments are moving abnormally [38]. A more systematic way to evaluate regional wall motion is to divide the ventricle into 8 or 16 segments, which relate the various segments to coronary artery distribution more conveniently [39–41]. The longitudinal views including anterior, septal, posterolateral, or inferior wall, may be divided into the basal (mitral valvular level), middle (papillary muscular level), and apical segments. The anterior wall and interventricular septum is supplied by the left anterior descending coronary artery, the posterolateral wall by the left circumflex, and the inferior wall by the right coronary artery.

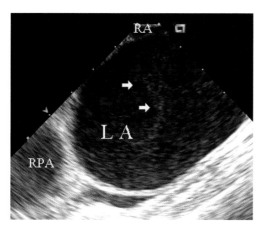

Figure 4.23 ICE image with the transducer placed in the right atrium (RA), showing spontaneous echocardiographic contrast (arrows) as slowly swirling nonhomogeneous amorphous echoes seen in the left atrium (LA). RPA: right pulmonary artery.

An isolated apical abnormality is interpreted as indicating coronary artery disease but is not used to localize disease to a specific coronary artery [39,40]. Left ventricular regional wall motion abnormalities may be evaluated by regional endocardial motion and wall thickening. Wall thickening (calculated as fractional shortening = End-systolic wall thickness − End-diastolic wall thickness/End-diastolic wall thickness) might be more sensitive to reductions of blood flow and myocardial perfusion. Unlike endocardial motion, wall-thickening measurements may be less affected by translational motion associated with heart contraction during systole, in which the heart rotates and moves in an inferior and anterior direction [40,42].

Spontaneous echocardiographic contrast

Spontaneous echocardiographic contrast defined as slowly swirling nonhomogeneous amorphous echoes seen in the left atrium (Figure 4.23), can be demonstrated with ICE imaging at 7.5 MHz. It is distinguishable from background noise or speckle by manipulation of gain settings. The presence of left atrial spontaneous echo contrast has been recognized as a major factor predisposing to the development of left atrial thrombus [43–45] and it may also predict future embolism and death [46]. Hematological

studies have shown that left atrial spontaneous echo contrast is a marker of a hypercoagulable state. Left atrial spontaneous echo contrast is a manifestation of red cell aggregation, arising from an interaction between red cells and plasma proteins such as fibrinogen, at low shear rates [47,48]. It does not require platelets [46]. The detection of left atrial spontaneous echo contrast on ultrasound imaging arises from the increased amplitude of the backscatter from red cell aggregates rather than single cells. To reduce left atrial thrombus formation, patients with atrial fibrillation and left atrial spontaneous echo contrast should be treated with intensified anticoagulation during transseptal catheterization and left atrial ablation procedures [49]. Increased intensity (full-dose) of intravenous heparin anticoagulation may suppress plasma prothrombin fragment 1 + 2 levels [50], which may diminish spontaneous contrast by a separate mechanism.

References

1 Netter FH, Yonkman FF. The CIBA collection of medical illustrations, Volume 5. *A Compilation of Paintings on the Normal and Pathologic Anatomy and Physiology, Embryology, and Diseases of the Heart.* Summit: CIBA, 1974: 8.

2 Werner JA, Chietlin MD, Cross BW, Speck SM, Ivey TD. Echocardiographic appearance of the Chiari network: differentiation from right heart pathology. *Circulation* 1981; **63**: 1104–1109.

3 Koenig PR. Abnormalities of the atria and atrial septum. In: St John Sutton M, Oldershaw P, Kotler MN, eds. *Textbook of Echocardiography and Doppler in Adults and Children*, 2nd edn. Blackwell Science, Inc., Cambridge, 1996: 765.

4 Prior JT. Lipomatous hypertrophy of cardiac interatrial septum: a lesion resembling hibernoma, lipoblastomatosis and infiltrating lipoma. *Arch Pathol* 1964; **78**: 11–15.

5 Fyke FE III, Tajik AJ, Edwards WD, Seward JB. Diagnosis of lipomatous hypertrophy of atrial septum by two-dimensional echocardiography. *J Am Coll Cardiol* 1983; **1**: 1352–1357.

6 Shirani J, Roberts WC. Clinical, electrographic and morphologic features of massive fatty deposits (lipomatous hypertrophy) in the atrial septum. *J Am Coll Cardiol* 1993; **22**: 226–238.

7 Ghods M, Lighty JGW, Ren JF, Constantinescu D, Garden JL, Elia EM. Lipomatous hypertrophy of the atrial septum. *Video J Echocardiogr* 1994; **4**: 21–26.

8 Hanley PC, Tajik AJ, Hynes JK, *et al.* Diagnosis and classification of atrial septal aneurysm by two-dimensional echocardiography: report of 80 consecutive cases. *J Am Coll Cardiol* 1985; **6**: 1370–1382.

9 Belkin RN, Waugh RA, Kisslo. Interatrial shunting in atrial septal aneurysm. *Am J Cardiol* 1986; **57**: 310–312.

10 Pearson AC, Nagelhout D, Castello R, Gomez CR, Labovitz AJ. Atrial septal aneurysm and stroke: a transesophageal echocardiographic study. *J Am Coll Cardiol* 1991; **18**: 1223–1229.

11 Click RL, Epinosa RE, Khandheria BK. Source of embolism: utility of transesophageal echocardiography, chapter 15. In: Freeman WK, Seward JB, Khandheria BK, Tajik AJ, eds. *Transesophageal Echocardiography*. Little, Brown and Co., Boston, 1994: 478–488.

12 Falk RH. PFO or UFO? The role of a patent foramen ovale in cryptogenic stroke (editorial). *Am Heart J* 1991; **121**: 1264–1266.

13 de Belder MA, Tourikis L, Leech G, Camm AJ. Risk of patent foramen ovale for thromboembolic events in all age group. *Am J Cardiol* 1992; **69**: 1316–1320.

14 Siostrzonek P, Lang W, Zangeneh M, *et al.* Significance of left-side heart disease for the detection of patent foramen ovale by transesophageal echocardiography. *J Am Coll Cardiol* 1992; **19**: 1192–1196.

15 Bridges ND, Hellenbrand W, Latson L, Filiano J, Newburger JW, Lock JE. Transcatheter closure of patent foramen ovale after presumed paradoxical embolism. *Circulation* 1992; **86**: 1902–1908.

16 Hijazi ZM, Wang Z, Cao Q, Koenig P, Waight D, Lang R. Transcatheter closure of atrial septal defects and patent foramen ovale under intracardiac echocardiographic guidance: feasibility and comparison with transesophageal echocardiography. *Catheter Cardiovasc Interv* 2001; **52**: 194–199.

17 Ren JF, Marchlinski FE, Callans DJ, Herrmann HC. Clinical use of AcuNav diagnostic ultrasound catheter imaging during left heart radio frequency ablation and transcatheter closure procedures. *J Am Soc Echocardiogr* 2002; **15**: 1301–1308.

18 Anderson R, Ho SY. Echocardiographic diagnosis and description of congenital heart disease: anatomic principles and philosophy. In: St John Sutton M, Oldershaw P, Kotler MN, eds. *Textbook of Echocardiography and Doppler in Adults and Children*, 2nd edn. Blackwell Science, Inc., Cambridge, 1996: 716–717.

19 Ryan T. Congenital heart disease, chapter 7. In: Feigenbaum H, ed. *Echocardiography*, 5th edn. Lea & Febiger, Philadelphia, 1994: 374–399.

20 Shiina A, Seward JB, Edwards WD, Hagler DJ, Tajik AJ. Two-dimensional echocardiographic spectrum of Ebstein's anomaly: detailed anatomic assessment. *J Am Coll Cardiol* 1984; **3**: 356–370.

21 Celermajer DS, Bull C, Till JA, *et al.* Ebstein's anomaly: presentation and outcome from fetus to adult. *J Am Coll Cardiol* 1994; **23**: 170–176.

22 Ren JF, Schwartzman D, Marchlinski FE, Brode SE, Lighty GW, Chaudhry FA. Intracardiac ultrasound catheter imaging in Ebstein's anomaly. *J Cardiovasc Diagnosis and Procedures* 1997; **14**: 173–176.

23 Kocheril AG, Rosenfeld LE. Radiofrequency ablation of an accessory pathway in a patient with corrected Ebstein's anomaly. *PACE* 1994; **17**: 986–900.

24 Ren JF, Hakki A-H, Kotler MN, Iskandrian AS. Exercise systolic blood pressure: a powerful determination of increased left ventricular mass in patients with hypertension. *J Am Coll Cardiol* 1985; **5**: 1224–1231.

25 Yock PB, Popp RL. Noninvasive estimation of right ventricular systolic pressure by Doppler ultrasound in patients with tricuspid regurgitation. *Circulation* 1984; **70**: 657–662.

26 Currie PJ, Seward JB, Chan KL, *et al.* Continuous wave Doppler determination of right ventricular pressure: a simultaneous Doppler catheterization study in 127 patients. *J Am Coll Cardiol* 1985; **6**: 750–756.

27 Chan KL, Currie PJ, Seward JB, Hagler DJ, Mair DD, Tajik AJ. Comparison of three Doppler ultrasound methods in the prediction of pulmonary artery pressure. *J Am Coll Cardiol* 1987; **9**: 549–554.

28 Maniet AR, DeGuise M, St John Sutton MG. Mitral and tricuspid valve disease. In: St John Sutton M, Oldershaw P, Kotler MN, eds. *Textbook of Echocardiography and Doppler in Adults and Children*, 2nd edn. Blackwell Science, Inc., Cambridge, 1996: 168–169.

29 Cooper JW, Nanda NC, Philpot EF, Fan P. Evaluation of valvular regurgitation by color Doppler. *J Am Soc Echocardiogr* 1989; **2**: 56–66.

30 Ren JF, Kotler MN, DePace NL, *et al.* Two-dimensional echocardiographic determination of left atrial emptying volume: a noninvasive index in quantifying the degree of nonrheumatic mitral regurgitation. *J Am Coll Cardiol* 1983; **2**: 729–736.

31 Wiegers SE, St John Sutton MG. Acquired aortic and pulmonary valve disease. In: St John Sutton M, Oldershaw P, Kotler MN, eds. *Textbook of Echocardiography and Doppler in Adults and Children*, 2nd edn. Blackwell Science, Inc., Cambridge, 1996: 245, 261.

32 Perry GJ, Helmcke F, Nanda NC, Byard C, Soto B. Evaluation of aortic insufficiency by Doppler color flow mapping. *J Am Coll Cardiol* 1987; **9**: 952–959.

33 Olson LJ, Freeman WK, Enriquez-Sarano M, Tajik AJ. Transesophageal echocardiographic evaluation of native valvular heart disease. In: Freeman WK, Seward JB,

Khandheria BK, Tajik AJ, eds. *Transesophageal echocardiography*, Little, Brown and Co., Boston, 1994: 226.

34 Weyman A. Normal cross-sectional echocardiographic measurements in adults. In: Weyman A, ed. *Cross-Sectional Echocardiography*, Lea & Febiger, Philadelphia, 1982: 497–508.

35 Kennedy JW, Trennolme SE, Kasser IS. Left ventricular volume and mass from single-plane cineangiography. A comparison of anterior/posterior and right anterior oblique methods. *Am Heart J* 1970; **80**: 343–352.

36 Ren JF, Kotler MN, DePace NL, *et al.* Comparison of left ventricular ejection fraction and volumes by two-dimensional echocardiography, radionuclide angiography and cineangiography. *J Cardiovasc Ultrasonogr* 1983; **2**: 213–222.

37 Kennedy JW, Baxley WA, Figley MM, Dodge HT, Blackman JR. Quantitative angiocardiography: the normal left ventricle in man. *Circulation* 1966; **34**: 272–278.

38 Feigenbaum H. *Echocardiography*, 5th edn. Lea & Febiger, Philadelphia, 1994: 147–151.

39 Edwards WD, Tajik AJ, Seward JB. Standardized nomenclature and anatomic basis for regional tomographic analysis of the heart. *Mayo Clin Proc* 1981; **56**: 479–497.

40 Ren JF, Kotler MN, Hakki A-H, Panidis IP, Mintz GS, Ross J. Quantitation of regional left ventricular function by two-dimensional echocardiography in normals and patients with coronary srtery disease. *Am Heart J* 1985; **110**: 552–560.

41 Schiller NB, Shah PM, Crawford M, *et al.* Recommendations for quantitation of the left ventricle by two-dimensional echocardiography. *J Am Soc Echocardiogr* 1989; **2**: 358–367.

42 McDonald JG. The shape and movements of the human left ventricle during systole. *Am J Cardiol* 1970; **26**: 221–230.

43 Fatkin D, Kelly RP, Feneley MP. Relations between left atrial appendage blood flow velocity, spontaneous echocardiographic contrast and thromboembolic risk *in vivo. J Am Coll Cardiol* 1994; **23**: 961–969.

44 Leung DY, Black IW, Cranney GB, Hopkins AP, Walsh WF. Prognostic implications of left atrial spontaneous echo contrast in nonvalvular atrial fibrillation. *J Am Coll Cardiol* 1994; **24**: 755–762.

45 Ren JF, Marchlinski FE, Callans DJ. Left atrial thrombus associated with ablation for atrial fibrillation: identification with intracardiac echocardiography. *J Am Coll Cardiol* 2004; **43**: 1861–1867.

46 Black IW. Spontaneous echo contrast: where there's smoke there's fire. *Echocardiography* 2000; **17**: 373–382.

47 Merino A, Hauptman P, Badimon L, *et al.* Echocardiographic "smoke" is produced by an interaction of erythrocytes and plasma proteins modulated by shear forces. *J Am Coll Cardiol* 1992; **20**: 1161–1168.

48 Rastegar R, Harnick DJ, Weidemenn P, *et al.* Spontaneous echo contrast videodensity is flow-related and is dependent on the relative concentrations of fibrinogen and red blood cells. *J Am Coll Cardiol* 2003; **41**: 603–610.

49 Ren JF, Marchlinski FE, Callans DJ, *et al.* Increased intensity of anticoagulation may reduce risk of thrombus during atrial fibrillation ablation procedure in patients with spontaneous echo contrast. *J Cardiovasc Electrophysiol* 2005; **16**: 474–477.

50 Amelsberg A, Zurborn KH, Gartner U, Kiehne KH, Preusse AK, Bruhn HD. Influence of heparin treatment on biochemical markers of an activation of the coagulation system. *Thromb Res* 1992; **66**: 121–131.

CHAPTER 5

Utility of Intracardiac Echocardiographic Imaging for Transseptal Catheterization

Jian-Fang Ren, MD*, & Francis E. Marchlinski,* MD

Transseptal catheterization was initially introduced by Ross [1] and Cope [2] in 1959 and later modified by Brockenbrough and Braunwald [3] and by Mullins [4] for measurement of left atrial and left ventricular pressure. After the introduction of the retrograde arterial approach for entering the left ventricle and the Swan-Ganz catheter for measuring the pulmonary artery wedge pressure, the use of transseptal catheterization had become an infrequent procedure. But it has again become a relatively common procedure since the advent of percutaneous mitral valvuloplasty [5] and left heart radiofrequency catheter ablation in the treatment of cardiac tachyarrhythmias [6,7]. Transseptal catheterization is also reserved for a failed retrograde left heart catheterization due to severe peripheral arterial disease, aortic stenosis or the presence of a certain type of mechanical prosthetic valve (e.g., Bjork-Shiley or St Jude valve) [8]. The procedure is technically challenging and requires experience and extreme caution because of the potentially devastating complications reportedly associated with puncture of structures other than the atrial septum [9–12]. Traditionally, it has relied on fluoroscopic guidance, in which anatomic structures are not visualized directly and the catheter was guided entirely by its position in cardiac silhouette. Two-dimensional transthoracic and transesophageal echocardiography may be helpful in performing transseptal catheterization by imaging the position of the catheter in relationship to the atrial septum [13–17]. However, difficulties encountered with transthoracic echocardiography in imaging critical intracardiac structures

from the thoracic cage and with transesophageal echocardiography and the need for heavy sedation and/or general anesthesia have hindered their routine use for imaging and monitoring during transseptal catheterization and interventional electrophysiologic procedures. The role of intracardiac echocardiography (ICE) during electrophysiologic procedures has been firmly established [18–20]. One of the major reasons for the clinical acceptance of the small-diameter, low-frequency ultrasound catheter placed in the right atrium is because it provides high-quality cardiac image monitoring and can remain in place for the entire procedure with excellent patient tolerance. With proper manipulation of the ICE catheter, imaging of the regional anatomy of the atrial septum can be rapidly established. The appropriate septal imaging shows the aortic root and left atrial appendage at its left anterior and superior aspect, and the lower left pulmonary vein ostium and the mitral annulus at its left inferior and posterior aspect. Interatrial septal puncture can be performed safely by direct ICE imaging [20–24].

Best cross-sectional imaging view of the interatrial septum (fossa ovalis) for guiding/monitoring of transseptal puncture

The optimum ICE image will demonstrate adequate space behind the interatrial septum on the left atrial side and clearly identify adjacent structures.

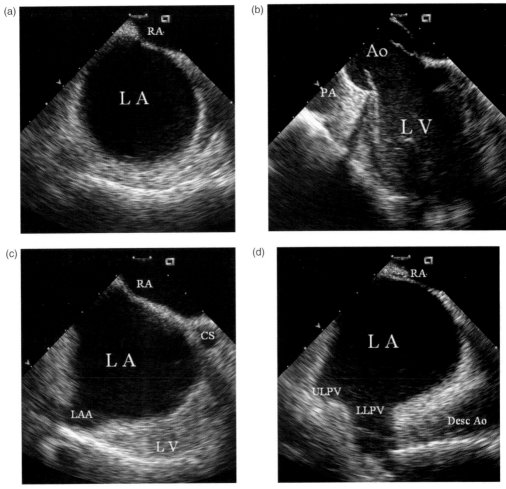

Figure 5.1 ICE images with the transducer placed near the superior limbus of the fossa ovalis in the high right atrium (RA), showing: (a) the best imaging view of the interatrial septum (fossa ovalis) for guiding transseptal puncture. Note the maximal space behind the septum on the left atrial (LA) side with this view. This best view is obtained by rotating the transducer clockwise; (b) the images pass through the left ventricular (LV) outflow tract with aortic root (Ao) visible; and (c) then through the LA at the level of the LA appendage (LAA) orifice. (d) Further clockwise rotation beyond the ideal view displays an image of the lower (LLPV) and upper left pulmonary vein (ULPV) ostia; counterclockwise rotation from this view will recreate the ideal image. CS: coronary sinus; Desc Ao: descending aorta; PA: pulmonary artery.

A cross-sectional view of the fossa ovalis is best provided with the AcuNav transducer placed near the interatrial septum in the right atrium and the catheter rotated clockwise to establish the best view (Figure 5.1a). The imaging view should pass through the aortic root (Figure 5.1b) and then the left atrial appendage orifice (Figure 5.1c). Further clockwise rotation beyond the ideal location will demonstrate images of the left pulmonary vein ostia (Figure 5.1d).

An optimal view will not include the aortic root structure since a cross-sectional view that includes the aortic root will be too anterior to be punctured safely. With an enlarged left atrium, a cross-sectional view which includes the atrial appendage is also optimal if an adequate space exists behind the atrial septum on the left atrial side. Mechanical radial ICE imaging can also provide satisfactory imaging of the fossa ovalis for guiding transseptal puncture viewed from the right

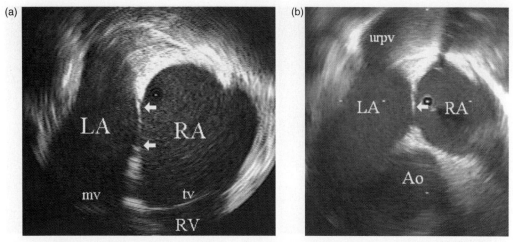

Figure 5.2 Mechanical radial ICE images: (a) with the transducer placed near the interatrial septum in the high right atrium (RA), showing the fossa ovalis with its superior and inferior limbus (arrows) and right (RV) and left ventricular inflow images; (b) with the transducer placed near the interatrial septum in the middle RA showing the fossa ovalis (arrow) at optimal site for transseptal puncture. Ao: aortic root; LA: left atrium; mv: mitral valve; tv: tricuspid valve; urpv: upper right pulmonary vein.

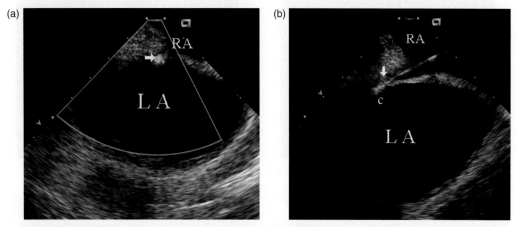

Figure 5.3 ICE images with the transducer placed in the right atrium (RA), showing: (a) a patent foramen ovale with left to right shunting (red color flow, arrow); and (b) the catheter (c) guided into the left atrium (LA) through the patent foramen ovale (arrow) after imaging region was expanded by a slightly posterior deflection of the imaging catheter transducer tip.

and left ventricular inflow (Figure 5.2a) or aortic root (Figure 5.2b).

Transseptal catheterization through a patent foramen ovale or atrial septal defect without needle puncture

With Doppler color flow imaging, a probe-patent foramen ovale, when it is present (Figure 5.3a), can be detected before transseptal catheterization. A mapping/ablation catheter can then be guided through the patent foramen into the left atrium (Figure 5.3b). As reported previously, in approximately 10% of patients, this maneuver is performed inadvertently during right heart catheterization with a woven Dacron catheter [8]. However, when a catheter crosses a patent foramen, the transseptal location is often at the superoanterior limbus of the fossa ovalis. Thus, it may be difficult to position such an anteriorly

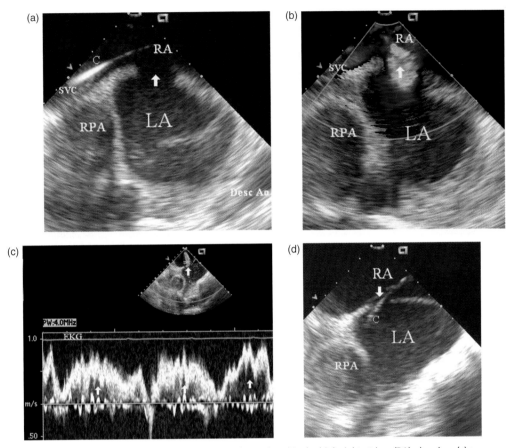

Figure 5.4 Doppler color flow ICE images with the transducer placed in the high right atrium (RA), showing: (a) a secundum atrial septum defect (arrow, diameter = 2.3cm); (b) color flow (red, arrow) toward the RA; and (c) pulsed-wave Doppler spectrum indicating a left atrium (LA) to RA shunt during systole and diastole; (d) an ablation catheter "C" through the defect (arrow) into the LA. C: catheter; Desc Ao: descending aorta; RPA: right pulmonary artery; SVC: superior vena cava.

displaced mapping/ablation catheter into the right pulmonary veins or even the upper left pulmonary vein ostium. Transseptal catheterization with needle puncture directed at middle portion of the fossa ovalis may need to be considered.

In contrast, in patients with a common type of the secundum septal defect (Figure 5.4a), ICE Doppler color flow imaging can accurately identify the defect's location, size and associated shunt flow (Figure 5.4b,c). The defect often involves the mid portion of the fossa ovalis. A mapping/ablation catheter can be easily guided through the septal defect into the left atrium (Figure 5.4d) and properly manipulated for the left atrial/pulmonary vein ostial ablation.

Transseptal puncture at the optimal site, optimum imaging techniques and confirmation of sheath placement in left atrium

Transseptal catheterization typically uses a Brockenbrough needle/stylet in conjunction with Mullins sheath/dilator unit [4] (or a Brockenbrough catheter). Prior to insertion, the needle and stylet are inserted into the dilator of the long vascular sheath so that the tip of the needle is just inside the dilator. When the needle/sheath/dilator unit is placed into the superior vena cava with pressure recorded through the needle, the needle is rotated toward the interatrial septum (4 o'clock when looking from below) and

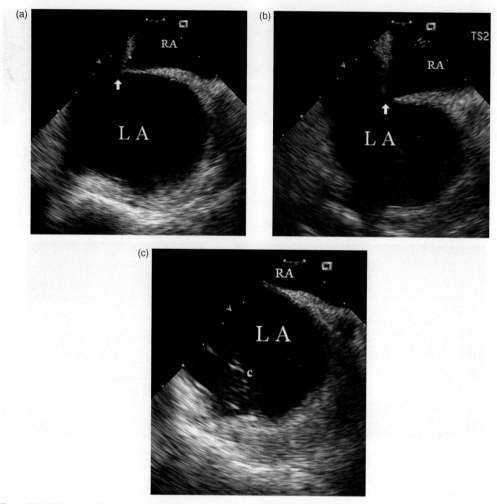

Figure 5.5 ICE images with the transducer placed in the right atrium (RA), showing: (a) transseptal needle tip tenting against the interatrial septum at the fossa ovalis (arrow), initially the needle tip location is at the top of the fossa ovalis; (b) proper location and direction of the puncture needle tip is obtained at the middle fossa ovalis (arrow) after pulling the needle tip slightly downward; (c) the echo bubbles are imaged in the left atrium (LA) during an injection with saline through the end of the sheath "c" confirming the location of the transseptal sheath in the LA.

slowly withdrawn until the tip is visible with ICE imaging. The unit is manipulated until the tip is resting against the fossa ovalis. After positioning in the middle portion of the fossa ovalis which is the optimal site of transseptal puncture, the unit is advanced gently to show the needle tip/dilator tenting of the fossa ovalis (Figure 5.5a). The needle is advanced beyond the tip of the dilator to puncture the septum. During this process, the proper direction and the depth of the puncture can be determined with imaging of the needle tip tenting (Figure 5.5b) and the crossing of the septum as the tenting is relieved. As the

dilator and sheath is sequentially advanced over the needle into the left atrium, transient "tenting" of the interatrial septum may be again observed. Successful entry into the left atrium should be confirmed by the recording of a left atrial pressure waveform. The needle and dilator are subsequently removed and echo micro bubbles are observed in the left atrium when the sheath is flushed with saline confirming the transseptal sheath location in the left atrium (Figure 5.5c).

Mechanical radial ICE imaging can also guide transseptal catheterization. Accurate anatomic imaging of

(a)
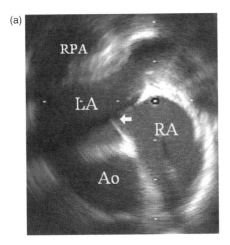

(b)
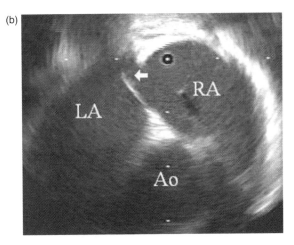

(c)
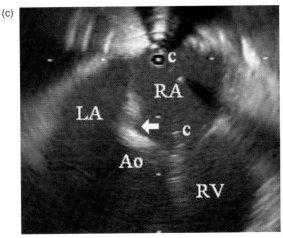

Figure 5.6 Mechanical radial ICE images with the transducer placed in the right atrium (RA), showing: (a) a transseptal needle properly positioned with tenting (arrow) against the mid-interatrial septum at the fossa ovalis. (b) Also shown as reference positions (arrow) are too high; and (c) too low on the septum. Each scale = 16 mm. Ao: aortic root; c: catheter; LA: left atrium; RPA: right pulmonary artery; RV: right ventricle.

the fossa ovalis of the interatrial septum, tenting transseptal needle tip and successful puncture can be identified (Figure 5.6a). Position, either too high (Figure 5.6b) or too low (Figure 5.6c) at the septum can be recognized and avoided. Importantly, ICE with a 9 MHz ultrasound transducer has a limited imaging depth and may be incapable of imaging the distal structures of an enlarged left atrium.

Under ICE guidance and monitoring needle tip or sheath movement may be effectively controlled to avoid damage to the adjacent structures, such as the aortic root, left atrial appendage, pulmonary veins, coronary sinus, mitral valve and annulus, or atrial wall.

Transseptal puncture at the optimal site may provide further optimal manipulation of catheters for mapping and ablation in the different region of the left heart during electrophysiologic procedure.

Guiding reinsertion of a catheter to the left atrium from the right atrium through the initial atrial septal puncture site

Manipulation of the mapping ablation catheter occasionally resulting in movement from left atrium back to the right atrium is not uncommon. With ICE

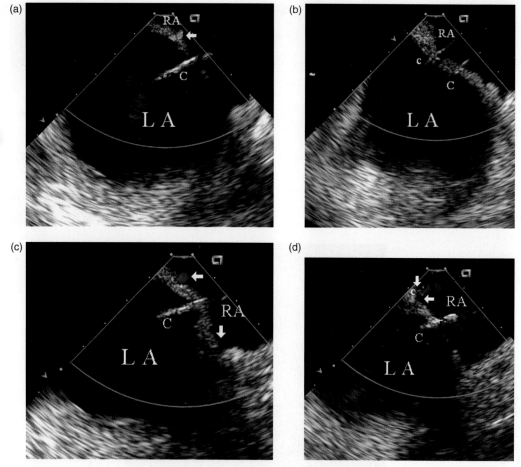

Figure 5.7 ICE Doppler color flow images with the transducer placed in the right atrium (RA), showing: (a) a residual atrial septal defect (2.5 mm) with tiny shunt flow toward RA (red mosaic color, horizontal arrow) after an unexpected withdrawal of an ablation catheter from left atrium (LA) into RA; (b) guided by ICE color flow imaging reinsertion of the ablation catheter "c" through the residual septal defect; (c) following correction of its tenting (vertical arrow) at a lower interatrial septal location; and (d) a location against the interatrial septum (c, vertical arrow) with a strong distal fan-shadow artifact just immediately above the initial residual defect (horizontal arrow) on the RA side. C: multipolar mapping catheter.

Doppler color flow imaging, an initial atrial septal puncture site with a residual septal defect may be easily detected (Figure 5.7a). Reinsertion of a catheter from the right atrium back to the left atrium may be considered as the first preferred choice. The catheter tip can be imaged and demonstrates tenting (Figure 5.7b) or a strong distal fan-shadow artifact when it is placed against the interatrial septum on the right atrial side (Figure 5.7c). The reinsertion across the residual septal defect at the previous transseptal puncture site can be performed with a high success rate under ICE Doppler color flow imaging guidance (Figure 5.7d) avoiding the need for additional needle puncture.

Abnormal atrial conditions that require caution during transseptal catheterization

A very large left atrium due to mitral stenosis and/or longstanding atrial fibrillation creates a challenging condition for transseptal catheterization and a

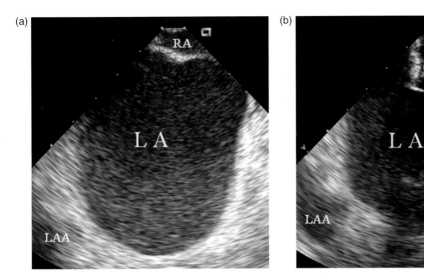

Figure 5.8 ICE images with the transducer placed in the high right atrium (RA), showing: (a) the interatrial septum in a significantly enlarged left atrium (LA) (diameter = 6.5 cm); and (b) transseptal puncture with needle tip (c) positioned and tenting at an optimal interatrial septum location under ICE imaging guidance. LAA: LA appendage.

potential high risk for cardiac perforation. Transseptal access close to the center of the septum is difficult since the center of the atrial septum projects notably toward the right in these patients [22,25]. ICE imaging can identify the actual location of the fossa ovalis (Figure 5.8a) and guide the transseptal puncture without any difficulty (Figure 5.8b).

The presence of an atrial septal aneurysm, especially with a normal atrial size, is a condition requiring careful transseptal catheterization. ICE imaging may detect an atrial septal aneurysm bulging toward the right atrium (Figure 5.9a), left atrium, or back and forth between the atria depending on the difference in the atrial pressure during the cardiac cycle. The transseptal puncture may be performed in the fossa ovalis where the aneurysm is located. During transseptal puncture a deep tenting and bulging of the aneurysm may be observed and penetration through the septum may be difficult (Figure 5.9b). Less space behind the septum with the bulging may indicate a higher potential risk of inadvertent puncture of adjacent structures. ICE imaging monitoring is necessary to control the needle direction and motion to avoid injury to the left atrial and adjacent structures (the aortic root, left atrial wall and appendage, or the pulmonary veins) when puncture is finally achieved (Figure 5.9c). To avoid an extensive dilatation of the punctured thin-walled

aneurysm (residual septal defect) due to repeated traction with manipulation of the catheter during the procedure, a puncture site caudal and lateral to the border of the aneurysm may be considered [26,27]. Such directed puncture can be safely performed under ICE imaging guidance [22].

Lipomatous hypertrophy of the atrial septum is commonly seen in aged patients with cardiac arrhythmias. Attempts at transseptal puncture are difficult in the thickened portion of the septum. ICE imaging can easily localize the thinner portion of the fossa ovalis to be penetrated (Figure 5.10) avoiding the hypertrophied atrial septum (Figure 5.11a,b).

In patients with a repaired patch or an "occluder" device (Figure 5.12a,b) in the atrial septum after closure of atrial septum defect, ICE imaging can provide accurate location of the occluding device and guide the transseptal puncture safely (Figure 5.12c). Placement of the catheter/sheath into the left atrium via a transseptal puncture avoids the closure material (Figure 12.5d).

In general, other distorted cardiac anatomy due to congenital heart disease, marked right atrial enlargement, significant chest or spine deformity, the inability to lie flat, the presence of a left atrial tumor, and ongoing anticoagulation make transseptal catheterization guided by fluoroscopy a higher risk

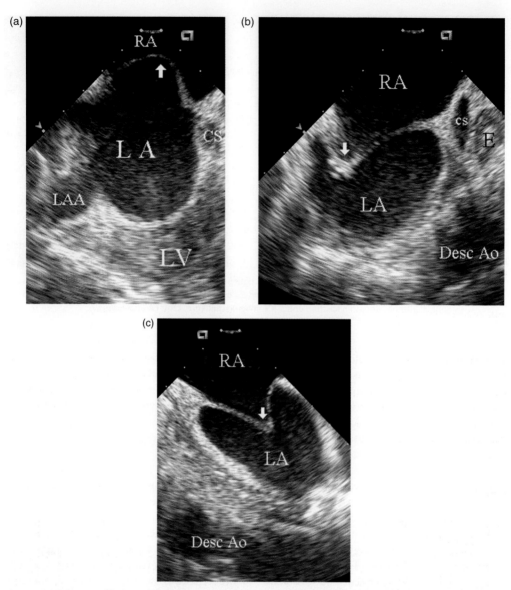

Figure 5.9 ICE images with the transducer placed in the right atrium (RA) and its tip deflected posteriorly, showing: (a) left atrial (LA) and ventricle (LV) in patient with interatrial septal aneurysm bulging (arrow, amplitude = 2 cm) to the right atrial side; (b) transseptal puncture with needle tip tenting (arrow) and small amount space behind the tented septum on the LA side. (c) With manipulation of the needle tip (arrow) in the posterior direction towards LA more space exists behind the tented septum (with imaging "L/R" marker changed). ICE imaging facilitated safe transseptal puncture in the patient with interatrial septal aneurysm. CS: coronary sinus; Desc Ao: descending aorta; E: esophagus; LAA: LA appendage; LV: left ventricle.

procedure [8]. However, with real-time ICE imaging guidance and monitoring, actual imaging of the puncture needle and catheter as it relates to the fossa ovalis and its adjacent structures makes the transseptal catheterization expeditious and safe even in these conditions.

Residual atrial septal defect following transseptal catheterization

Dual transseptal catheterization has been routinely performed in left atrial radiofrequency ablation for

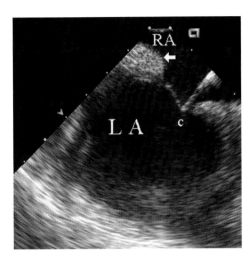

Figure 5.10 ICE image with the transducer placed in the high right atrium (RA), showing lipomatous hypertrophy of the atrial septum (arrow, thickness = 13 mm) and transseptal puncture with needle tip tenting (c) at the fossa ovalis. LA: left atrium.

atrial fibrillation. It creates atrial septal defects with interatrial shunting immediately after withdrawal of the catheters from left atrium following a left atrial ablation procedure. Residual flow through the interatrial septal defect can be detected (Figure 5.13) and the size of atrial septal defect resulting from dual transseptal catheterization (with two 8 Fr Mullins sheaths) can be quantified using ICE with Doppler color flow imaging (Figure 5.14). Out of 53 patients, residual

atrial septal defect with interatrial septal shunt was measured in 85% of the patients with dual transseptal catheterization immediately following left atrial ablation procedure [28]. Atrial septal defects with left to right shunting measured 2.0 ± 0.7 mm (range 1.0–4.4) in size following dual transseptal catheterization [28]. The size measures <4 mm in 98% of the atrial septal defects detected and appears to be clinically insignificant.

The characteristics and resolution of such residual atrial septal defect have been further studied [29]. The study was performed using ICE imaging in 33 patients to characterize the magnitude, time course and regression of the residual atrial septal defect immediately after (procedure duration 225 ± 94 min) and at repeat atrial fibrillation ablation. Acute changes in atrial septal defect size after transseptal catheterization (left atrial ablation procedure) (Figure 5.15a,b) are listed in Table 5.1. There was no significant change in atrial septal defect size from 6 to 30 min immediately after removal of transseptal catheters. The residual atrial septal defect after transseptal catheterization appears to reduce in size (all <4 mm) during follow-up (3 days to 13 months) and typically resolves completely by 6 months [29].

Potential complications

Complications of transseptal catheterization are generally infrequent if performed by experienced

(a)

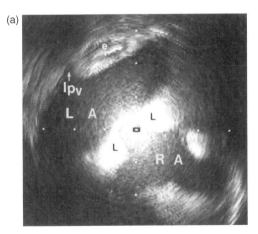

(b)

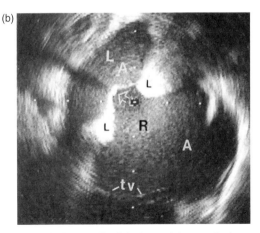

Figure 5.11 Mechanical radial ICE images with the transducer placed at the fossa ovalis of the interatrial septum in the right atrium (RA), showing: (a) lipomatous hypertrophy of the interatrial septum (L, thickness = 1.5 cm); and (b) transseptal puncture with needle tip tenting at the fossa ovalis (arrow). Scale = 16 mm; e: esophagus; LA: left atrium; lpv: upper left pulmonary vein; tv: tricuspid valve.

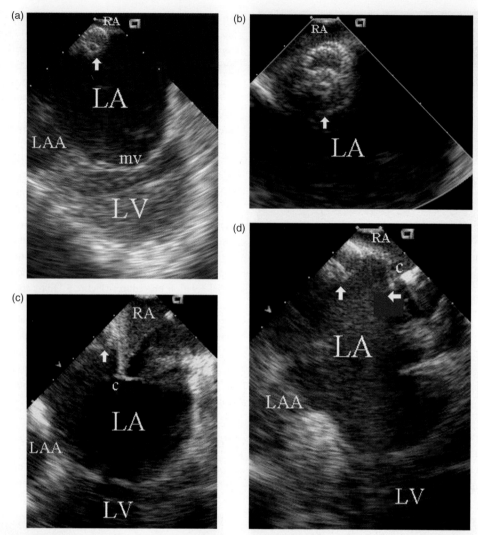

Figure 5.12 ICE images with the transducer placed in the high right atrium (RA), showing transseptal puncture in a patient who had percutaneous transcatheter repaired secundum atrial septal defect: (a) with an Amplatzer occluder device (upward arrow); and (b) emphasizing the Amplatzer occluder at the septum (upward arrow); (c) puncture needle "c" tenting toward the left atrium (LA) at a distance from the Amplatzer (upward arrow) during transseptal puncture; and (d) transseptal catheter/sheath "C" positioned properly at the atrial septum (leftward arrow) and through the septum into the LA, avoiding damage to the occluder device (upward arrow). LAA: LA appendage; LV: left ventricle; mv: mitral valve.

Table 5.1 Acute changes in atrial septal defect (ASD) size following transseptal catheterization (TC) after left atrial ablation procedure.

	Post-TC	2 min	4 min	6 min	10 min	15–30 min
ASD (mm)	$3.5 \pm 12^*$	$2.9 \pm 0.6^{**}$	$2.9 \pm 0.5^{**}$	2.6 ± 0.5	2.6 ± 0.6	2.5 ± 0.5
Range (mm)	2.2–4.7	2.1–3.9	2.2–3.9	1.9–3.4	1.6–3.6	1.6–3.6

$^*p < 0.05$: versus all others; $^{**}p < 0.05$: versus 15–30 min.

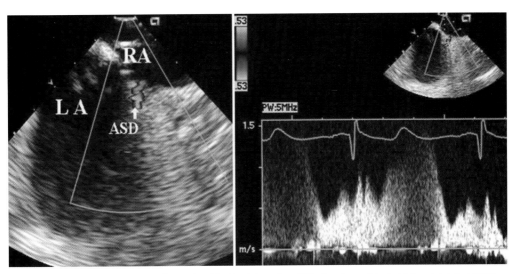

Figure 5.13 ICE images with the transducer placed in the right atrium (RA), showing residual atrial septal defect (ASD) with Doppler color flow imaging (left panel) and pulsed-wave Doppler spectral recording of left-to-right shunting flow during systole and diastole (right panel). LA: left atrium.

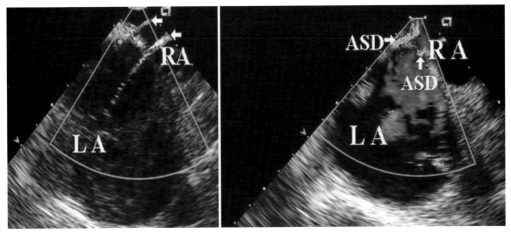

Figure 5.14 ICE images with the transducer placed in the right atrium (RA), showing the dual transseptal catheters (arrows) across the interatrial septum in the left atrium (LA) pre-radiofrequency (RF) ablation (left panel) and residual atrial septal defects (ASD) with Doppler color flow imaging of flow across septum (arrows) post-RF after catheter removal from LA (right panel).

operators. They are more common and serious early in an operator's experience or in high-risk patients. Complications associated with transseptal catheterization included "needle tip" perforation (<3%), pericardial tamponade (<1%); and death (<0.5%) [8,12,25,30]. It is believed, but not yet documented that ICE imaging guidance would reduce serious complications (such as "needle tip" perforation of aortic wall, Figure 5.16) by real-time imaging of aortic root, coronary sinus, and other important anatomic landmarks.

ICE imaging may also allow for early detection and optimal management of some complications, such as pericardial effusion, damage to the mitral

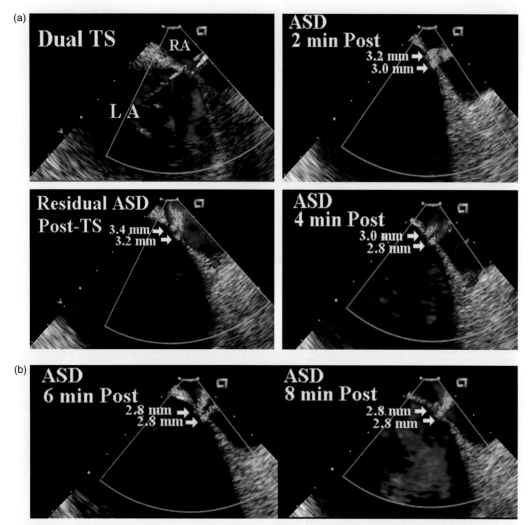

Figure 5.15 ICE images with the transducer placed in the right atrium (RA), showing: (a) dual transseptal catheters across the septum in the left atrium (LA) (left upper panel), size of residual atrial septal defect (ASD) immediately Post-transseptal catheterization (TS) (left lower panel) and acute changes in residual ASD size at 2 min (the right upper panel) and 4 min Post-TS; and (b) residual ASD size at 6 min (left panel) and 8 min Post-TS (right panel). Persistency of ASD over this short time course is documented.

valve, and right and left atrial thrombus formation. When a mild or mild-to-moderate pericardial effusion is detected with ICE imaging immediately following puncture (Figure 5.17a,b), careful monitoring of change in fluid amount (pericardial echo-free space), and reversal of the anticoagulation status may prevent temponade. The mitral valve may be damaged when transseptal catheter/sheath advances into the left ventricle during transseptal catheterization. ICE with Doppler color flow imaging can reveal entry of a catheter/sheath into the left ventricle (Figure 5.18a) and detect the development of mitral regurgitant flow (Figure 5.18b). Doppler color flow imaging may also help to determine if damage of the mitral valve exists after withdrawal of the catheter/sheath from the left ventricle (Figure 5.18c). ICE imaging can easily detect atrial thrombus in the right atrium or left atrium. A significant incidence (32%) of right atrial thrombus detected by mechanical radial ICE (9 MHz) imaging has been reported in 136 patients when long catheter sheath was used during transseptal catheterization and/or cardiac ablation procedures [31]. Right atrial thrombus is usually single, linear, and mobile in a small size (maximal 22 ± 8 mm $\times$ 2.2 ± 0.5 mm), and typically is found attached to

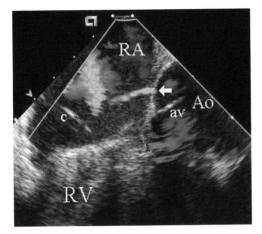

Figure 5.16 ICE Doppler color flow image with the transducer placed near the aortic root in the middle anterior right atrium (RA), identifying a tiny flow jet (arrow, diameter $= 2.7$ mm) from aortic root (Ao) to RA during systole, induced by an inadvertent transseptal puncture. av: aortic valve; c: catheter; RV: right ventricle (provided by AcuNav peer training course).

a long sheath (Figure 5.19a,b) or occasionally to the interatrial septum at the transseptal puncture point (Figure 5.20a–c). None of the patients in the study cohort suffered clinical intra/post-procedural thromboembolic complications. ICE becomes even more important in its capability to detect left atrial thrombus formation since clinical consequence of left atrial thrombus may be more serious than that of right. The incidence of left atrial thrombus has been reported as high as 10.3% associated with dual transseptal catheterization and left atrial ablation guided by a multipolar Lasso catheter for atrial fibrillation [32]. Importantly, the left atrial thrombus can occur early following needle/catheter/sheath puncture into the left atrium (Figure 5.21a). The characteristics of such thrombus is single, generally small (size 13 ± 11 mm $\times 2 \pm 1$ mm), linear, mobile, and firmly attached to the catheter/sheath. It can be successfully withdrawn from the left atrium by careful withdrawal of the catheter/sheath with the thrombus as a unit across the interatrial septum (Figure 5.21b) into the right atrium (Figure 5.21c) under ICE imaging monitoring [32]. In patients with atrial fibrillation and spontaneous echo contrast (Figure 5.22) in the left atrium detected before transseptal puncture, increased intensity of

(a)

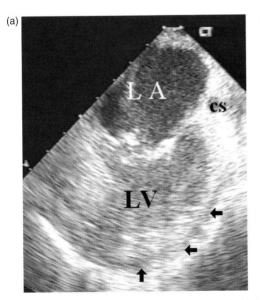

(b)

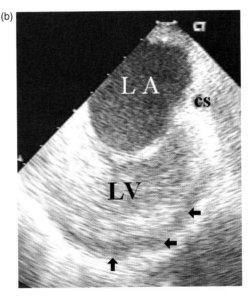

Figure 5.17 ICE images with the transducer placed in the high right atrium, showing: (a) an echo-free space (arrows) around left ventricular (LV) apex and posterior wall at end-diastole (echo- free space 2–6 mm); and (b) end-systole (4–9 mm), consistent with a mild-to-moderate pericardial effusion. CS: coronary sinus. LA: left atrium.

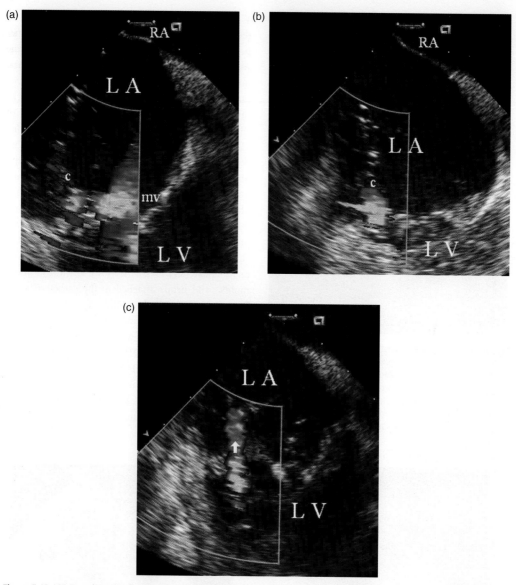

Figure 5.18 ICE Doppler color flow images with the transducer placed in the right atrium (RA), showing: (a) a transseptal sheath (c) entering into left ventricle (LV) through the mitral valve (mv) with two regurgitant flow jets from the sheath position (red mosaic color) and the orifice (red color) imaged immediately after sheath placement. (b) Mitral regurgitant flow (red mosaic color) was continuously imaged with the sheath (c) through the mitral valve during systole; and (c) final mitral regurgitant flow (red mosaic color, arrow) persisting during systole after withdrawal of the transseptal sheath from the LV indicating some structural damage to the mitral valve.

anticoagulation with activated clotting time >300 s, may reduce the incidence of the left atrial thrombus formation during transseptal catheterization and left atrial ablation procedure [33]. It has become our routine policy to initiate anticoagulation with a bolus of intravenous heparin prior to transseptal puncture to avoid early thrombus formation and to maintain activated clotting time between 325 and 375 s during the procedure. ICE imaging has thus provided a greater comfort level with aggressive anticoagulation aimed at avoiding thromboembolic events.

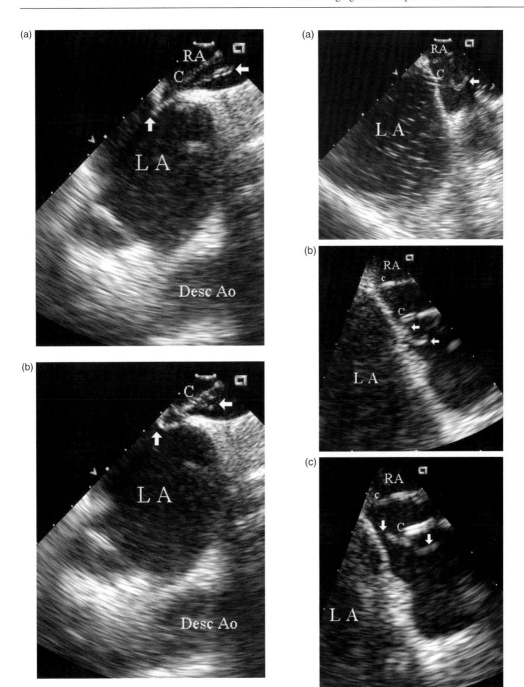

Figure 5.19 ICE images with the transducer placed in the right atrium (RA), showing: (a) RA thrombus (arrow, looped linear, size = 20 × 0.8 mm²) attached to a transseptal sheath (C) identified at the time of needle tip tenting against the interatrial septum during transseptal catherization; (b) the thrombus (arrow) attached to the sheath (C) incompletely imaged. Desc Ao: descending aorta; LA: left atrium.

Figure 5.20 ICE images with the transducer placed in the right atrium (RA), showing: (a) right atrial thrombus (arrow, linear, size = 22 × 2.0 mm²) developed immediately following dual transseptal punctures with bubbles (flushing the sheath) imaged in the left atrium (LA); and (b and c) the thrombus (arrows) attached to the interatrial septum at the transseptal punctural point.

(a)

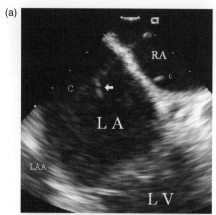

(b)

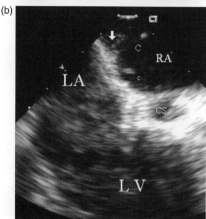

(c)

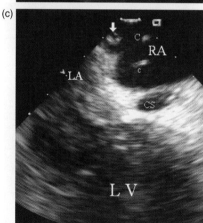

Figure 5.21 ICE images with the transducer placed in the right atrium (RA), showing: (a) a linear thrombus (arrow, size = 11 × 2 mm²) attached to the transseptal catheter sheath (C) in the left atrium (LA); and (b) withdrawal of the thrombus by pulling back the sheath with the thrombus (arrow) from the LA, through the atrial septum; (c) into the RA under ICE guidance and monitoring. c: catheter; CS: coronary sinus; LAA: LA appendage; LV: left ventricle.

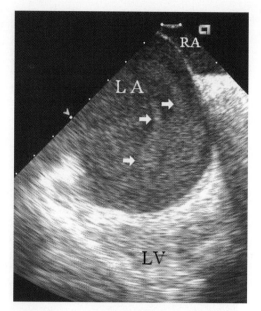

Figure 5.22 ICE image with the transducer (7.5 MHz) placed in the right atrium (RA), showing spontaneous echo contrast, as slowly swirling nonhomogeneous echoes (arrows) in an enlarged (diameter = 5.7 cm) left atrium (LA). LV: left ventricle.

References

1 Ross J Jr. Transseptal left heart catheterization: a new method of left atrial puncture. *Ann Surg* 1959; **149**: 395–401.

2 Cope C. Technique for transseptal catheterization of the left atrium: preliminary report. *J Thorac Surg* 1959; **37**: 482–486.

3 Brockenbrough EC, Braunwald E. A new technique for left ventricular angiocardiography and transseptal left heart catheterization. *Am J Cardiol* 1960; **6**: 1062–1064.

4 Mullins CE. Transseptal left heart catheterization: experience with a new technique in 520 pediatric and adult patients. *Pediatr Cardiol* 1983; **4**: 239–246.

5 O'Keefe JH, Vlietstra RE, Hanley PC, Seward JB. Revival of the transseptal approach for catheterization of the left atrium and ventricle. *Mayo Clin Proc* 1985; **60**: 790–795.

6 Morady F, Harvey M, Kalbfleisch SJ, EL-Atassi R, Calkins H, Langberg J. Radiofrequency catheter ablation of ventricular tachycardia in patients with coronary artery disease. *Circulation* 1993; **87**: 363–372.

7 Haissaguerre M, Jais P, Shah DC, *et al.* Electrophysiological end point for catheter ablation of atrial fibrillation initiated from multiple pulmonary venous foci. *Circulation* 2000; **101**: 1409–1417.

8 Baim DS. Percutaneous approach, including transseptal and apical puncture, chapter 4. In: Baim DS,

Grossman W, eds. *Grossman's Cardiac Catheterization, Angiography, and Intervention*, 6th edn. Lippincott Williams & Wilkins, Philadelphia, 2000: 92–97.

9 Adrouny ZA, Sutherland DW, Griswold HE, Ritzmann LW. Complications with transseptal left heart catheterization. *Am Heart J* 1963; **65**: 327–333.

10 Lindeneg O, Hansen AT. Complications in transseptal left heart catheterization. *Acta Med Scand* 1966; **180**: 395–399.

11 B-Lundqvist C, Olsson SB, Varnauskas E. Transseptal left heart catheterization: a review of 278 studies. *Clin Cardiol* 1986; **9**: 21–26.

12 Roelke M, Smith AJ, Palacios IF. The technique and safety of transseptal left heart catheterization: the Massachusetts General Hospital experience with 1279 procedures. *Cathet Cardiovasc Diagn* 1994; **32**: 332–339.

13 Kronzou I, Glassman E, Cohn M, Winer H. Use of two-dimensional echocardiography during transseptal cardiac catheterization. *J Am Coll Cardiol* 1984; **4**: 425–428.

14 Ballal RS, Mahan EF III, Nanda NC, Dean LS. Utility of transesophageal echocardiography in interatrial septal puncture during percutaneous mitral balloon commissurotomy. *Am J Cardiol* 1990; **66**: 230–232.

15 Vilacosta I, Iturralde E, San Roman JA, *et al*. Transesophageal echocardiographic monitoring of percutaneous mitral balloon valvulotomy. *Am J Cardiol* 1992; **70**: 1040–1044.

16 Hahn K, Gal R, Sarnoski J, Kubota J, Schmidt DH, Bajwa TK. Transesophageal echocardiographically guided atrial transseptal catheterization in patients with normal-sized atria: incidence of complications. *Clin Cardiol* 1995; **18**: 217–220.

17 Hurrell DG, Nishimura RA, Symanski JD, Holmes DR Jr. Echocardiography in the invasive laboratory: utility of two-dimensional echocardiography in performing transseptal catheterization. *Mayo Clin Proc* 1998; **73**: 126–131.

18 Chu E, Fitzpatrick AP, Chin MC, Sudhir K, Yock P, Lesh MD. Radiofrequency catheter ablation guided by intracardiac echocardiography. *Circulation* 1994; **89**: 1301–1305.

19 Kalman JM, Olgin JE, Karch MR, Lesh MD. Use of intracardiac echocardiography in interventional electrophysiology. *PACE* 1997; **20**: 2248–2262.

20 Ren JF, Schwartzman D, Callans D, Marchlinski FE, Gottlieb CD, Chaudhry FA. Imaging technique and clinical utility for electrophysiologic procedures of lower frequency (9 MHz) intracardiac echocardiography. *Am J Cardiol* 1998; **82**: 1557–1560.

21 Hung JS, Fu M, Yeh KH, Chua S, Wu JJ, Chen YC. Usefulness of intracardiac echocardiography in transseptal puncture during percutaneous transvenous mitral commissurotomy. *Am J Cardiol* 1993; **72**: 853–854.

22 Hung J-S, Fu M, Yeh K-H, Wu C-J, Wong P. Usefulness of intracardiac echocardiography in complex transseptal catheterization during percutaneous transvenous mitral commissurotomy. *Mayo Clin Proc* 1996; **71**: 134–140.

23 Daoud EG, Kalbfleisch SJ, Hummel JD. Intracardiac echocardiography to guide transseptal left heart catheterization for radiofrequency catheter ablation. *J Cardiovasc Electrophysiol* 1999; **10**: 358–363.

24 Ren JF, Schwartzman D, Callans DJ, Brode SE, Gottlieb CD, Marchlinski FE. Intracardiac echocardiography (9 MHz) in humans: methods, imaging views and clinical utility. *Ultrasound in Med & Biol* 1999; **25**: 1077–1086.

25 Hung JS. Atrial septal puncture technique in percutaneous transvenous mitral commissurotomy: mitral valvuloplasty using the Inoue balloon catheter technique. *Cath Cardiovasc Diagn* 1992; **26**: 275–284.

26 Yeh KH, Fu M, Wu CJ, Chua SO, Chen YC, Hung JS. Transseptal balloon mitral valvuloplasty in mitral stenosis with atrial septal aneurysm. *Am Heart J* 1993; **126**: 474–475.

27 Lau KW, Ding ZP, Johan A. Percutaneous transseptal mitral valvuloplasty in the presence of atrial septal aneurysm. *Cath Cardiovasc Diagn* 1994; **31**: 337–340.

28 Ren JF, Marchlinski FE, Callans DJ. Quantitative evaluation of atrial septal defect resulting from dual transseptal catheterization for ablation of atrial fibrillation: a Doppler color flow imaging study (abstr). *PACE* 2002; **24**: 559.

29 Ren JF, Marchlinski FE, Callans DJ. Residual atrial septal defect following dual transseptal catheterization: a Doppler color flow imaging follow-up (abstr). *J Am Coll Cardiol* 2003; **41**: 95A.

30 Clugston R, Lau FYK, Ruiz C. Transseptal catheterization update 1992. *Cathet Cardiovasc Diagn* 1992; **26**: 266–274.

31 Ren JF, Callans DJ, Schwartzman D, Marchlinski FE. Significant incidence of right atrial thrombus associated with long catheter sheath during cardiac ablation procedures (abstr). *PACE* 2001; **24**: 603.

32 Ren JF, Marchlinski FE, Callans DJ. Left atrial thrombus associated with ablation for atrial fibrillation: identification with intracardiac echocardiography. *J Am Coll Cardiol* 2004; **43**: 1861–1867.

33 Ren JF, Marchlinski FE, Callans DJ, *et al*. Increased intensity of anticoagulation may reduce risk of thrombus during atrial fibrillation ablation procedures in patients with spontaneous echo contrast. *J Cardiovasc Electrophysiol* 2005; **16**: 474–477.

CHAPTER 6

Intracardiac Echocardiographic Imaging in Radiofrequency Catheter Ablation for Inappropriate Sinus Tachycardia and Atrial Tachycardias

Jian-Fang Ren, MD, *& David J. Callans,* MD

Introduction

Inappropriate sinus tachycardia is a clinical syndrome characterized by an increased resting heart rate accompanied by exaggerated response to exercise or stress. The mechanism may involve a primary abnormality of the sinus node demonstrating enhanced automaticity or a primary autonomic disturbance [1]. Radiofrequency catheter ablation of the superior portion of the sinus node can be helpful in patients with drug-refractory symptoms [2–4]. These results indicate that radiofrequency ablation of inappropriate sinus tachycardia can be conceptualized as an anatomically based procedure. Intracardiac echocardiography (ICE) has been used to assist ablation catheter positioning at the anatomic location of the sinus node [4–7] and for monitoring potential complications [6,7]. Despite ICE imaging guidance, catheter ablation of inappropriate sinus tachycardia often is difficult and requires multiple ablation lesions, typically delivered within a very small area [2–7]. The need for repeated lesion applications coupled with the known epicardial location of the sinus node led us to hypothesize that catheter ablation of inappropriate sinus tachycardia may be successful only when the lesion extends to the epicardium opposite the superolateral crista terminalis. Furthermore, we have defined a characteristic echocardiographic signature that signifies when transmural/epicardial damage is present, which correlates with successful heart rate reduction when using this anatomic echocardiographically based approach [8].

Electrophysiologic study and catheter ablation

The patient is studied in the postabsorptive state under conditions of conscious sedation obtained by intravenous infusion of midazolam and a short-acting narcotic agent. Catheters are inserted through the femoral veins and positioned under fluoroscopic and ICE guidance to the high right atrium, atrioventricular junction and right ventricular apex. A steerable thermistor-equipped catheter with either a 4- or 8-mm tip electrode is used for mapping and ablation [7,8] (EP Technologies, San Jose, California); the 8-mm tip is used preferentially to facilitate visualization with ICE imaging. Surface leads and intracardiac electrograms filtered from 30 to 250 Hz are displayed and recorded using a digital amplifier/recorder system. Episodes of inappropriate sinus tachycardia, if not present spontaneously, are induced with graded infusion of isoproterenol. Although the mapping and ablation procedure is primarily anatomically based, electrophysiologic mapping of the earliest atrial activation during episodes of inappropriate sinus tachycardia is performed for confirmation of the appropriateness of ablation site targets using one or more of the following techniques: (1) sequential multisite mapping using the ablation catheter; (2) multisite simultaneous mapping using a multipolar "crista" catheter (Webster Laboratories, Baldwin Park, CA), or (3) nonfluoroscopic, electroanatomic mapping for right atrial activation (CARTO™, Biosense Ltd., Israel).

Radiofrequency energy is delivered in a unipolar fashion to areas of the superior lateral crista terminalis, demonstrating earliest activation during sinus tachycardia. High output pacing (10 mA, 2 ms pulse width) is performed at all prospective radiofrequency target sites to ensure that diaphragmatic stimulation does not occur, indicating the potential for radiofrequency-induced damage to the phrenic nerve. Radiofrequency power output is adjusted to achieve a tip temperature of 50° to 55°C and/or a specified impedance drop from baseline (measured at 5 W output, 10 Ω drop with a 4-mm tip electrode and 7–8 Ω with an 8-mm tip), and applied for 120 s. Procedural success is defined by the following: (1) an abrupt decrease ($\geq$30 bpm) in sinus rate following radiofrequency energy delivery; (2) the sudden appearance of superiorly directed P-wave morphology (negative P-wave in lead III); and (3) the persistence of these features despite infusion of isoproterenol (up to 4 μg/min) for at least 30 min following the delivery of the final radiofrequency lesion.

Imaging of the superolateral crista terminalis – the sinus node

The sinus node lies immediately subepicardially within the terminal groove (sulcus terminalis) of the right atrium. In most cases, the node lies lateral to the crest of the right atrial appendage and has a tail extending down toward the inferior vena cava [1,9]. Sympathetic activation causes an increase in heart rate accompanied by a shift in earlier activation to the superior portion of the sinus node, whereas vagal stimulation results in a decrease with a more inferior focus [1,10,11]. Thus, ablation targeted at the higher rate, to superior portion of the sinus node could result in slowing of the dominant pacemaker while retaining chronotropic competence [1]. A mechanical radial ICE imaging catheter or AcuNav ultrasound catheter is advanced to the high right atrium via a femoral venous approach using an 11-Fr Mullins sheath. The cross-sectional imaging view

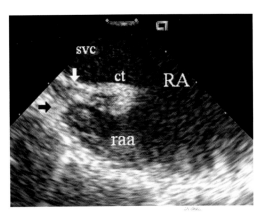

Figure 6.1 ICE image with the transducer placed at the junction of the superior vena cava (svc) and right atrial (RA) appendage (raa), showing the superolateral crista terminalis (ct) and the area for ablation and modification of sinus node (between arrows). Pectinate muscles are seen in the raa.

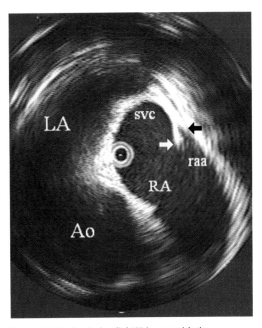

Figure 6.2 Mechanical radial ICE image with the transducer placed at the superior vena cava (svc)-right atrial (RA) appendage (raa) junction level, showing the superolateral crista terminalis region with its endocardium (white arrow) and epicardium (black arrow) for ablation and modification of sinus node. The superolateral crista terminalis wall thickness (between the arrows) measured 5 mm, and lateral svc wall measured 2.1 mm. The radius of the image = 40 mm. Ao: aorta; LA: left atrium.

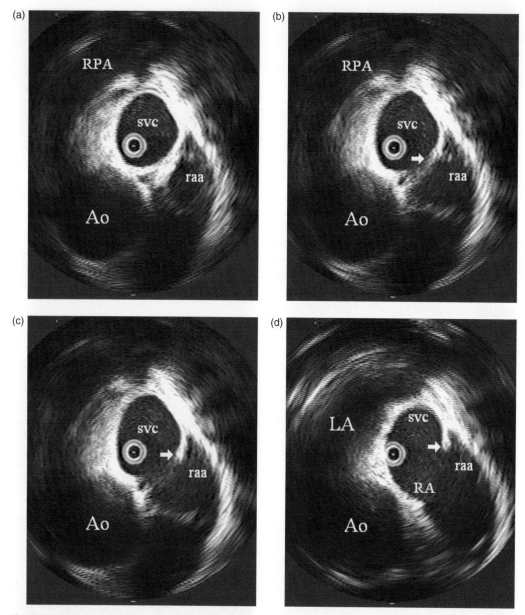

Figure 6.3 Mechanical radial ICE images with the transducer placed at the superior vena cava (svc)-right atrial (RA) appendage (raa) junction region, showing the imaging level of the svc-raa junction (arrow) orifice: (a) closing; (b and c) to opening partially; and (d) fully, representative of the superolateral crista terminalis level. Ao: aorta; LA: left atrium; RPA: right pulmonary artery.

used for guiding and monitoring of inappropriate sinus tachycardia ablation is at the level of the superior vena cava-right atrial appendage junction, which demonstrates the superolateral crista terminalis, representative of the area of the sinus node location (Figures 6.1 and 6.2).

The endocardium and epicardium of the crista terminalis area can be imaged clearly. ICE imaging is used during the procedure to guide catheter positioning and maintain optimal catheter contact. ICE imaging is used to confirm that the ablation catheter is positioned at the superior aspect of the crista

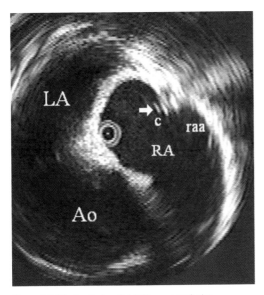

Figure 6.4 Mechanical radial ICE image with the transducer placed at the superior vena cava-right atrial (RA) appendage (raa) junction level, showing the ablation catheter (c) positioned at the superolateral crista terminalis (arrow) with distal fan-shaped shadow artifact. Ao: aorta; LA: left atrium.

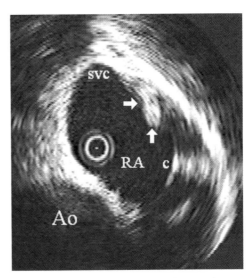

Figure 6.6 Mechanical radial ICE image showing the crista terminalis (upward arrow) wall thickness with swelling/dimpling (horizontal arrow) after the 11th radiofrequency lesion, increased to 7.5 mm, including 3.5-mm increased inhomogeneous echodensity and 4-mm unchanged zone, and superior vena cava (svc) wall to 3.1 mm. The radius of the image = 30 mm. Ao: aorta; c: catheter; RA: right atrium.

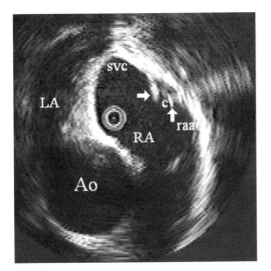

Figure 6.5 Mechanical radial ICE image with the transducer placed at the superior vena cava (svc)-right atrial (RA) appendage (raa) junction level, showing an ablation catheter (c) shifting within the raa (upward arrow) rather than the intended position at the superolateral crista terminalis (horizontal arrow). Ao: aorta; LA: left atrium.

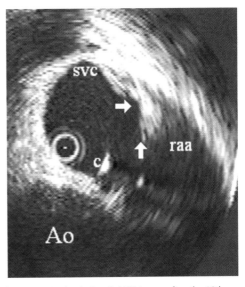

Figure 6.7 Mechanical radial ICE image after the 16th lesion showing the crista terminalis (upward arrow) wall thickness increased to 9 mm, including 7.0-mm increased echodensity and 2-mm less changed zone, and superior vena cava wall (svc) to 4.1 mm. In addition, a crater has formed at the endocardial surface (horizontal arrow). The radius of the image = 30 mm. Ao: aorta; c: catheter; raa: right atrial appendage.

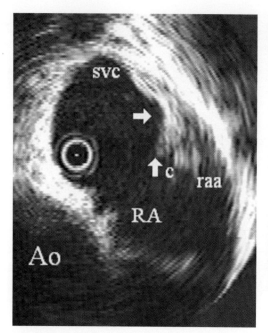

Figure 6.8 Mechanical radial ICE image after the 24th lesion showing deepening crater formation (horizontal arrow); the crista terminalis (upward arrow) wall thickness has increased to 9.5 mm, and inhomogeneous increases in echogenicity are now partially reaching the epicardium. The wall thickness of the superior vena cava (svc) wall has increased to 4.3 mm. At this point, the heart rate decreased transiently from 100 to 75 beat/min, and the P-wave in lead III started to change from a positive to a flat direction. The radius of the image = 30 mm. Ao: aorta; c: catheter; raa: right atrial appendage.

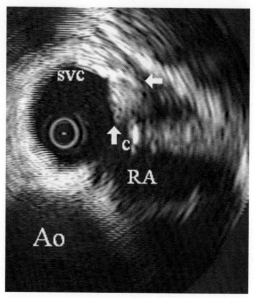

Figure 6.9 Mechanical radial ICE image after the last (52nd) lesion showing the crista terminalis wall thickness (arrows) was 9.2 mm, with echogenicity changes directly reaching to the epicardium with a trivial linear interstitial space (horizontal arrow). The lateral superior vena cava (svc) wall was 5.1 mm thick. The heart rate was reduced to 60 beat/min, with a negative P-wave in lead III. The radius of the image = 30 mm. Ao: aorta; c: catheter; RA: right atrium.

terminalis just at the level of the superior vena cava-right atrial appendage junction orifice. In this view, the junction orifice opens and closes as the heart moves through systole and diastole (Figure 6.3a–d). This is important, as the crista terminalis is a continuous structure extending from the superior vena cava orifice level down to near the inferior vena cava orifice. ICE is also used to monitor the stability of ablation catheter electrode-tissue contact (Figure 6.4) and to recognize and prevent sudden shifting of the ablation catheter within the right atrial appendage (Figure 6.5) during radiofrequency ablation.

Lesion morphologic changes

On-line monitoring for ablation lesion morphologic changes is important in creating anatomically based lesions. From *in vivo* validation and clinical observations, lesion morphologic changes including wall thickness, echodensity, and crater formation, can be assessed during and following radiofrequency energy delivery. With the delivery of serial radiofrequency energy applications, morphologic evolution of the local right atrial wall with three phases occurs in the lesion area as imaged by ICE imaging [12]. Imaging features and pathophysiological responses in the three phases are: (1) Phase I – increased wall thickness to 120% baseline, increase in echogenicity, swelling and edema; (2) Phase II – endocardial dimple formation, further increase in wall thickness to 150% baseline, further increases in echogenicity, edema; (3) Phase III – crater formation, increased wall thickness, shaggy appearance of the endocardial surface and/or thrombus formation, increased central and decreased peripheral echogenicity, coagulative necrosis, and edema. Using on-line (or videotape) ICE imaging, wall thickness, echogenicity and their changes at the crista terminalis lesion site are

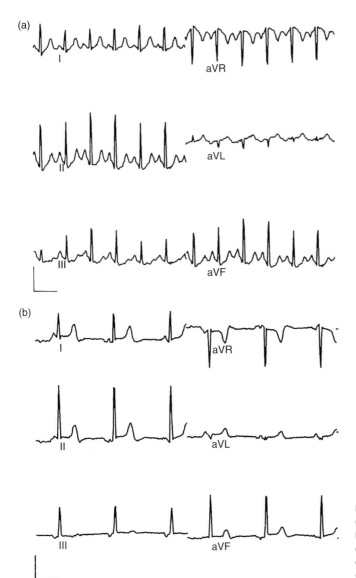

Figure 6.10 Surface electrocardiogram (limb leads) demonstrating a decrease in heart rate with changes in the P-wave, especially in lead III: (a) from a positive direction Pre-ablation; (b) to a negative direction post-ablation.

assessed at baseline, after each radiofrequency lesion, and with the lesion that produces a reduction in heart rate. Special attention is directed to changes in echogenicity which reach the epicardium at the lesion site during or after radiofrequency energy delivery. Serial lesion morphologic changes during repeat radiofrequency energy delivery at the superolateral crista terminalis area can be regularly observed with ICE imaging. As compared to the baseline crista terminalis wall (Figure 6.2), increased wall thickness with swelling/dimpling (Figure 6.6), followed by crater formation (Figure 6.7) is observed at lesion site during

initial and repeated lesion applications. Increased inhomogeneous echogenicity within the endocardium at the superolateral crista terminalis area gradually expands to near the epicardium with serial lesion applications. Wall thickness with further deepening crater formation and increasing swelling expanding to the wall of the superior vena cava can also be imaged. With further radiofrequency lesion applications, wall thickness markedly increases and when inhomogeneously increased echogenicity partially reaches the epicardium (Figure 6.8), intermittent decrease in heart rate and change in the P-wave from a positive to a flat direction in lead III may be observed. After the effective radiofrequency lesion, wall thickness at the crista terminalis may increase 48 ± 33% compared with baseline and the adjacent proximal superior vena cava lateral wall thickness may increase to 6.1±1.9 mm from 2.6 ± 0.9 mm at baseline. Multiple craters may reach to 5.7 ± 1.8 mm in width and 1.9 ± 0.7 mm in depth. With the final radiofrequency lesion, echogenicity changes may directly reach to the epicardium with development of a complete trivial linear interstitial echo-free (or low echodensity) space (Figure 6.9) and a reduced heart rate with further change in the P-wave from a flat to negative direction in lead III (Figure 6.10).

Imaging features for procedural endpoints

When radiofrequency lesion-induced echogenicity reaches to the epicardium, a complete trivial linear interstitial echo-free space at the superolateral crista terminalis lesion area is observed (Figure 6.11). This characteristic echocardiographic signature suggesting transmural/epicardial damage appears to be present at the time of successful heart rate reduction and the P-wave change into flat or negative direction in lead III. When this echocardiographic sign is not present, additional radiofrequency applications are delivered even if the heart rate has decreased. Multiple applications of radiofrequency energy in this region guided by a purely anatomic approach using ICE usually result first in slowing and then in abrupt termination of tachycardia. Wall swelling and thickness increases with multiple radiofrequency applications. However, the degree of swelling and thickening alone varies among patients and is not directly proportional to the number of radiofrequency applications; also this alone does not predict a positive heart rate response. Importantly, the development of a trivial linear echo-free space more reliably identified an effective heart rate reduction response. Thus, it appears that a characteristic imaging signature, suggesting transmural lesion damage reaching to the epicardium is present at the time of successful heart rate reduction. Acute procedural success, that is, successful heart rate reduction reported in 15 patients, required 41±31 (range 5–110, and median 40) radiofrequency applications (4 mm tip electrode, up to 40 W, 52°C, and 90 s) [8].

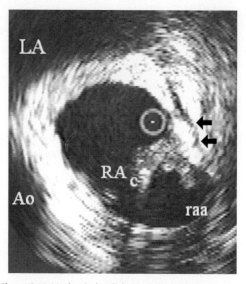

Figure 6.11 Mechanical radial ICE image with the transducer placed at the superior vena cava (svc)-right atrial (RA) appendage (raa) level, showing ablation (echogenic) lesions with multiple craters reaching the epicardium at the superolateral crista terminalis and development of a linear interstitial echo-free space (arrows), representative of procedural anatomic-imaging endpoint with transmural/epicardial damage.

Repeat ablation

Repeat radiofrequency catheter ablation of inappropriate sinus tachycardia is required for initial failure or recurrent symptoms. In patients without successful acute outcome and heart rate reduction, an increased/changed echogenicity does not reach the epicardium, and the linear interstitial echo-free space between the epicardium and the pericardium does not develop (Figure 6.12a,b). Patients undergoing repeat ablation procedures (required in 30% in our series [8]) all had a successful acute outcome, defined by abrupt slowing of the sinus rate and transition to a superiorly directed P-wave morphology in lead III, and the above mentioned echocardiographic changes (Figure 6.13a,b). The effective radiofrequency has been observed starting with the 23rd ± 31st lesion in repeat procedures (range 6th to 92nd, median 12th). Ablation response and echocardiographic imaging changes after effective radiofrequency lesions are similar to those with initial ablation procedure. The predictive value of this echo signature for long-term inappropriate sinus tachycardia control at mean 32 ± 17 months (range 6–54) was 12 of 17 patients (70%).

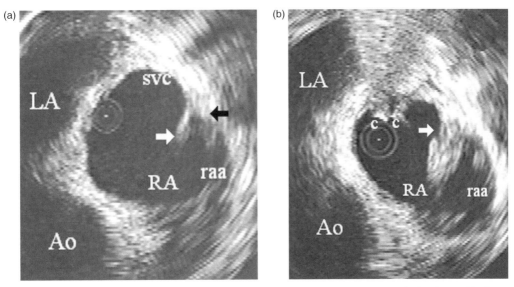

Figure 6.12 Mechanical radial ICE imaging with the transducer placed at the superior vena cava (svc)-right atrial (RA) appendage (raa) level, showing: (a) patient with inappropriate sinus tachycardia undergoing radiofrequency ablation with initial failure. The crista terminalis wall thickness (between arrows) measured 7.6 mm, and the lateral svc wall measured 1.6 mm at baseline; and (b) after the last ablation lesion the wall thickness with crater formation (arrow) increased to 18 mm, including enhanced inhomogeneous echodensity near the epicardium without development of an echo-free space, and the svc wall increased to 5 mm. Despite these changes, heart rate remained at 102 beat/min without significant change in P-wave morphology. The radius of the image = 40 mm. Ao: aorta; c: catheter; LA: left atrium.

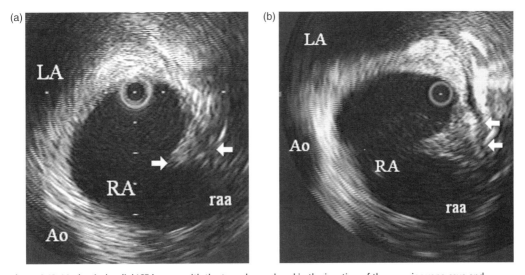

Figure 6.13 Mechanical radial ICE images with the transducer placed in the junction of the superior vena cava and right atrial (RA) appendage (raa), showing: (a) at the repeat ablation procedure the crista terminalis wall thickness (between arrows) was 8 mm and lateral superior vena cava wall 1.8 mm before lesion application (each scale = 5 mm); (b) after the 27th ablation lesion the wall thickness was 13.1 mm, with the enhanced echodensity zone reaching the epicardium and development of a linear interstitial echo-free space (arrows), and the lateral superior vena cava wall was 3.7 mm (the radius of the image = 30 mm). With this lesion, heart rate decreased from 100 to 60 beat/min. Ao: aorta; LA: left atrium.

(a)

(b)

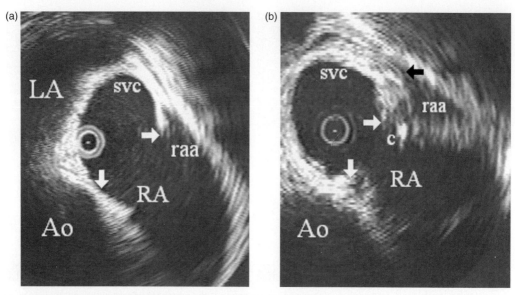

Figure 6.14 Mechanical radial ICE images with the transducer placed at the superior vena cava (svc)-right atrial (RA) appendage (raa) junction level, showing change in the svc-raa junction orifice: (a) from 17 mm (between arrows) at baseline (the radius of the image = 40 mm); (b) to 9 mm (between white arrows) post-ablation lesions (47% reduction), with the echogenic lesions reaching to the epicardium and development of the linear interstitial space between the epicardium and pericardium (black arrow) (the radius of the image = 30 mm). c: catheter; Ao: aorta; LA: left atrium.

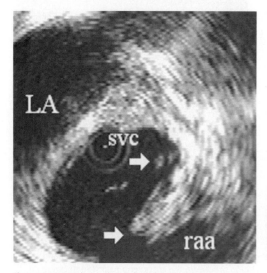

Figure 6.15 Mechanical radial ICE image showing a thickened crista terminalis wall (lower arrow) ablated with a thrombus attached at a deeper crater (upper arrow). LA: left atrium; raa: right atrial appendage; svc: superior vena cava.

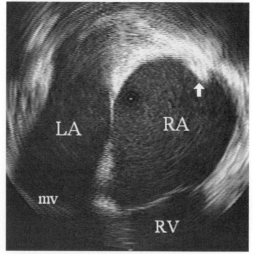

Figure 6.16 Mechanical radial ICE image with the transducer placed near the interatrial septum in the middle right atrium (RA), showing the left atrium (LA), RA and the middle portion of the crista terminalis (arrow). The radius of the image = 60 mm. mv: mitral valve; RV: right ventricle.

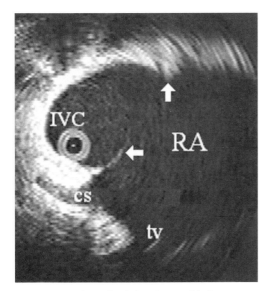

Figure 6.17 Mechanical radial ICE image with the transducer placed at the orifice of the inferior vena cava (IVC), showing the right atrium (RA) and the inferior portion of the crista terminalis (upward arrow) and eustachian valve (horizontal arrow). cs: coronary sinus; tv: tricuspid valve.

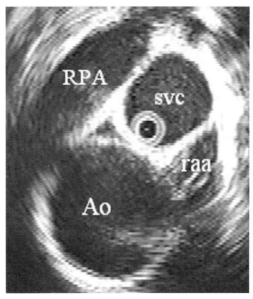

Figure 6.19 Mechanical radial ICE image with the transducer placed just above the orifice of the superior vena cava (svc), showing the svc at a proximal level with its immediately adjacent structures including the right pulmonary artery (RPA), ascending aorta (Ao), and right atrial appendage (raa).

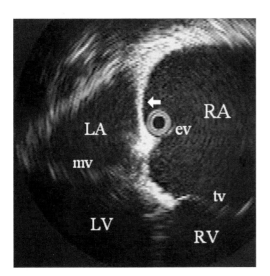

Figure 6.18 Mechanical radial ICE image with the transducer placed just above the orifice of the inferior vena cava, showing the left (LA) and right atrium (RA) with a lower portion of the interatrial septum (arrow). ev: eustachian valve; LV and RV: left and right ventricle; mv: mitral valve; tv: tricuspid valve.

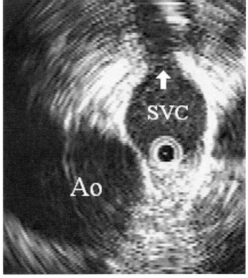

Figure 6.20 Mechanical radial ICE image with the transducer placed at the azygos vein orifice (arrow) level of the superior vena cava (svc), showing the distal svc just at/below the orifice of the azygos vein. Ao: ascending aorta.

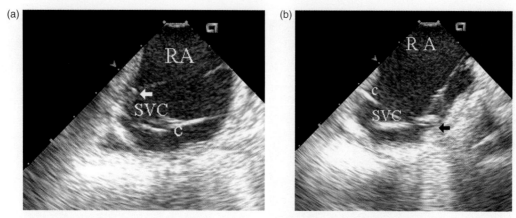

Figure 6.21 ICE image of superior vena cava (SVC) with the transducer placed in the middle right atrium (RA) with its tip directed slightly posteriorly, showing the ablation catheter electrode (arrow) with a strong distal fan-shaped shadow artifact, positioned at: (a) the SVC posterior; and (b) anterior wall just above the SVC-RA junction, a multipolar mapping catheter (c) seen in the SVC.

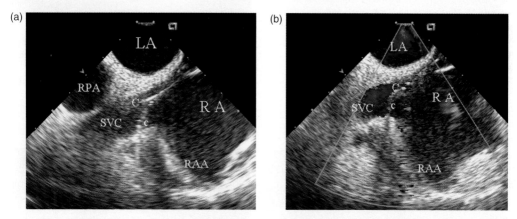

Figure 6.22 ICE images of superior vena cava (SVC) with the transducer placed in the left atrium (LA) through a patent foramen ovale, showing: (a) a multipolar mapping catheter (C) and ablation catheter (c) positioned in the SVC lumen with adjacent structures including the right pulmonary artery (RPA) and the right atrial appendage (RAA). (b) The color flow imaging shows the blood flow (red color) from SVC into the right atrium (RA).

Potential complications

Transient superior vena cava occlusion or superior vena cava syndrome has been reported following catheter ablation for inappropriate sinus tachycardia [4,13]. Presumably, venous occlusion could occur on the basis of radiofrequency lesion-induced tissue swelling and/or development of thrombus. Under ICE imaging guidance and monitoring of the ablation procedure, increased wall thickness and multiple craters are often observed at the superolateral crista terminalis lesion site during repeat lesion applications. The radiofrequency energy delivery causes tissue swelling at the site of catheter contact as well as circumferential swelling around the superior vena cava-right atrium junction orifice. With ICE imaging monitoring, a reduction of the superior vena cava-right atrium junction orifice diameter of 22% (range 11–47%) has been detected as compared with baseline (Figure 6.14a,b) [7–8]. Narrowing of the junction orifice >50% was not identified. Recovery of tissue swelling within the superior vena cava-right atrium junction has not been observed during ICE imaging monitoring for 30 min following the delivery of the final radiofrequency lesion. In the patients who

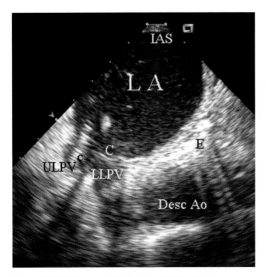

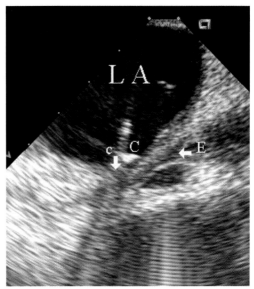

Figure 6.23 ICE image of left atrium (LA) with the transducer placed near the interatrial septum (IAS) in the right atrium (RA), showing multipolar mapping catheter (C) at the ostium of the lower (L) left pulmonary vein (LPV) and ablation catheter (c) at the upper (U) LPV ostium. LA posterior wall is partially contiguous to the esophagus (E). Desc Ao: descending aorta.

Figure 6.24 ICE image of left atrium (LA) with the transducer placed in the right atrium, showing ablation catheter electrode (c, downward arrow) with a strong distal fan-shaped shadow artifact, at the LA posterior wall near the lower right pulmonary vein ostium (C, multipolar mapping catheter) adjacent to the esophagus (E). During radiofrequency energy delivery, another distal fan-shaped shadow artifact is seen from the center of the transducer down to the distal field (horizontal arrow), with the interference of energy delivery electronic device.

require repeat procedures (range 1–8 months between procedures), no evidence of persistent tissue swelling at the superior vena cava-right atrium junction has been observed [7].

Small adherent thrombi have been generally identified within crater lesions (Figure 6.15) in 35% patients, but do not appear to contribute significantly to superior vena cava-right atrium junction orifice reduction under ICE imaging monitoring [7,8].

The other potential complications related to catheter ablation procedures, such as pericardial effusion and damage to adjacent cardiovascular structures or the phrenic nerve may be reduced or prevented by using currently available ICE imaging guidance and monitoring.

The need for pacemaker implantation after sinus node modification has been noted in up to 20% of patients; however, using an anatomic approach, this complication appears to be much more infrequent.

Identifying common sites of origin for atrial tachycardias

Atrial tachycardia is a rhythm that may originate from either left or right atrium and may be caused

by reentry, triggered, or abnormal automaticity [14]. Surface electrocardiography can be useful to determine the arrhythmia site of origin. A positive or biphasic P-wave in surface lead in aVL suggests a right atrial origin, whereas a positive P-wave in V_1 and a negative P-wave in aVL indicate a left atrial arrhythmia origin [15]. Because the right pulmonary veins are located posterior and toward right of the right atrial septum, the surface P-wave morphology can sometimes be inaccurate in predicting the arrhythmia site of origin. Mapping of atrial tachycardia is best achieved with activation mapping to identify local atrial activity before onset of the surface P-wave, pace mapping to identify a site where the paced P-wave is identical to the spontaneous tachycardia P-wave, and paced activation sequence mapping where the relative activation timing from multiple atrial recording sites is identical between pacing and spontaneous tachycardia [14]. Using this approach atrial tachycardia sites can be determined and successfully ablated [16].

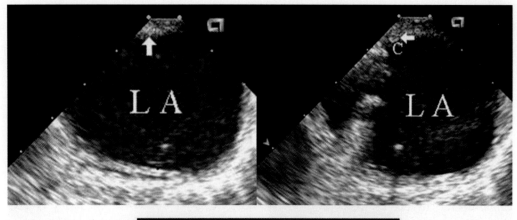

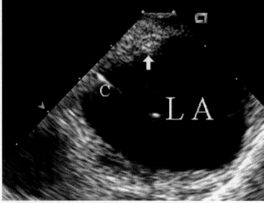

Figure 6.25 ICE images of left atrium (LA) with the transducer placed in the right atrium, showing pre- (left upper panel), during (right upper panel) and post-radiofrequency lesion (lower panel) in the left interatrial septum (arrow). The thickness of the septum is 3.5 mm pre- and 8 mm post-lesion. During ablation, the ablation catheter (C) is placed at the left interatrial septum (arrow) with a strong distal fan-shaped shadow artifact.

Common sites of origin for right atrial tachycardias include the superior (Figure 6.2), middle (Figure 6.16) or lower portion (Figure 6.17) of the crista terminalis, the low atrial septum (Figure 6.18), right atrial appendage (Figure 6.1), and the proximal (Figure 6.19) and distal portion (Figure 6.20) of the superior vena cava [17]. The superior vena cava can be imaged using mechanical radial catheter or AcuNav ICE imaging (Figure 6.21). In patients with patent foramen ovale, the imaging catheter can be positioned in the left atrium parallel to the superior vena cava lumen and its adjacent structures in guiding catheter location during ablation procedure (Figure 6.22a,b). Atrial tachycardia originating in the left atrium is most often from the origins of the pulmonary vein ostia (Figure 6.23), although the posterior wall (Figure 6.24) and the left interatrial septum (Figure 6.25) are also common sites of origin. AcuNav ICE imaging is preferred during left atrial ablation procedures, as mechanical radial ICE with 9 MHz ultrasound has insufficient imaging depth to resolve lateral left atrial structures (such as left pulmonary vein ostia) when the transducer is placed in the right atrium.

References

1 Krahn AD, Yee R, Klein GJ, Morillo C. Inappropriate sinus tachycardia: evaluation and therapy. *J Cardiovasc Electrophysiol* 1995; **6**: 1124–1128.
2 Sanders WE, Sorrentino RA, Greenfield RA, Shenasa H, Hamer ME, Wharton JM. Catheter ablation of sinoatrial reentrant tachycardia. *J Am Coll Cardiol* 1994; **23**: 926–934.
3 Waspe LE, Chien WW, Merrillat JC, Stark SI. Sinus node modification using radiofrequency current in a patient with persistent inappropriate sinus tachycardia. *PACE* 1994; **17**: 1569–1576.

4 Lee RJ, Kalman JM, Fitzpatrick AP, *et al.* Radiofrequency catheter modification of the sinus node for "inappropriate" sinus tachycardia. *Circulation* 1995; **92**: 2919–2928.

5 Kalman JM, Olgin JE, Karch MR, Hamdan M, Lee RJ, Lesh MD. "Crista tachycardias": origin of right atrial tachycardias from the crista terminalis identified by intracardiac echocardiography. *J Am Coll Cardiol* 1998; **31**: 451–459.

6 Ren JF, Schwartzman D, Callans DJ, Marchlinski FE, Gottlieb CD, Chaudhry FA. Imaging technique and clinical utility for electrophysiologic procedures of lower frequency (9 MHz) intracardiac echocardiography. *Am J Cardiol* 1998; **82**: 1557–1560.

7 Callans DJ, Ren JF, Schwartzman D, Gottlieb CD, Chaudhry FA, Marchlinski FE. Narrowing of the superior vena cava-right atrium junction during radiofrequency catheter ablation for inappropriate sinus tachycardia: analysis with intracardiac echocardiography. *J Am Coll Cardiol* 1999; **33**: 1667–1670.

8 Ren JF, Marchlinski FE, Callans DJ, Zado ES. Echocardiographic lesion characteristics associated with successful ablation of inappropriate sinus tachycardia. *J Cardiovasc Electrophysiol* 2001; **12**: 814–818.

9 Anderson KR, Ho SY, Anderson RH. The location and vascular supply of the sinus node in the human heart. *Br Heart J* 1979; **41**: 28–32.

10 Boineau JP, Schuessler RB, Hackel DB, Miller CB, Brockus CW, Wylds AC. Widespread distribution and rate differentiation of the atrial pacemaker complex. *Am J Physiol* 1980; **239**: H406–H415.

11 Randall WC, Rinkema LE, Jones SB, Moran JF, Brynjolfsson G. Functional characterization of atrial pacemaker activity. *Am J Physiol* 1982; **242**: H98–H106.

12 Ren JF, Schwartzman DS, Brode SE, *et al.* Intracardiac echocardiographic monitoring for morphologic changes in radiofrequency ablation atrial lesions: *in vivo* validation and clinical observations (abstr). *Circulation* 1997; **96**: I-22.

13 Leonelli FM, Pisano E, Requarth JA, *et al.* Frequency of superior vena cava syndrome following radiofrequency modification of the sinus node and its management. *Am J Cardiol* 2000; **85**: 771–774.

14 Haines DE. Catheter ablation therapy for arrhythmias. In: Topol EJ, ed. *Textbook of Cardiovascular Medicine*, 2nd edn. Lippincott Williams & Wilkins, Philadephia, 2002: 1559.

15 Tang CM, Scheinman MM, Van Hare GF, *et al.* Use of P wave configuration during atrial tachycardia to predict site of origin. *J Am Coll Cardiol* 1995; **26**: 1315–1324.

16 Tracy CM, Swartz JF, Fletcher RD, *et al.* Radiofrequency catheter ablation of ectopic atrial tachycardia using paced activation sequence mapping. *J Am Coll Cardiol* 1993; **21**: 910–917.

17 Gerstenfeld EP, Ren JF, Marchlinski FE. Atrial tachycardia successfully treated by electrical isolation of the superior vena cava. *PACE* 2003; **26**(Pt.I): 906–910.

CHAPTER 7

Intracardiac Echocardiographic Imaging in Radiofrequency Catheter Ablation for Atrial Fibrillation

Jian-Fang Ren, MD, *& Francis E. Marchlinski,* MD

Introduction

Atrial fibrillation is the most common sustained arrhythmia affecting humans. It may occur in paroxysmal (self-terminating), persistent (terminating with treatment), or permanent (sinus rhythm cannot be restored) form [1]. Maintenance of atrial fibrillation likely depends on reentry, with multiple wavelets occurring simultaneously [2]. The initiation of atrial fibrillation in many patients may be caused by a rapidly firing focus, often in the pulmonary veins [3–5]. Anatomic studies have confirmed that cardiac muscle extends onto the pulmonary veins in humans [6] and have found automaticity in an experimental model [7]. Atrial fibrillation is characterized by rapidly irregular and chaotic atrial fibrillatory waves at a rate of >300–600 beats per min. Pathologic studies have found loss of atrial myocardium with fibrosis and fatty infiltration, but many similar changes can occur as a result of aging. A variety of cardiac disease is associated with atrial fibrillation, most frequently hypertension, coronary artery disease, valvular heart disease, and hyperthyroidism. Many patients with apparently normal structural hearts have idiopathic, or lone, atrial fibrillation.

Radiofrequency catheter ablation of pulmonary veins has been used for the treatment of paroxysmal atrial fibrillation [3–5]. The efficacy

and safety have improved using pulmonary vein electrical isolation/ablation coupled with the use of three-dimensional electroanatomic mapping systems, intracardiac echocardiography (ICE), and special mapping catheters [8]. ICE imaging may play an important role in guiding transseptal catheterization (see Chapter 5), imaging pulmonary vein ostia, assisting accurate placement of mapping and ablation catheter, monitoring lesion morphology and flow changes at an ablated pulmonary vein orifice following ablation, and instantly detecting procedural complications [9].

Imaging and quantitative measurement of pulmonary vein ostium

It becomes of critical importance to identify pulmonary vein anatomic features and to determine ostial diameter to optimize the pulmonary vein ostial isolation/ablation strategy and select the appropriate sized circular multipolar mapping catheter (e.g. LASSO™). From our AcuNav imaging data of more than 600 patients undergoing pulmonary vein ostial isolation/ablation, the left pulmonary vein ostia demonstrate a shared common ostium (Figure 7.1a,b) in the majority of patients and less commonly

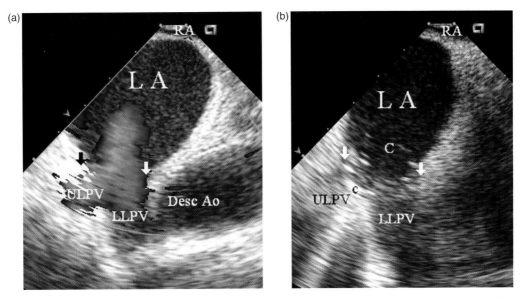

Figure 7.1 ICE images with the transducer placed in the right atrium (RA), showing: (a) the common left pulmonary vein ostium (between arrows) with confluence of red color flow directed to the left atrium (LA) from both the upper (ULPV) and the lower (LLPV) left pulmonary veins; (b) circular multipolar mapping (C) and ablation (c) catheters positioned at the common left pulmonary vein (between arrows). Desc Ao: descending aorta.

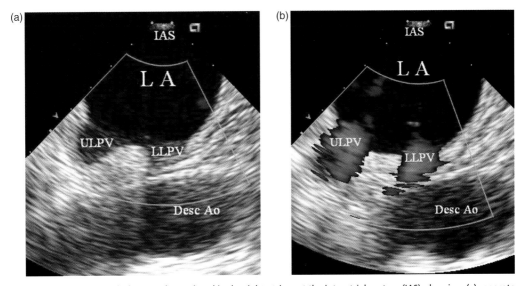

Figure 7.2 ICE images with the transducer placed in the right atrium at the interatrial septum (IAS), showing: (a) separate upper (ULPV) and lower left pulmonary vein (LLPV) ostia; (b) color flow (red) directed to the left atrium (LA) from separate ostia. Desc Ao: descending aorta.

completely separate ostia (Figure 7.2a,b). The right pulmonary veins generally have the upper, middle, and lower pulmonary veins. For the isolation and ablation technology, the upper and middle right pulmonary veins may be recognized as a shared common upper right pulmonary vein ostium since a carina commonly exists between the middle and lower right pulmonary vein (Figure 7.3). In variant anatomy of the right pulmonary veins, a separate middle right pulmonary vein or the right middle vein may be more closely

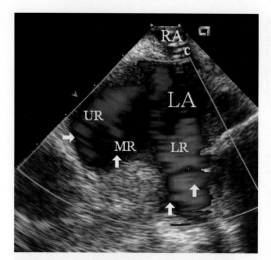

Figure 7.3 ICE image with the transducer placed in the right atrium (RA), showing the color flow (arrows) directed to the left atrium (LA) with shared ostium of the upper (UR) and middle right (MR) pulmonary vein, and a carina seen between the MR and lower right (LR) pulmonary vein ostia. C: catheter.

aligned to the lower right pulmonary vein (Figure 7.4). First degree pulmonary vein branches, especially of both left and right lower pulmonary veins, are often visualized with color flow imaging (Figure 7.5).

In 143 patients (113 men; age 55 ± 11 years) with atrial fibrillation undergoing radiofrequency ablation, the upper and lower left pulmonary vein ostial diameters measured 15.7 ± 2.3 and 16.1 ± 2.8 mm, and the upper and lower right pulmonary vein ostial diameters measured 15.6 ± 2.0 and 16.2 ± 1.4 mm before ablation, respectively [10,11]. No significant differences were found for individual ostial diameters. Left-shared common ostium measured 25.5 ± 4.5 mm [11].

Guiding mapping and ablation catheter placement at pulmonary vein ostium

After dual transseptal catheterization (see Chapter 5), a circular multipolar mapping catheter (LASSO™) and a mapping/ablation catheter (NAVISTAR™, Biosense Webster, Diamond Bar, CA, USA) are positioned through the sheaths within the left atrium and deployed at different pulmonary vein ostia under ICE imaging guidance. Based on the size measured with ICE Doppler color flow imaging, an appropriate

circular multipolar catheter can be applied at the shared (Figures 7.1b and 7.6) or individual upper and lower left pulmonary vein ostium (Figure 7.7a–c) and right pulmonary vein ostia (Figure 7.8a,b), respectively. When the shared ostial diameter is larger than that of the circular mapping catheter used, the latter may be positioned at the top portion of the ostium and then moved to the bottom under ICE imaging guidance (Figure 7.9). With ICE imaging of the ablation catheter, radiofrequency energy is always delivered proximal to the LASSO, and lesion inside the pulmonary vein ostium avoided (Figure 7.10).

Changes in ostial flow velocity during initial pulmonary vein ablation

The effectiveness of the ICE with Doppler color flow imaging in detecting pulmonary vein ostial flow velocity, for monitoring pulmonary vein ostial narrowing during focal atrial fibrillation ablation, has been described [10]. Peak flow velocity of the pulmonary vein ostium is measured at systole and diastole before and after the ablation (Figure 7.11). From a technical viewpoint it is important to adjust the imaging catheter position optimally. The ultrasound beam and the pulsed Doppler sampling gate (3–5 mm) should be aligned at an angle ≤25° and directed within 1 cm of the pulmonary vein ostium. The peak pressure gradient can be estimated using the simplified Bernoulli equation ($\Delta P = 4V^2$) where flow acceleration, viscous friction factors, and proximal velocity are ignored [12]. From our early experience radiofrequency energy was deployed at a total of 219 pulmonary vein ostia and changes in pulmonary vein ostial peak flow velocities/pressure gradients after ablation were noted (Table 7.1) [10]. The peak velocity of pulmonary vein ostial flow measured 56 ± 12 cm/s (range 21–98) before and 101 ± 22 cm/s (range 47–211) after ablation ($p < 0.001$). Peak velocities >100 cm/s (pressure gradient >4 mmHg) after ablation were detected in 103 (47%) of 219 ablated pulmonary veins. Significant turbulent flow features with spectral broadening of Doppler signal recorded at the ablated pulmonary veins have been observed when the peak velocity was >130 cm/s after ablation (Figures 7.11 and 7.12). An abrupt increase in peak flow velocities at the atrial ostium has been

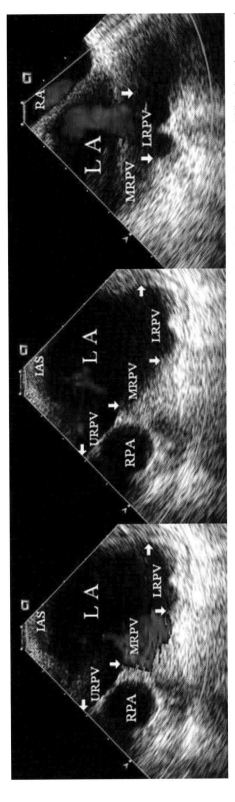

Figure 7.4 ICE images with optimal alignment of the catheter transducer placed in the right atrium (RA), showing Doppler color flow imaging from the middle right pulmonary vein (MRPV) ostium (left panel), separate (arrows) from the upper right (URPV) (middle panel) and lower right pulmonary vein (LRPV) ostial flow (right panel). Two proximal branches of the LRPV are also imaged. IAS: interatrial septum; LA: left atrium; RPA: right pulmonary artery.

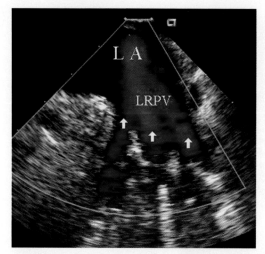

Figure 7.5 ICE image with the transducer placed in the right atrium, showing the color flow (arrows) directed to the left atrium (LA) from proximal branches of the lower right pulmonary vein (LRPV).

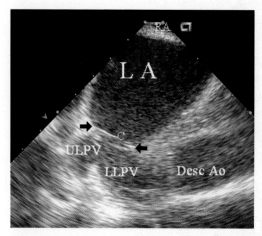

Figure 7.6 ICE image with the transducer placed in the right atrium (RA), showing the common left pulmonary vein ostium (arrows) shared with upper (ULPV) and lower left pulmonary veins (LLPV) and the circular multipolar mapping catheter (C) positioned at the shared common ostium. Desc Ao: descending aorta; LA: left atrium.

detected compared with pulmonary vein flow before the lesions, indicative of narrowing effects of the ostial lesions after ablation (Figure 7.13).

Follow-up and resolution of increased pulmonary vein flow velocity: based on the observed maximal pulmonary vein flow velocities, magnetic resonance imaging or contrast-enhanced computed tomography

follow-up, and the absence of symptoms consistent with pulmonary vein stenosis during follow-up of 6 to 18 months, our clinical experience suggests that an acute increase in pulmonary vein peak velocity up to 158 cm/s appears to be well tolerated. However, the seriousness of pulmonary vein stenosis has resulted in a much more conservative approach by our group. We typically target pulmonary vein flow velocities of <100 cm/s. A flow velocity change of >100 cm/s will warrant a more proximal approach to lesion deployment if possible. A maximal flow velocity of up to 120 cm/s for left side pulmonary veins has appeared to be associated with a low risk of significant narrowing on follow-up imaging studies. Our clinical observation with a Doppler color flow imaging also established a time-dependent reversal of the acute increase in pulmonary vein velocity during follow-up. An average reduction of 22 ± 14 cm/s in pulmonary vein peak velocity was noted at repeat ablation study (Figure 7.12), with over 88% of ablated pulmonary veins demonstrating values that approximated baseline values when measurements were made >3 months after initial procedure (Table 7.2, Figure 7.14).

Monitoring ostial flow velocity during repeat ablation at previously ablated pulmonary veins

Repeat pulmonary vein ablation noted in patients with increased pulmonary vein ostial flow velocities may induce further increases in pulmonary vein flow velocity and the development of persistent clinically meaningful changes in pulmonary vein flow. A cautious approach is warranted in such cases. We reported the outcome of our first 13 patients undergoing repeat ablation procedures for recurrent atrial fibrillation after an initial ablation (0.1–13 months after the initial procedure) [10]. There were two patients with pulmonary vein flow velocities >100 cm/s before repeat ablation with three pulmonary vein ostial velocities increasing to >158 cm/s after repeat ablation. In one patient, the upper left pulmonary vein flow velocity increased from 116 to 194 cm/s (15.1 mmHg); in another patient, the upper left pulmonary vein flow velocity increased from 118 to 172 cm/s and lower left pulmonary vein from 83 to 176 cm/s.

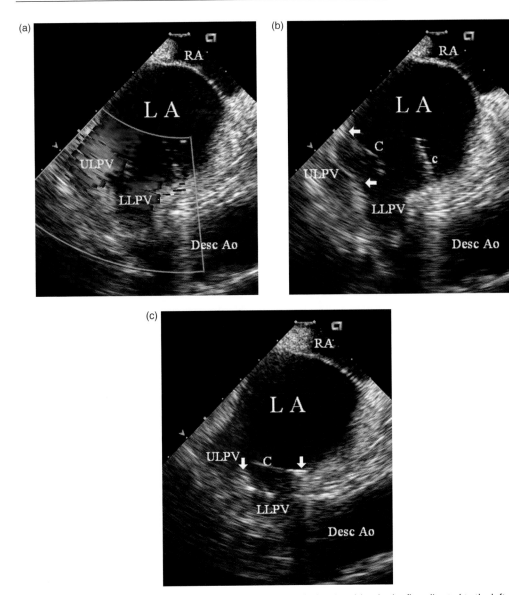

Figure 7.7 ICE images with transducer placed in the right atrium (RA), showing: (a) red color flow directed to the left atrium (LA) from separate upper (ULPV) and lower left pulmonary vein (LLPV); (b) circular multipolar mapping catheter (C) positioned at the ostium of the ULPV (between arrows); (c) circular multipolar mapping catheter (C) positioned at the ostium of the LLPV (between arrows). Desc Ao: descending aorta.

In these two patients with pulmonary vein ostial flow >158 cm/s, magnetic resonance imaging was performed at 2 to 4 months follow-up. Mild-to-moderate pulmonary vein stenosis (50–60%) was noted, and symptoms of exertional dyspnea developed at 4 months after the repeat ablation procedure in the patient with two veins with pulmonary vein velocities >158 cm/s. The other patient had no symptoms or significant stenosis (<50%) with late magnetic resonance imaging. No patient with pulmonary vein flow velocity <158 cm/s has been found to develop any symptoms consistent with pulmonary vein stenosis after repeat ablation [10]. Nevertheless, these data resulted in our taking a conservative approach to acceptable flow changes with repeat procedures. Repeated acute assessment of flow with flow velocity ≥120 cm/s

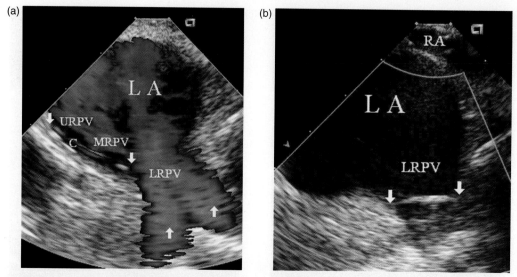

Figure 7.8 ICE images with the transducer in the right atrium (RA), showing: (a) red confluent flow directed to the left atrium (LA), one confluence from the upper (URPV) and middle (MRPV) right pulmonary veins and the other from the lower right pulmonary vein (LRPV) branches (two upward-arrows), and a circular multipolar mapping catheter positioned at the shared URPV and MRPV ostium (between two downward-arrows); (b) circular mapping catheter at the LRPV ostium (between arrows).

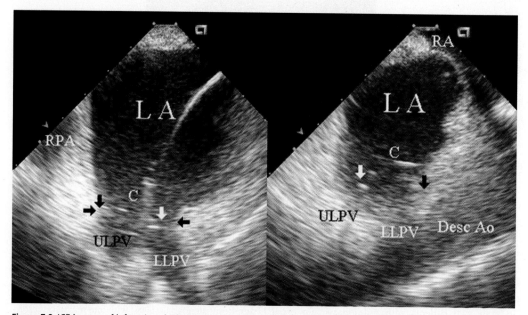

Figure 7.9 ICE images of left atrium (LA) with the transducer placed in the right atrium (RA), showing circular multipolar mapping catheter (vertical arrows) first at the top portion of the shared left pulmonary vein (LPV) ostium (horizontal arrows, left panel), then at the bottom portion of the shared ostium (right panel). C: catheter; Desc Ao: descending aorta; RPA: right pulmonary artery; ULPV and LLPV: upper and lower LPV.

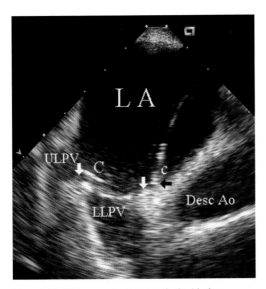

Figure 7.10 ICE image of left atrium (LA) with the transducer placed in the right atrium, showing the ablation catheter electrode (horizontal black arrow) placed near LA wall proximal to the LASSO poles (between two vertical arrows) just at the lower (L) left pulmonary vein (LPV) ostium. C: Lasso catheter; c: ablation catheter; Desc Ao: descending aorta; ULPV: upper LPV.

warrants redirection of the ablation approach to avoid further changes.

Effect of heart rate and isoproterenol on pulmonary vein flow velocity

Isoproterenol infusion is one of the most useful provocative maneuvers for potentiating firing of both pulmonary vein and non-pulmonary triggers for atrial fibrillation. Effect of isoproterenol (up to 20 μg/min) on pulmonary vein ostial flow velocity has been studied using ICE with Doppler color flow imaging in 31 patients (24 men, age 51±12 years) with paroxysmal atrial fibrillation [13]. The findings demonstrated that isoproterenol may increase ostial peak flow velocity of non-ablated pulmonary veins (Figure 7.15) and induce significantly additional increase in ostial velocity of ablated pulmonary veins (Figure 7.16, Table 7.3). This effect of isoproterenol appears to be independent of the heart rate effect since there was no significantly additional increase in pulmonary vein flow velocity with similar heart rate increase during atrial pacing (Figures 7.15

and 7.16, Table 7.3). Typical Doppler color flow imaging findings in true pulmonary ostial stenosis may include an increased pulmonary vein ostial peak flow velocity (turbulent jet) with a blunted systolic velocity and a prolonged elevated diastolic velocity with a long pressure-half time, and/or the systolic and diastolic components fused [10,12,14,15]. Although isoproterenol-induced peak velocity of pulmonary vein ostial flow may reach 190 cm/s post-ablation, the pulsed Doppler spectral imaging mimics a biphasic variation pattern without imaging features indicating ostial flow obstruction (Figure 7.16). Isoproterenol is a nonglycoside (sympathomimetic) inotropic agent and its effect on pulmonary vein flow may be related to its increasing cardiac output and also its stimulating β_2-adrenoceptors in the systemic vascular bed [16]. In clinical hemodynamic studies in patients with normal cardiac output (>2.2 L/min/m^2), isoproterenol increased both cardiac output and pulmonary vein flow velocity in parallel [17,18]. These isoproterenol effects are important to recognize when peak velocity of pulmonary vein flow is used as an index for interpreting the impact of pulmonary vein ostial lesions on functionally significant pulmonary vein narrowing. The clinical implication is that an "isoproterenol effect" on pulmonary vein ostial flow may be misinterpreted as clinically significant pulmonary vein stenosis due to the ablation procedure itself.

Characteristic lesion morphological changes

Radiofrequency energy delivered at left atrial wall adjacent to the pulmonary vein ostium induces lesion morphologic changes including wall thickening, echodensity, and crater formation. Left atrial wall thickness can be assessed by ICE two-dimensional or M-mode imaging (Figure 7.17). In 34 patients (age 54 ± 10 years) with atrial fibrillation left atrial wall measured 2.8 ± 0.6 mm baseline and increased its thickness (4.4 ± 1.2 mm) and echogenecity at the lesion area following radiofrequency energy ablation (4-mm electrode, up to 40 W, 52°C, 90 s) (Figure 7.18) [19]. The ligament of Marshall tissue (see Chapter 3) is an important target of ablation for atrial fibrillation-inducing triggers. The thickness of ligament of Marshall tissue area is usually

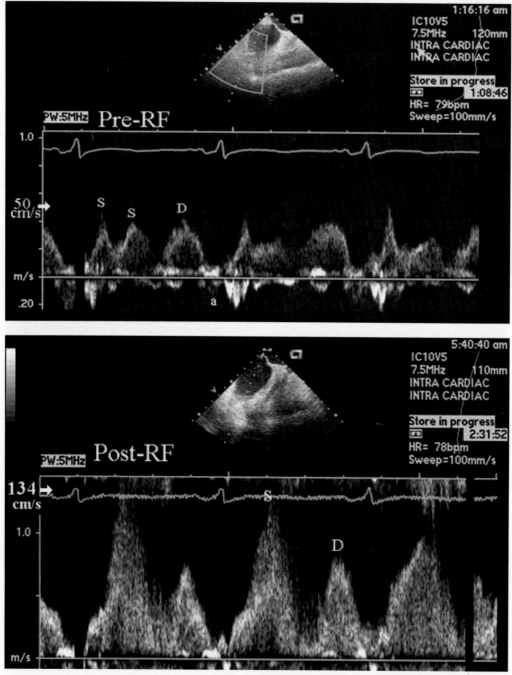

Figure 7.11 Pulsed Doppler spectrum recorded peak flow velocity of the upper left pulmonary vein (ULPV) ostium shows the maximal velocity measured 50 cm/s with two systolic components (S), as well as early diastolic (D) and late reversal (a) waves before ablation (Pre-RF), the ostial peak flow velocity increased to 134 cm/s (7.2 mmHg) with turbulence after lesions deployed at the ostium after ablation (Post-RF).

Table 7.1 Changes in pulmonary vein ostial flow velocities/pressure gradients after radiofrequency ablation.

	ULPV	URPV	LLPV	LRPV
n	81	73	43	22
Ostial diameter (mm)	15.6 ± 2.0	15.3 ± 1.9	15.6 ± 2.0	16.2 ± 1.4
Pre-ablation V (cm/s)	59 ± 12	54 ± 11	58 ± 13	44 ± 10
PG (mmHg)	1.5 ± 0.6	1.2 ± 0.5	1.5 ± 0.6	0.8 ± 0.3
HR (bpm)	76 ± 17	81 ± 20	76 ± 15	84 ± 16
Lesions/PV	14 ± 7	12 ± 6	11 ± 5	15 ± 9
Post-ablation V (cm/s)*	109 ± 21	97 ± 20	101 ± 25	79 ± 22
PG (mmHg)*	5.0 ± 3.4	4.0 ± 1.5	4.5 ± 2.3	2.8 ± 1.4
HR (bmp)	81 ± 15	83 ± 15	79 ± 15	81 ± 16

* All $p < 0.001$: post- versus pre-ablation. LLPV and LRPV: lower left and right pulmonary vein; PG: pressure gradient; ULPV and URPV: upper left and right pulmonary vein; V: peak flow velocity. Reproduced with permission [10].

greater and echogenecity is higher, indicating it is prominently fibrosed as compared to the other left atrial wall [19]. During radiofrequency ablation (4-mm electrode, up to 40 W, 52°C, and 90 s), catheter tip location is readily identified and small bubbles were observed in 25% lesions of the ligament of Marshall tissue area (Figure 7.19), and the echogenic thickness was significantly increased [19]. The thickness of the Marshall ligament tissue area measured 6.5 ± 1.9 mm pre-ablation and 11.9 ± 2.9 mm post-ablation (Figure 7.20). Repeat (≥ 5 lesions) radiofrequency energy (67.4%) is always needed and the number of lesions delivered is higher than that of the other locations of pulmonary vein ostial-left atrial wall indicating difficulty in isolating left pulmonary vein at ligament of Marshall tissue.

Using an 8-mm electrode (up to 70 W, 50–52°C, 60 s) or irrigated tip catheter (up to 40°C by power control) radiofrequency ablation, the lesion morphologic changes in the left atrial wall adjacent to the pulmonary vein ostium become more significant than those using 4-mm electrode ablation (up to 50 W, 52°C, 90 s) with more dramatic swelling, and possible dimpling or frank crater formation (Figures 7.21 and 7.22). Morphologic changes in the left atrial wall adjacent to the pulmonary vein ostium resulted in a "cauliflower or multi-ring" sign (Figure 7.23) or with mobile thrombus formation at the lesion (Figure 7.24) during repeated radiofrequency energy delivery have been identified, and should be avoided. ICE imaging monitoring of lesion morphologic changes marked by

the development of significantly accelerated bubble formation and transmural echodensity may reduce, or even prevent intramural superheating and sudden "popping" (Figure 7.25a–c). The popping results in crater-like lesions with a small but real risk of wall perforation at the ablated site during radiofrequency delivery.

Using ICE imaging the cross-sectional area of the pulmonary vein ostia has been observed to change with lesion applying. An increase in wall thickness and decrease in static and phasic cross-sectional area following radiofrequency ablation at the entire circumference of the left atrium bordering the veno-atrial junction is characteristic [20]. In addition to the swelling and thickened wall, shrinkage due to heat-induced contraction of support proteins [21] may also account for the cross-sectional area reduction and increased pulmonary vein ostial velocity or pressure gradient following pulmonary vein ostial ablation.

Monitoring to detect procedural complications

Potential complications during left atrial ablation procedure for atrial fibrillation include those occurring during transseptal catheterization (see Chapter 5) and left atrial mapping and ablation. Major potential complications documented by ICE imaging during left atrial ablation are left atrial thrombus formation, pulmonary vein stenosis, esophagus injury, and pericardial effusion.

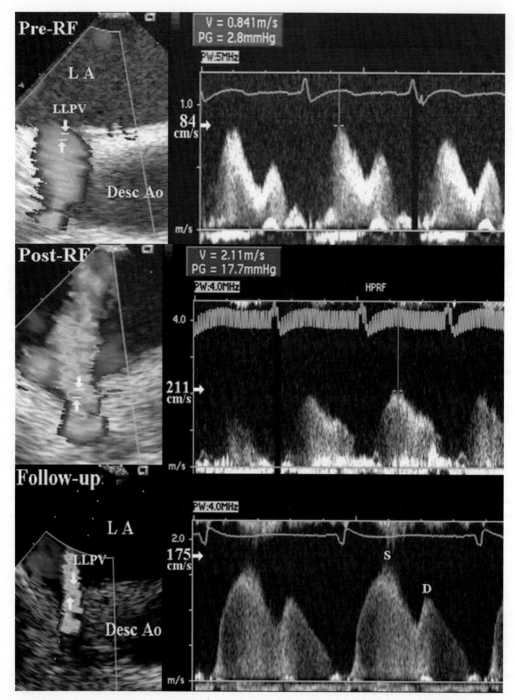

Figure 7.12 Color flow image and pulsed Doppler spectrum recorded peak flow velocities of the lower left pulmonary vein (LLPV) ostium (sampling gate, arrows) show a maximal velocity of 84 cm/s with phasic wave during systole and diastole before ablation (upper panels). After ablation, the ostial peak flow velocity increased to 211 cm/s with increased turbulent duration and little phasic variation, which is recorded with no aliasing by high pulse repetition frequency pulsed Doppler after ablation (middle panels). Ostial velocity follow-up after 1.6 months shows the maximal velocity decreased to 175 cm/s with phasic variation indicative of improved flow features (lower panels). Desc Ao: descending aorta; LA: left atrium. Reproduced by the permission [10].

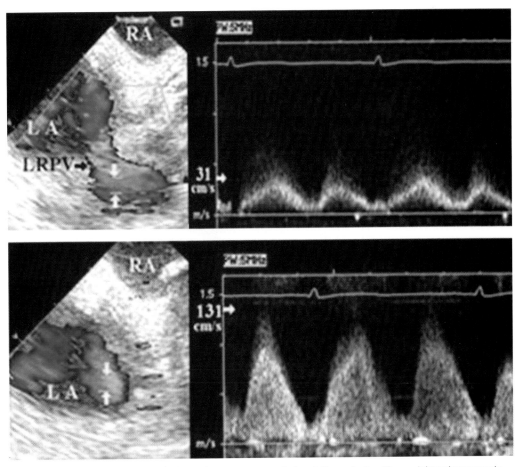

Figure 7.13 Color flow image and pulsed Doppler spectrum recorded peak flow velocity of lower right pulmonary vein (LRPV) after ablation (14 lesions) shows the maximal velocity measured 31 cm/s with sampling gate placed proximal (two white arrows) to the lesion area with narrowing color flow (black arrow) (upper panels) and 131 cm/s near the ostium in the left atrium (LA), that is, distal (two white arrows) to the lesion area (lower panels), indicative of lesion narrowing effects. RA: right atrium. Reproduced with permission [10].

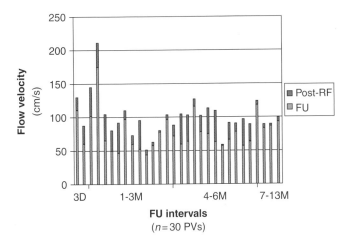

Figure 7.14 Changes in Doppler measurements of individual pulmonary vein (PV) ostial peak flow velocity after initial ablation (Post-RF) on the order of follow-up (FU) intervals. D: days; M: months. Reproduced with permission [10].

Table **7.2** Follow-up changes in pulmonary vein ostial peak flow velocity (cm/s) and estimated pressure gradient (mmHg).

Follow-up interval	Ablated PVs (n)	Previous ablation		Follow-up*
		Before	After	
3 days	2	58 ± 3(1.4 ± 0.2)	108 ± 21(4.8 ± 1.8)	86 ± 24(3.2 ± 1.6)
1–3 months	12	60 ± 14(1.5 ± 0.5)	107 ± 25(5.1 ± 2.7)	75 ± 21(2.7 ± 1.8)
4–6 months	12	53 ± 8(1.1 ± 0.3)	88 ± 16(3.2 ± 1.1)	78 ± 17(2.6 ± 1.1)
7–13 months	4	55 ± 6(1.2 ± 0.3)	109 ± 9(4.8 ± 0.8)	79 ± 18(2.7 ± 1.4)

Pressure gradient is given in parentheses. * All $p < 0.05$: versus previous after-ablation.
PV: pulmonary vein. Reproduced with permission [10].

Left atrial thrombus

The incidence of systemic thromboembolic complications associated with radiofrequency catheter ablation in the left heart unrelated to atrial fibrillation has been reported to be as high as 2% [22,23]. The risk of embolic stroke has been reported to be even high, maybe as high as 5% in targeting the triggers for atrial fibrillation with ablation [24]. Thrombus formation may be due to activation of coagulation cascade related to the placement of intravascular catheters and the duration of the ablation procedure [25]. Recently, left atrial thrombus formation has been reported with ICE imaging-documented incidence of 10.3% (24/232) in patients undergoing left atrial ablation procedure when anticoagulation is maintained with an activated clotting time >250 s after dual transseptal catheterization [26]. These left atrial thrombi tend to be single, linear, and mobile. The thrombi are typically attached firmly to the transseptal sheath (Figure 7.26) or circular mapping catheter (Figure 7.27) and not directly attached to the ablation catheter or to the pulmonary vein ostia at the site of the ablation lesions. The size of thrombi reported is 12.9 ± 11.1 mm (range 3–40 mm) in maximal length and 2.2 ± 1.3 mm (range 0.5–5.8 mm) in maximal width.

After ICE imaging recognition of left atrial thrombus the following management strategy is suggested [26]: (1) Anticoagulation status is confirmed and additional heparin is administrated as a bolus and continuous infusion of heparin is maintained to achieve an activated clotting time >350 s; (2) The sheath and catheter on which a thrombus is identified are immediately withdrawn as a single unit into the right atrium under careful ICE monitoring; (3) If successful complete withdrawal into the right atrium is noted, the catheter and/or sheath are removed from the body under careful hemodynamic and oxygen saturation monitoring; (4) The sheath and/or catheter is usually replaced and readvanced into the right atrium and catheters (without sheath support) are readvanced into the left atrium using appropriate catheter exchange and manipulation techniques and the procedure may be continued; (5) A decision to abort the ablation procedure and not recross into the left atrium is left to the electrophysiologist, but is typically based on failure to remove thrombus completely into the right atrium or recurrence of thrombus after continuing procedure. In our experience, most thrombi (27/30, 90%) are immediately eliminated by withdrawal of the sheath and catheter from the left atrium into the right atrium under ICE imaging monitoring (Figures 7.26 and 7.27). Two thrombi became wedged in the interatrial septum with a small residual end in the left atrium as a result of attempted withdrawal into the right atrium. Reassessment with ICE imaging at 24 h after maintaining activated clotting time >300 s documented resolution of wedged thrombus in one and marked reduction in size with the second (Figure 7.28) with no overt complications.

Patients with left atrial thrombus more commonly have an increased left atrial diameter (>4.5 cm), spontaneous echo contrast in the left atrium (Figure 7.29), and a history of persistent atrial fibrillation. From multivariate discriminant analysis we found that spontaneous echo contrast was the most important determinant of left atrial thrombus formation [26].

Pulmonary vein stenosis

Pulmonary vein stenosis can be accurately evaluated and monitored using ICE Doppler and color flow

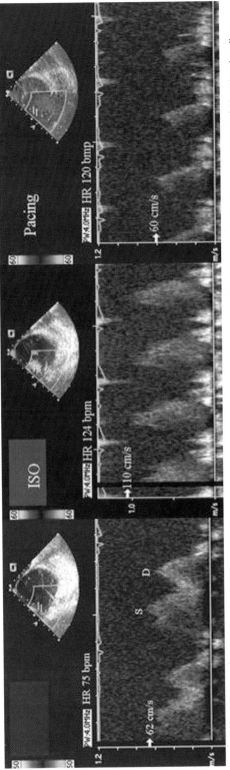

Figure 7.15 ICE Doppler spectra with sampling volume at and recorded from a non-ablated ostium of upper left pulmonary vein. Peak velocity measured 62 cm/s at baseline heart rate (HR) of 75 bpm (left panel); during isoproterenol (ISO) infusion (6 µg/min), peak velocity reached 110 cm/s at HR 124 bpm (middle panel) and during atrial pacing at HR 120 bpm matching with ISO, peak velocity measured 60 cm/s similar to the baseline level (right panel). Reproduced with permission [13].

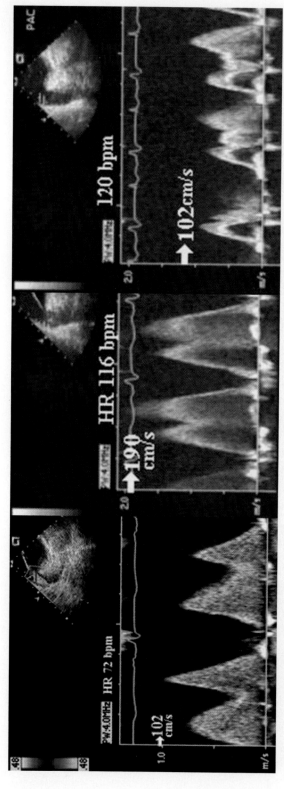

Figure 7.16 ICE Doppler spectra with sampling volume at and recorded from an ablated ostium of upper left pulmonary vein. Peak velocity measured 102 cm/s Post-RF (radiofrequency ablation) at heart rate (HR) 72 bpm (left panel); during isoproterenol (ISO) infusion (10 μg/min), peak velocity increased to 190 cm/s at HR 116 bpm (middle panel) and during atrial pacing at HR 120 bpm matching with ISO, peak velocity measured 102 cm/s similar to the post-RF level (right panel). Reproduced with permission [13].

Table 7.3 Changes in pulmonary vein (PV) ostial flow velocities pre-, post-ablation, during isoproterenol (ISO) or pacing.

	Pre-	Post-	ISO	Matched heart rate	
				Atrial pacing	ISO
Non-ablated PVs					
Heart rate (bpm)	84 ± 13	—	132 ± 26	116 ± 20	(92–150)
Velocity (cm/s)	70 ± 11	—	118 ± 35*	78 ± 26	117 ± 42**
Range (cm/s)	55–92	—	58–190	58–114	58–190
Ablated PVs					
Heart rate (bpm)	68 ± 14	76 ± 13	128 ± 6	116 ± 14	(92–130)
Velocity (cm/s)	59 ± 17	95 ± 25***	122 ± 40*	96 ± 37	118 ± 34**
Range (cm/s)	30–95	58–136	65–187	54–128	63–186

***$p < 0.001$: versus pre-ablation; *$p < 0.01$: versus pre- or post-ablation; **$p < 0.03$: versus atrial pacing, pre- or post-ablation. Reproduced with permission [13].

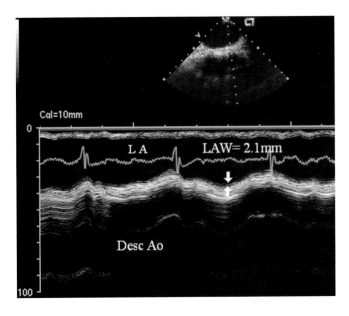

Figure 7.17 ICE M-mode image of left atrial (LA) wall (LAW) guided by two-dimensional imaging, showing atrial wall motion during cardiac cycle and the wall thickness measured 2.1 mm baseline at end-systole. Desc Ao: descending aorta.

imaging. The simplified Bernoulli equation relates fluid convective energy derived from flow velocities to a pressure gradient and is commonly used in clinical echocardiography to determine pressure differences across stenotic orifices. Its application to pulmonary vein flow has been studied with simultaneous high-fidelity pulmonary vein and left atrial pressure measurements and pulmonary vein pulsed Doppler echocardiography performed in humans during cardiac surgery [27]. These results showed that the pressure gradients for the systolic and diastolic phases of pulmonary vein flow determined using the simplified Bernoulli equation correlated ($r = 0.82$ and 0.81)

with measured actual pressure differences. *In vitro* experiments also have shown that the relation between pressure gradient and velocity is valid for orifices having a diameter ≥ 8 mm (area ≥ 0.5 m^2) [28]. With very smaller orifices (diameters of 1.5 and 3.5 mm; area ≤ 0.1 cm^2), velocity measurements significantly underestimate the pressure gradients because inertial and viscous losses become more important [27–29]. Hence, the importance of continuous monitoring is to avoid missing progression of stenosis to a severe state.

Recently, using ICE Doppler and color flow imaging our clinical observation suggests that pulmonary vein

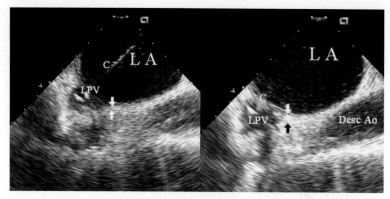

Figure 7.18 ICE images of left atrium (LA) with the transducer placed in the right atrium, showing the atrial wall thickness adjacent to the left pulmonary vein (LPV) ostium measured 3 mm pre-ablation (between arrows, left panel) and 5.5 mm with increased echodensity post-ablation (between arrows, right panel). C: catheter; Desc Ao: descending aorta.

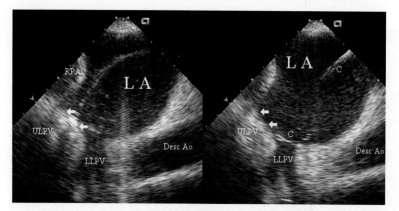

Figure 7.19 ICE images of left atrium (LA) with the transducer placed in the right atrium, showing increased echodensity and small bubbles around the lesion during radiofrequency ablation at the ligament of Marshall tissue area (arrows, left panel) and increased thickness post-radiofrequency lesion (arrows, right panel). C: catheter; Desc Ao: descending aorta; LLPV and ULPV: lower and upper left pulmonary vein; RPA: right pulmonary artery.

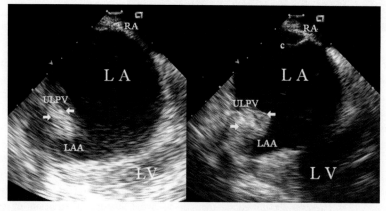

Figure 7.20 ICE images of left atrium (LA) with the transducer placed in the right atrium (RA), showing the thickness of the ligament of Marshall tissue area measured 7 mm pre-radiofrequency (RF) ablation (arrows, left panel) and increased to 16 mm with echodensity post-RF (arrows, right panel). C: catheter; LAA: LA appendage; LV: left ventricle; ULPV: upper left pulmonary vein.

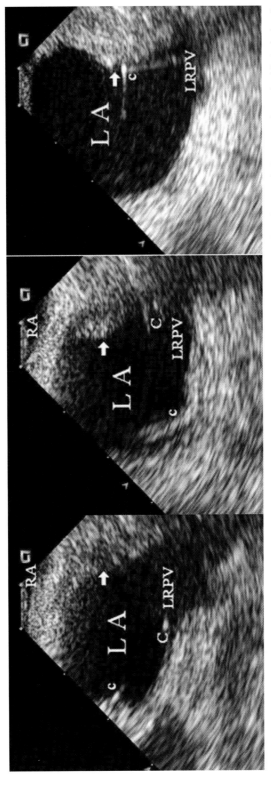

Figure 7.21 ICE images of lesion morphologic changes in the left atrial (LA) wall adjacent to the lower right pulmonary vein (LRPV) ostium (using 8 mm electrode ablation), showing LA wall thickness (3 mm, arrow) before ablation (left panel), swelling and increased wall thickness (6.8 mm) and echogenecity (arrow) after a lesion delivered (middle panel) and further wall thickening (12 mm) and crater formation (arrow) with repeat radiofrequency energy delivered (right panel). C: catheter; RA: right atrium.

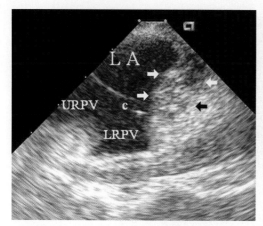

Figure 7.22 ICE image of lesion morphology in the left atrial (LA) wall adjacent to the lower right pulmonary vein (LRPV) ostium (using cooling tip catheter ablation), showing LA wall with severe swelling (13.5 mm), hetero-echogenecity and transmural lesions (arrows) following repeat radiofrequency energy delivery. C: catheter; URPV: upper right pulmonary vein.

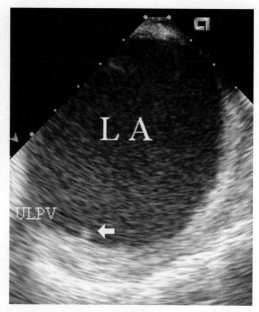

Figure 7.24 ICE image of lesion morphology in the left atrial (LA) wall adjacent to the left pulmonary vein (LPV) ostium (using cooling tip catheter ablation), showing LA wall with severe swelling (12 mm), hetero-echogenecity and small mobile thrombus (arrow) at the lesions. ULPV: upper LPV.

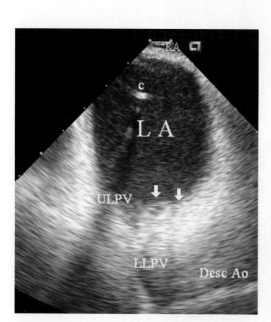

Figure 7.23 ICE image of lesion morphology in the left atrial (LA) wall adjacent to the lower left pulmonary vein (LLPV) ostium (using 8 mm electrode ablation), showing LA wall with severe swelling (15 mm), hetero-echogenecity and "cauliflower or multi-ring" sign (arrows). C: catheter; Desc Ao: descending aorta; RA: right atrium; ULPV: upper left pulmonary vein.

ostial peak flow velocity increasing to >158 cm/s (pressure gradient >10 mmHg) with Doppler spectral patterns of turbulent, more continuous and showing little phasic variation (Figure 7.12) indicate a moderate narrowing effect. Clinical symptoms/signs of stenosis may be present in patients with multiple pulmonary veins demonstrating flow increases and abnormal patterns of ostial flow velocities [10]. A clinical study evaluating obstruction to pulmonary venous blood flow return based on catheterization and transthoracic Doppler echocardiographic data demonstrated that patients without significant obstruction had a lower Doppler velocity, and none had a maximal Doppler velocity ≥200 cm/s (estimated pressure gradient 16 mmHg) [30]. The complication of pulmonary vein stenosis with resultant severe pulmonary hypertension was reported after extensive linear catheter ablation of chronic atrial fibrillation [31]. One patient in that previous report demonstrated a peak flow velocity of 250 cm/s detected near the ostia of both upper pulmonary veins and an estimated pulmonary arterial systolic pressure of 88 mmHg by transesophageal echocardiography at

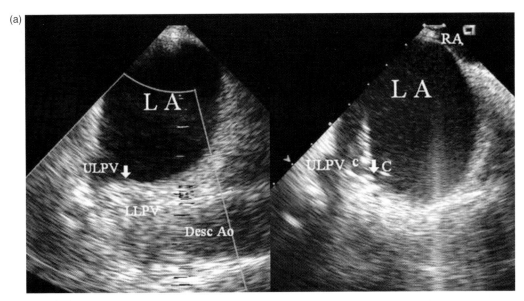

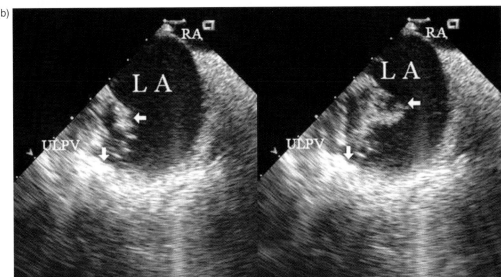

Figure 7.25 ICE serial images with the transducer placed in the high interatrial septum of right atrium (RA), showing: (a) the carina (arrow) between the upper (ULPV) and lower left pulmonary vein (LLPV) ostia in the left atrium (LA) pre-radiofrequency ablation (RF) using 8 mm electrode (70 W, up to 50°C, 60 s) (left panel) and increased echodensity at the ablated site (arrow) during initial RF (right panel); (b) initially accelerated bubbles (horizontal arrow) ejected from the ablated site (vertical arrow) during continuous RF (left panel) and becoming more significantly accelerated bubbles (right panel).

8 month follow-up. Using transesophageal echocardiography, another study reported a significant increase in pulmonary vein peak flow velocity in 59 ablated pulmonary veins measured within 3 days after pulmonary vein ablation procedure (125 ± 10 cm/s versus 65 ± 7 cm/s baseline) [32]. In these patients, two had pulmonary vein stenosis with mild exertional dyspnea. Pressure gradients within both upper pulmonary veins of 12 and 18 mmHg, respectively, were noted in one of the patients. Although pulmonary vein stenosis when presented can be treated with percutaneous pulmonary vein angioplasty and stent implantation, it is one of

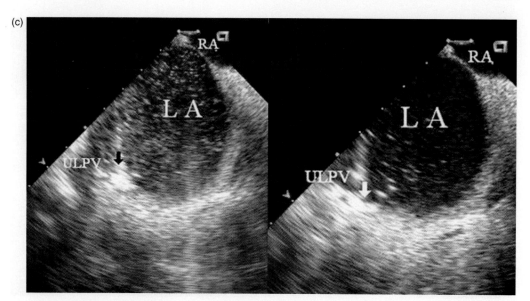

Figure 7.25 *Continued.* (c) subsequently sudden burst into "popping" with echogenic response at the lesion site (arrow) (left panel) and a transmural lesion developed with a crate-like morphology (right panel). c and C: ablation and multipolar mapping catheters; Desc Ao: descending aorta.

the serious complications associated with pulmonary vein ablation and pulmonary vein isolation for atrial fibrillation. Using advanced mapping and ablation techniques under ICE with Doppler and color flow imaging monitoring, pulmonary vein stenosis can be prevented by an experienced operator by avoiding any lesion deployed inside the pulmonary vein ostium and insuring proximal lesion placement at the antrum of the pulmonary vein. Also, monitoring for changes in flow velocity becomes critical when targeting the left pulmonary veins. This is because the anterior margin of these pulmonary veins is marked by the opening of the left atrial appendage. This forces lesion deployment of the true ostium of the pulmonary vein anteriorly.

Esophageal injury

With increased use of novel catheter designs and new energy sources, the depth and volume of left atrial wall injury may increase with catheter ablation for atrial fibrillation. The esophagus is immediately contiguous to the left atrial posterior wall. Esophageal injury with left atrio-esophageal fistula associated with a high mortality has been reported following left atrial intraoperative and percutaneous transcatheter ablation procedures for atrial fibrillation [33–35]. ICE

real-time imaging monitoring of this anatomic region and lesion development during radiofrequency energy application may reduce the risk of and avoid significant injury of the esophagus (see Chapter 11). With AcuNav ICE transducer placed in the right atrium close to the interatrial septum and scanning between the lower right and left pulmonary vein ostia, the maximal longitudinal bordering region of left atrial posterior wall contiguous to the esophagus can be imaged (Figure 7.30). The esophagus can be visualized to the right and anterior to the descending aorta (Figure 7.31). The maximal longitudinal length of left atrio-esophageal contiguous region (26.5 ± 6.5 mm) and the atrial (2.7 ± 0.5 mm) and esophageal wall thickness (3.4 ± 0.5 mm) were measured in patients ($n = 42$, 33 men) undergoing radiofrequency left atrial pulmonary vein electric isolation and ablation [36]. The radiofrequency lesions delivered at this region ($n = 44$) close to the lower right or left pulmonary vein ostium demonstrated an echogenic depth of 10.8 ± 2.2 mm (7.0–15.0) when using an 8-mm electrode (70 W, up to 50–52°C, 60 s) or cooled tip (up to 40°C, 60 s) ablation [37]. Echogenic lesion formation at the left atrial posterior wall extending to the esophageal anterior wall may be observed following repeat radiofrequency lesions (Figure 7.32a–c). An incomplete echo-free

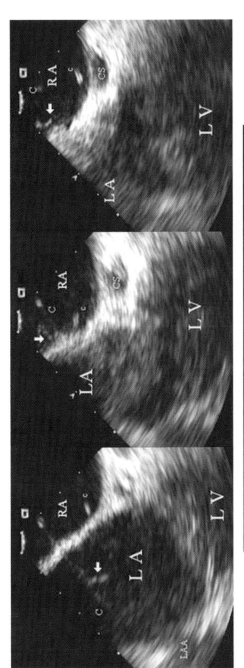

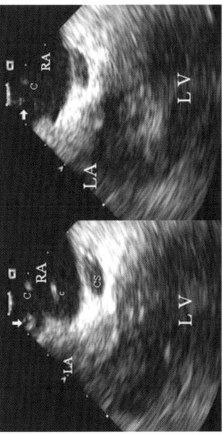

Figure 7.26 ICE serial images with the transducer placed in the right atrium (RA), showing a single, linear and mobile thrombus (arrow, size 9.8 × 2.1 mm²) attached at the sheath of Lasso (left upper panel), pulling of the sheath/Lasso with thrombus from the left atrium (LA) through the interatrial septum (middle upper panel) into the RA (right upper and two lower panels). C: catheter/sheath; CS: coronary sinus; LAA: LA appendage; LV: left ventricle.

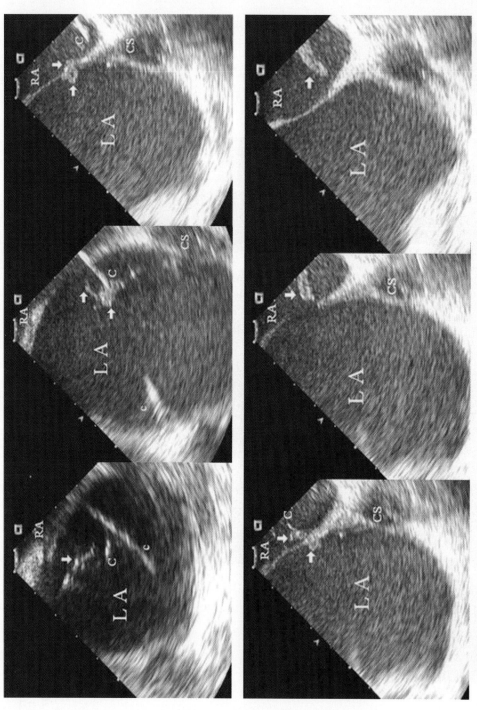

Figure 7.27 ICE serial images with the transducer placed in the right atrium (RA), showing a single, linear, and mobile thrombus (arrow, size 18 × 1.8 mm²) attached at distal shaft of Lasso (left upper panel), pulling of the sheath/Lasso with thrombus (middle upper panel) from the left atrium (LA) through the interatrial septum (right upper and left lower panel) into the RA (middle and left lower panel). C: catheter/sheath; CS: coronary sinus.

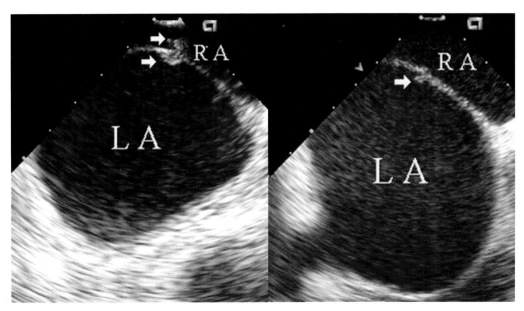

Figure 7.28 ICE images with the transducer placed in the right atrium (RA), showing left atrial (LA) thrombus (size 4.0×3.9 mm^2) wedged in the interatrial septum (left panel) and reduced in size (2.8×2.0 mm^2) with aggressive anticoagulation during follow-up images after 24 h (right panel). Reproduced with permission [26].

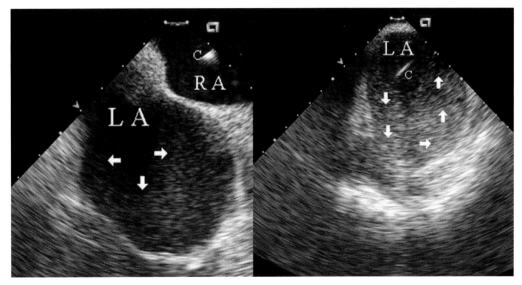

Figure 7.29 ICE image with the transducer (7.5 MHz) placed in the right atrium (RA), showing spontaneous echo contrast, as slowly swirling amorphous echoes in a dilated (diameter = 5.2 cm) left atrium (LA) (left panel) and slowly swirling echoes more prominent during sheath flushing with heparinized solution (right panel). Reproduced with permission [26].

space may occasionally develop between left atrial posterior wall and esophagus (as an interstitial exudate form in the oblique sinus) (Figure 7.33a–c) following numerous lesions at left atrial posterior wall in proximity to the middle/lower right pulmonary vein

ostia. Radiofrequency lesions in the posterior/lateral aspect of the middle/lower right, or posterior/medial aspect of the left pulmonary vein ostium are within proximity to the esophagus. ICE can provide imaging capability to identify the region of left atrial

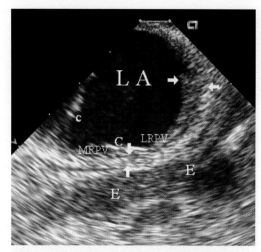

Figure 7.30 ICE image with the transducer placed in the right atrium, showing left atrial (LA) posterior wall contiguous to the esophagus (E). The thickness of both contiguous wall is 4.2 mm (vertical arrows). Swelling of the septal aspect (horizontal arrows) near the lower right pulmonary vein (LRPV) ostium occurred following multiple radiofrequency lesions with an 8 mm electrode ablation. C: catheter; MRPV: projected location of the middle right pulmonary vein ostium.

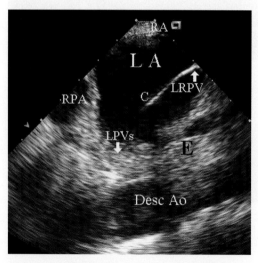

Figure 7.31 ICE image with the transducer placed in the higher right atrium (RA), showing left atrial (LA) posterior wall close to the left pulmonary vein ostia (LPVs), contiguous to the esophagus (E) and right/anterior to the descending aorta (Desc Ao). C: catheter; LRPV: lower right pulmonary vein ostium; RPA: right pulmonary artery.

(a)
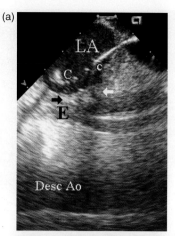

(b)
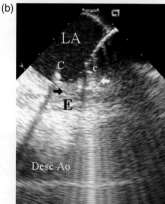

(c)
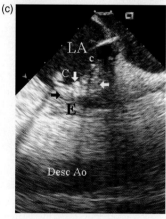

Figure 7.32 ICE images with the transducer placed in the right atrium, showing: (a) left atrial (LA) posterior wall contiguous to the esophageal anterior wall (E) (between arrows) pre-radiofrequency lesion; (b) during lesion delivery; (c) post-repeat lesions at this LA posterior wall region (between horizontal arrows), the echogenic inhomogeneous lesions extended from LA wall to the anterior E wall (vertical arrow). C: multipolar mapping catheter; c: ablation catheter; Desc Ao: descending aorta.

(a)
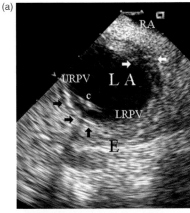

(b)
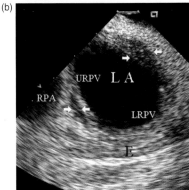

(c)
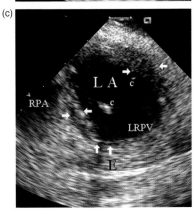

(a)
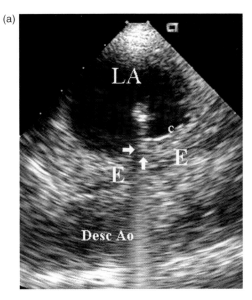

(b)
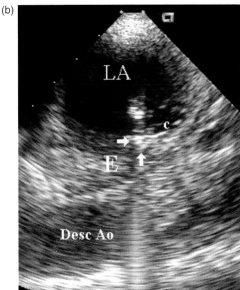

Figure 7.34 ICE images with the transducer placed in the right atrium, showing: (a) an ablation catheter positioned at the left atrial (LA) posterior wall (arrows) in the posterior/lateral aspect of the lower right pulmonary vein ostium, contiguous to the esophagus (E), a multipolar mapping catheter (c) positioned near the ostium and a strong sector artifact observed during initial delivery of the radiofrequency energy; (b) ICE imaging monitoring of the echogenic lesion (arrows) with development of slightly accelerated bubbles and power titrating for echogenic lesion depth limited to the LA wall to avoid E injury during continuous energy delivery. Desc Ao: descending aorta.

Figure 7.33 ICE images of the left atrium (LA) wall contiguous to the esophagus (E) with the transducer placed in the high right atrium (RA), showing: (a) swelling of the LA septal (between horizontal arrows) and posterior wall around the lower (LRPV) and middle right pulmonary vein ostia. A trivial echo-free space (serial black arrows) was observed posteriorly; (b) with time this space increased (between the lower horizontal arrows); and (c) expanded to the oblique sinus (vertical arrows) adjacent to the anterior E wall following numerous radiofrequency lesions delivered around the upper (URPV), middle and LRPV ostia. c: multipolar mapping or ablation catheter.

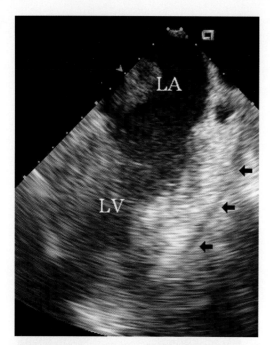

Figure 7.35 ICE image with the transducer placed in the high right atrium, showing an early detected small (echo-free space 3 mm) pericardial effusion (arrows) only along left ventricular (LV) posterior wall. LA: left atrium.

(a)
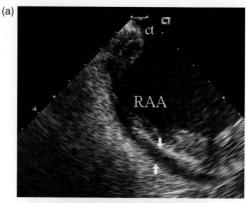

(b)
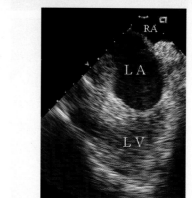

Figure 7.36 ICE images of right atrial appendage (RAA) and left atrium (LA) and ventricle (LV) with the transducer placed in the junction of RA-superior vena cava and high RA, respectively, showing: (a) small echo-free space (6 mm, arrows) around the RAA (A); (b) before any significant pericardial effusion seen around the LV posterior wall (B).

posterior wall contiguous to the esophagus and guide/monitor radiofrequency lesions in this region. Careful ICE imaging monitoring and power titration should permit the middle/lower right or left pulmonary vein ostial isolation while avoiding esophageal injury (Figure 7.34a,b) [37].

Pericardial effusion

Pericardial effusion is one of serious complications associated with catheter ablation procedure for atrial fibrillation. It may occur immediately following inadvertent catheter perforation of cardiac structure during transseptal puncture (see Chapter 5) or catheter manipulation for mapping and ablation. ICE imaging during the catheter ablation procedure may provide early and immediate diagnosis of pericardial effusion prior to significant changes in arterial blood pressure and other hemodynamic parameters. ICE diagnosis of pericardial effusion (see Chapter 11) has focuses on the detection of pericardial fluid posterior to the left ventricle (Figure 7.35), since relatively echo-free spaces anteriorly may represent epicardial fat, which can be mistaken for pericardial effusion.

Based on patient's supine position, small amount of pericardial effusion may be detected easily with ICE imaging in the posteriorly cardiac base surrounding the right atrial appendage (Figure 7.36a,b). ICE early detection of a small pericardial effusion should trigger stopping and possibly reversing of anticoagulation and may prevent further deterioration and the serious consequence of tamponade requiring urgent pericardiocentesis. ICE imaging may be helpful to guide transthoracic subxyphoid needle placement in selected patients with cardiac compression syndrome.

References

1 Fuster V, Ryden LE, Asinger RW, *et al.* ACC/AHA/ESC guidelines for the management of patients with atrial fibrillation. *J Am Coll Cardiol* 2001; **38**: 1231–1266.

2 Prystowsky EN, Katz A. Atrial fibrillation. In: Topol EJ, ed. *Textbook of Cardiovascular Medicine*, 2nd edn. Lippincott Williams & Wilkins, Philadelphia, 2002: 1403.

3 Jais P, Haissaguerre M, Shah DC. A focal source of atrial fibrillation treated by discrete radiofrequency ablation. *Circulation* 1997; **95**: 572–576.

4 Haissaguerre M, Jais P, Shah DC, *et al.* Spontaneous initiation of atrial fibrillation by ectopic beats originating in the pulmonary veins. *N Engl J Med* 1998; **339**: 659–666.

5 Chen SA, Hsieh MH, Tai CT, *et al.* Initiation of atrial fibrillation by ectopic beats originating from the pulmonary veins: electrophysiological characteristics, pharmacological responses, and effects of radiofrequency ablation. *Circulation* 1999; **100**: 1879–1886.

6 Nathan H, Eliakim M. The junction between the left atrium and the pulmonary veins: an anatomic study of human hearts. *Circulation* 1966; **34**: 412–422.

7 Cheung DW. Pulmonary vein as an ectopic focus in digitalis-induced arrhythmia. *Nature* 1981; **294**: 582–584.

8 Marchlinski FE, Callans D, Dixit S, *et al.* Efficacy and safety of targeted focal ablation versus PV isolation assisted by magnetic electroanatomic mapping. *J Cardiovasc Electrophysiol* 2003; **14**: 358–365.

9 Ren JF, Marchlinski FE, Callans DJ, Herrmann HC. Clinical use of AcuNav diagnostic ultrasound catheter imaging during left heart radiofrequency ablation and transcatheter closure procedures. *J Am Soc Echocardiogr* 2002; **15**: 1301–1308.

10 Ren JF, Marchlinski FE, Callans DJ, Zado ES. Intracardiac Doppler echocardiographic quantification of pulmonary vein flow velocity: an effective technique for monitoring pulmonary vein ostia narrowing during focal atrial fibrillation ablation. *J Cardiovasc Electrophysiol* 2002; **13**: 1076–1081.

11 Ren JF, Callans DJ, Marchlinski FE. Decreased ostial narrowing effect following pulmonary vein ostial ablation for atrial fibrillation: combined versus individual ostia (abstr). *PACE* 2003; **26**: 1074.

12 Feigenbaum H. *Echocardiography*. Lea & Febiger, Philadelphia, 1994: 195–196, 357–359, 556–557.

13 Ren JF, Marchlinski FE, Callans DJ. Effect of heart rate and isoproterenol on pulmonary vein flow velocity following radiofrequency ablation: a Doppler color flow imaging study. *J Interventional Cardiac Electrophysiol* 2004; **10**: 265–269.

14 Samdarshi TE, Morrow R, Helmcke FR, Nanda NC, Bargeron LM, Pacifico AD. Assessment of pulmonary vein stenosis by transesophageal echocardiography. *Am Heart J* 1991; **122**: 1495–1498.

15 Seshadri N, Novaro GM, Prieto L, *et al.* Pulmonary vein stenosis after catheter ablation of atrial arrhythmia. *Circulation* 2002; **105**: 2571–2572.

16 Smith TW, Braunwald E, Kelly RA. The management of heart failure. In: Braunwald E, ed. *Heart Disease*, 3rd edn. WB Saunders, Philadelphia, 1988: 524.

17 Nishimura RA, Abel MD, Hatle LK, Tajik AJ. Relation of pulmonary vein to mitral flow velocities by transesophageal Doppler echocardiography: effect of different loading conditions. *Circulation* 1990; **81**: 1488–1497.

18 Castello R, Vaughn M, Dressler FA, *et al.* Relation between pulmonary venous flow and pulmonary wedge pressure: influence of cardiac output. *Am Heart J* 1995; **130**: 127–134.

19 Ren JF, Lin D, Gerstenfeld EP, Lewkowiez L, Callans DJ. Ligament of Marshall tissue related to pulmonary vein ostial ablation: an intracardiac echocardiographic imaging study (abstr). *Circulation* 2003; **108**: IV-646.

20 Schwartzman D, Kanzaki H, Bazaz R, Gorcsan J 3rd. Impact of catheter ablation on pulmonary vein morphology and mechanical function. *J Cardiovasc Electrophysiol* 2004; **15**: 161–167.

21 Chen SS, Wright NT, Humphrey JD. Heat-induced changes in the mechanics of collagenous tissue: isothermal free shrinkage. *J Biomech Eng* 1997; **119**: 372–378.

22 Thakur RK, Klein GJ, Yee R, Zardini M. Embolic complications after radiofrequency catheter ablation. *Am J Cardiol* 1994; **74**: 278–279.

23 Zhou L, Keane D, Reed G, Ruskin J. Thromboembolic complications of cardiac radiofrequency catheter ablation: a review of the reported incidence, pathogenesis and current research directions. *J Cardiovasc Electrophysiol* 1999; **10**: 611–620.

24 Kok LC, Mangrum JM, Haines DE, Mounsey JP. Cerebrovascular complication associated with pulmonary vein ablation. *J Cardiovasc Electrophysiol* 2002; **13**: 764–767.

25 Dorbala S, Cohen AJ, Hutchison LA, Menchavez-Tan E, Steinberg JS. Does radiofrequency ablation induce a prethrombotic state? Analysis of coagulation system activation and comparison to electrophysiologic study. *J Cardiovasc Electrophysiol* 1998; **9**: 1152–1160.

26 Ren JF, Marchlinski FE, Callans DC. Left atrial thrombus associated with ablation for atrial fibrillation: identification with intracardiac echocardiography. *J Am Coll Cardiol* 2004; **43**: 1861–1867.

27 Firstenberg MS, Greenberg NL, Smedira NG, *et al.* Doppler echo evaluation of pulmonary venous-left atrial pressure gradients: human and numerical model studies. *Am J Physiol* 2000; **279**: H594–H600.

28 Holen J, Aaslid R, Landmark K, Simonson S, Ostrem T. Determination of effective orifice area in mitral stenosis from noninvasive ultrasound Doppler data and mitral flow rate. *Acta Med Scand* 1977; **201**: 83–88.

29 Hatle L, Angelsen B. *Doppler Ultrasound in Cardiology*. Lea & Febiger, Philadelphia, 1985: 104–108.

30 Vick GW 3rd, Murphy DJ Jr, Ludomirsky A, *et al.* Pulmonary venous and systemic ventricular inflow obstruction in patients with congenital heart disease: detection by combined two-dimensional and Doppler echocardiography. *J Am Coll Cardiol* 1987; **9**: 580–587.

31 Robbins IM, Colvin EV, Doyle TP, *et al.* Pulmonary vein stenosis after catheter ablation of atrial fibrillation. *Circulation* 1998; **98**: 1769–1775.

32 Chen S-A, Hsieh M-H, Tai C-T, *et al.* Initiation of atrial fibrillation by ectopic beats originating from the pulmonary veins: electrophysiological characteristics, pharmacological responses, and effects of radiofrequency ablation. *Circulation* 1999; **100**: 1879–1886.

33 Gillinov AM, Pettersson G, Rice TW. Esophageal injury during radiofrequency ablation for atrial fibrillation. *J Thorac Cardiovasc Surg* 2001; **122**: 1239–1240.

34 Mohr FW, Fabicius AM, Falk V, *et al.* Curative treatment of atrial fibrillation with intraoperative radiofrequency ablation: short-term and midterm results. *J Thorac Cardiovasc Surg* 2002; **123**: 919–927.

35 Pappone C, Oral H, Santinelli V, *et al.* Atrio-esophageal fistula as a complication of percutaneous transcatheter ablation of atrial fibrillation. *Circulation* 2004; **109**: 2724–2726.

36 Ren JF, Marchlinski FE, Callans DJ. Esophageal imaging characteristics and structural measurement during left atrial ablation for atrial fibrillation: an intracardiac echocardiographic study (abstr). *J Am Coll Cardiol* 2005; **45**: 114A.

37 Ren JF, Callans DJ, Marchlinski FE, Nayak H, Lin D, Gerstenfeld EP. Avoiding esophageal injury with power titrating during left atrial ablation for atrial fibrillation: an intracardiac echocardiographic imaging study (abstr). *J Am Coll Cardiol* 2005; **45**: 114A.

CHAPTER 8

Left Heart Transducer Position

David Schwartzman, MD

Introduction

Recent years have witnessed an expanding volume of endocardium-based interventions targeting the left heart. As is demonstrated in the preceding chapters, intracardiac echocardiography (ICE) using a right heart transducer position has become an important adjunct for these interventions [1]. However, there may be significant limitations to the right heart transducer position, including diminished image quality and restricted windows. In this chapter, we describe our experience with the left heart transducer position. The chapter begins with a review of anatomic windows, emphasizing those which are unique to left heart transducer position and concludes with a discussion of the role that left heart ICE has played as an adjunct to ablation in the posterior left atrium, which will serve to illustrate its utility. To promote comprehension the ICE images are supplemented with computed tomographic-based images (figures that present both ICE and computed tomographic images were each generated from the same patient), as well as with schematic illustrations.

Imaging technique and anatomic views

Access and sheath support for transducer positioning

Access to the left heart is gained via atrial transseptal puncture (see Chapter 5). The initial puncture is performed using a standard 8 Fr Mullins sheath and Brockenbrough needle. The specific puncture site is selected using mechanical radial ICE, depending on the primary imaging target. For ablation in the posterior left atrium, we puncture the fossa ovalis as close to Waterston's groove as possible, just beneath the apical region of the limbus [2]. Subsequently, the

8 Fr sheath is removed over a standard 0.035 inch exchange-length wire, and is replaced by an 11 Fr Mullins sheath (Cook, Bloomington, IN, USA). The AcuNav transducer is advanced into the left atrium through the 11 Fr sheath, which is then withdrawn into the right atrium. Imaging is performed by rotating and/or deflecting the catheter. Herein we provide no manual of catheter deflection or transducer rotation angles as a map for locating various cardiac structures because we have found this not to be possible, likely due in part to variation in heart position and catheter entry orientation into the left atrium. For the mechanical radial ICE transducer (UltraICE, 9 Fr), a 10 Fr sheath (Boston Scientific) is advanced through the 11 Fr sheath, which is then withdrawn into the inferior caval vein. This sheath is used in either its unmodified form (90° angle) or after modification to provide greater angulation by immersion in boiling water and traction (Figure 8.1). The stiffness of the imaging catheter demanded marked overangulation of the sheath relative to that of the desired imaging target. The unmodified sheath is used to image central and lateral aspects of the left atrium including left pulmonary veins, isthmus, and appendage, whereas the modified sheath is used to image left atrial paraseptal structures including right pulmonary vein complex, mitral–aortic continuity, and proximal coronary sinus. The distance between the distal end of the sheath and ICE catheter is varied as needed, as is torque placed on the sheath. It is important that the transducer be unsheathed to avoid image degradation (see Chapter 2).

Posterior left atrium
Left pulmonary vein complex
Vestibule

The left pulmonary venous vestibule can be defined proximally (e.g., toward the center of the left atrial

117

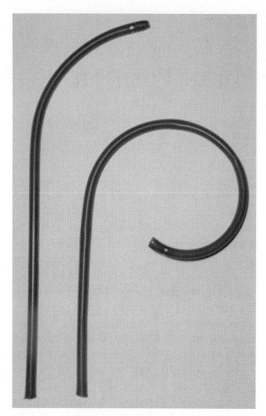

Figure 8.1 Modified (right) and unmodified (90°) Boston Scientific sheaths for left atrial ICE imaging. Note that the modified sheath has severe in-plane, as well as lesser out-of-plane (toward the reader) angulation.

an ovoid shape. Maximal dimensions of the roof–floor distance measured 2.9–5.1 cm and the ridge–posterior wall distance 1.5–3.9 cm. The cross-sectional area measured 4.1–6.2 cm^2. It was highly motile, with a maximum change in cross-sectional area of 20–40% during the cardiac mechanical cycle [3]. There was significant regional heterogeneity as to the magnitude and type of motion. For example, the ridge, roof, and floor walls moved to a significantly greater degree than the posterior wall, which appeared to be relatively tethered. In addition, unlike the other walls the ridge wall often had a distinct "shudder" or vibration which corresponded to peak transpulmonary venous flow velocity. Wall thickness also varied by region: posterior wall 1–3 mm, roof wall 5–12 mm, ridge wall 4–10 mm, and floor wall 2–5 mm. However, it is important not to necessarily equate echocardiographic wall thickness with that of myocardial investiture. For example, the ridge wall is comprised of venous and appendage vestibule walls in contiguity, but their investitures are anatomically separate. The venous vestibule myocardial thickness in this area was 2–3 mm. It is also worth noting that, in most patients, the left atrium has a subendocardial layer of fibrous tissue 1–2 mm thick. Peak blood flow velocity in the vestibule was 30–60 cm/s; flow was somewhat turbulent in the region of the intervenous saddle. Peak velocity fell rapidly once in the body of the left atrium. An important element of left vestibule anatomy is the close proximity of nonatrial structures, including esophagus (Figure 8.6), descending aorta (Figure 8.7), and pulmonary artery (Figure 8.8). The location, proximity, and extent of these relationships are variable between patients. By not more than 5 mm distal to the apex of the Marshall ridge, the wall common to venous and appendage vestibules separates (Figures 8.9 and 8.10). By not more than 10 mm distal to the Marshall ridge, the roof wall of the vestibule is echocardiographically distinct from Bachmann's bundle; a tissue "bridge" usually connects the two structures. This is a region of importance during catheter ablation (see below).

cavity) by the "Marshall Ridge" (the endocardial corroborate of the Marshall ligament) and distally by the intervenous "saddle" (Figure 8.2). We define the vestibule as having four walls: ridge, posterior, roof, and floor. Using mechanical radial ICE, the apex of the ridge wall is defined by loss of continuity during catheter pullback from within the left veins, whereas using AcuNav, it is viewed on edge (Figure 8.3). The ridge wall is shared by both left venous and atrial appendage vestibules (Figures 8.4 and 8.5). The roof wall abuts Bachmann's bundle, an epicardial structure (see below). There are no distinct anatomical features of the other walls: interpatient differences in transducer angulation may likely produce variation as to their precise anatomic locations. Note that angulation often prevents capture of the entire vestibule in a single image plane; the catheter is thus angulated and/or rotated as necessary. The vestibule has

Common vein

In a significant minority of patients, the left pulmonary vein is common, defined as a merger of the superior and inferior veins distal to the pericardial reflection (Figures 8.11 and 8.12) [4]. As noted above, the surface area of the left vestibule is

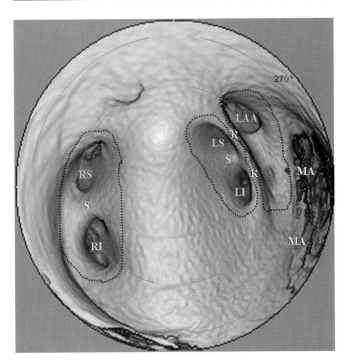

Figure 8.2 Computed tomography-derived endocardial view of the posterior left atrium. The right superior (RS) and inferior (RI) and left superior (LS) and inferior (LI) pulmonary venoatrial junctions, and left atrial appendage ostium (LAA) are demarcated by red. Lines demarcate approximate borders of the respective vestibules. The atrial wall between the pulmonary venous vestibules protrudes into the cavity due to compression by the descending aorta. MA: mitral annulus; R: ridge; S: saddle.

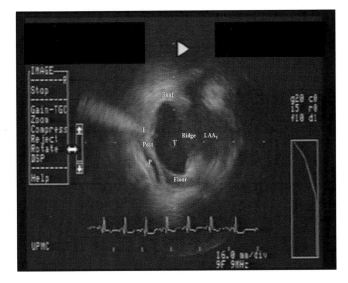

Figure 8.3 Mechanical radial ICE image of typical left pulmonary venous vestibule, demonstrating four "walls" (Roof, posterior [Post], Ridge, and Floor). The ultrasound transducer is seen as an artifact in the center of the figure. The mitral annulus is to the right of the left atrial appendage vestibule (LAAv) (not seen). Each scale = 16 mm. E: acoustic shadow cast be catheter electrode, shown abutting the contiguous endocardial surface; P: pericardial sinus with physiological fluid.

larger than when there is no common vein segment. Dimensions of the common vein are generally larger than either the superior or inferior vein [5]. It also demonstrates a high degree of motility during the cardiac mechanical cycle, with a maximum change in cross-sectional area of 15–35%. Wall thickness varies markedly depending on specific circumferential site and distance from the ridge, but always measured <5 mm. It is invested confluently with myocardium. Apart from the superior/inferior vein bifurcation, we have not observed branching of this vessel. The common left pulmonary vein may be in intimate proximity with extracardiac structures including descending aorta and esophagus.

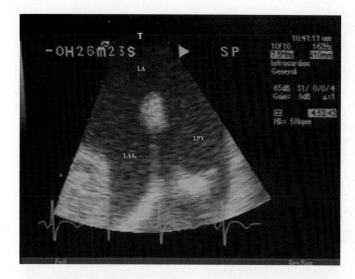

Figure 8.4 AcuNav ICE image with the transducer placed in the left atrium (LA) through a transseptal sheath, showing Marshall ridge (MR). Each scale = 1 cm. LPV: left pulmonary venous vestibule. LAA_V: appendage vestibule.

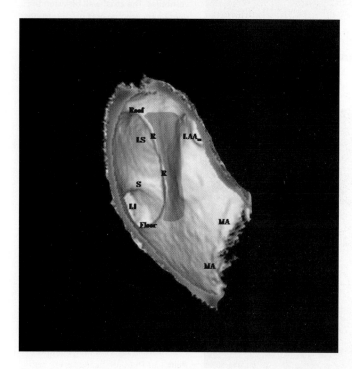

Figure 8.5 Computed tomography-derived cutaway endocardial view of lateral region of the left atrium (LA), demonstrating vein and appendage vestibules. The vestibules share a common "ridge" (R) wall (shaded) LAA_{os}: appendage orifice; LI and LS: left inferior and superior pulmonary vein; MA: mitral annulus; S: intervenous saddle.

Superior vein

When not emanating from a common left vein trunk, the orifice of the superior vein is apparent in approximately same imaging plane as the apex of the ridge and the intervenous saddle (Figures 8.11 and 8.12). In the setting of a common left vein, it can be defined by the plane of the saddle alone (Figure 8.13). Wall thickness is variable but always measured <3 mm. It is motile [3]. Branches may be seen proximally, but are generally not apparent until >5 mm distal to the orifice. It is asymmetrically invested with myocardium for a variable distance.

Approximately 1 cm distal to the orifice, the lateral wall of this vessel comes into proximity with the distal aspect of the left atrial appendage vestibule and the base of the left atrial appendage. This proximity

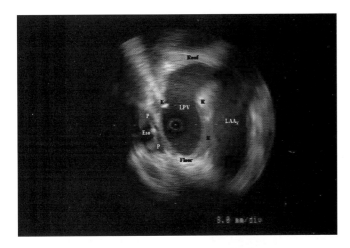

Figure 8.6 Mechanical radial ICE image of left pulmonary venous (LPV) vestibule demonstrating contiguity of esophagus (Eso). Each scale = 8 mm. E: electrode; LAA$_V$: left atrial appendage vestibule; P: pericardial oblique sinus; R: ridge.

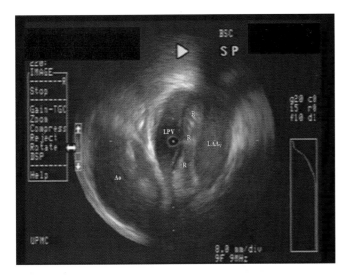

Figure 8.7 Mechanical radial ICE image of left pulmonary venous vestibule (LPV) demonstrating contiguity of descending aorta (Ao). Each scale = 8 mm. LAA$_V$: left atrial appendage vestibule; R: ridge.

is important because large "not-so-far-field" electrical potentials generated by the appendage are routinely recorded from this zone, which can create confusion during an ablation procedure (see below). The left superior vein is also in intimate proximity with extra-cardiac structures including left pulmonary artery and aorta.

Inferior vein

When not emanating from a common left vein trunk, the orifice of the inferior vein is apparent in approximately same imaging plane as the apex of the ridge and the intervenous saddle (Figure 8.14). In the setting of a common left vein, it can be defined by the plane of

the saddle alone (Figure 8.13). Wall thickness is variable but always measured <3 mm. It is motile [3]. Branches may be seen proximally, but are generally not apparent until >5 mm distal to the orifice. It is asymmetrically invested with myocardium for a variable distance, generally less than for the superior vein. The left inferior vein is also intimately adjacent to the aorta.

Right pulmonary vein complex

Vestibule

Unlike the left pulmonary vein vestibule, there are no echocardiographically distinct anatomic features to demarcate the proximal border of the right

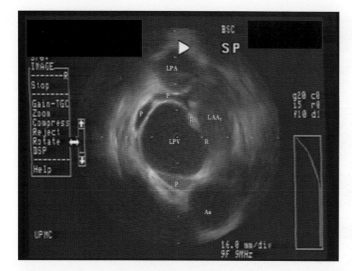

Figure 8.8 Mechanical ICE image of left pulmonary venous vestibule (LPV) demonstrating proximity of aorta (Ao) and left pulmonary artery (LPA). Each scale = 16 mm. LAA_V: left atrial appendage vestibule; P: pericardial sinus; R: ridge.

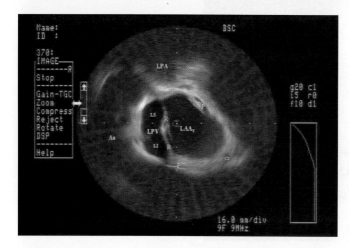

Figure 8.9 Mechanical radial ICE image of left vestibule viewed with the transducer in appendage vestibule. Each scale = 16 mm. Ao: aorta; CS: coronary sinus; LAA_V: left atrial appendage vestibule; LI and LS: left inferior and superior pulmonary vein; LPA: left pulmonary artery; LPV: left pulmonary vein vestibule; P: pericardial sinus; R: ridge.

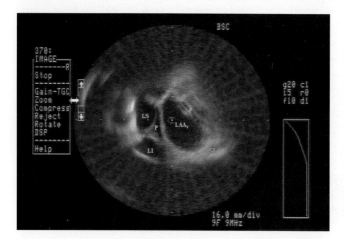

Figure 8.10 Mechanical radial ICE image of left pulmonary venous vestibule with the transducer in left atrial appendage vestibule (LAA_V), a few millimeters distal to the position shown in Figure 8.9. Separation of common ridge wall into distinct vein and LAA_V walls is demonstrated. Each scale = 16 mm. CS: coronary sinus; LI and LS: left inferior and superior pulmonary vein; P: pericardial sinus; S: saddle.

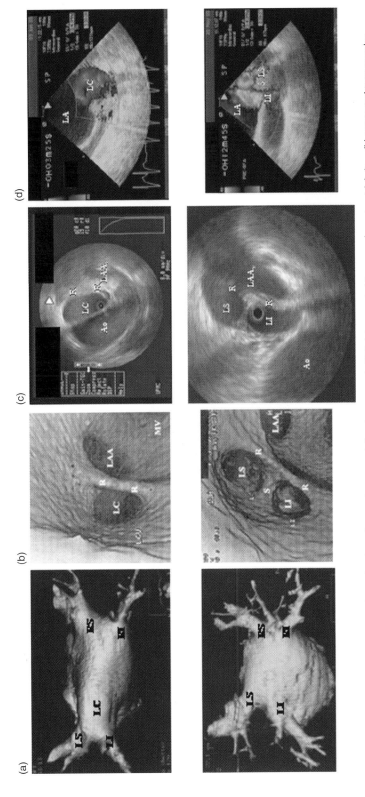

Figure 8.11 Images from patient with (top) and without (bottom) common left pulmonary vein (LC): (a) computed tomography, intraatrial view; (b) computed tomography, extraatrial view; (c) mechanical radial ICE; (d) AcuNAV. Ao: descending aorta; LA: left atrium; LAA: LA appendage and LAA vestibule; LI: left inferior; LS: left superior; MV: mitral valve; R: ridge; RI: right inferior; RS: right superior; S: saddle.

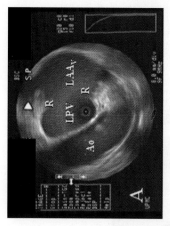

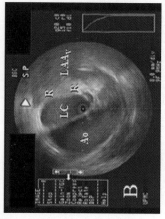

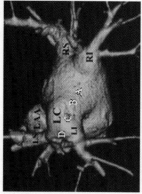

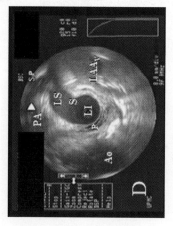

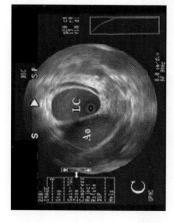

Figure 8.12 Computed tomographic image of LA demonstrating left common (LC) pulmonary vein (LPV) (central panel). The white letters (A, B, C, D) on this CT image correspond to the approximate location of the mechanical radial ICE transducer when the ICE images (panels A, B, C, and D) were obtained. Ao = descending aorta; LAA and LAAv: left atrial appendage and LAA vestibule; LCV: LC vestibule; LI: left inferior; LS: left superior; PA: pulmonary artery; R: ridge; RI: right inferior; RS: right superior; S: saddle.

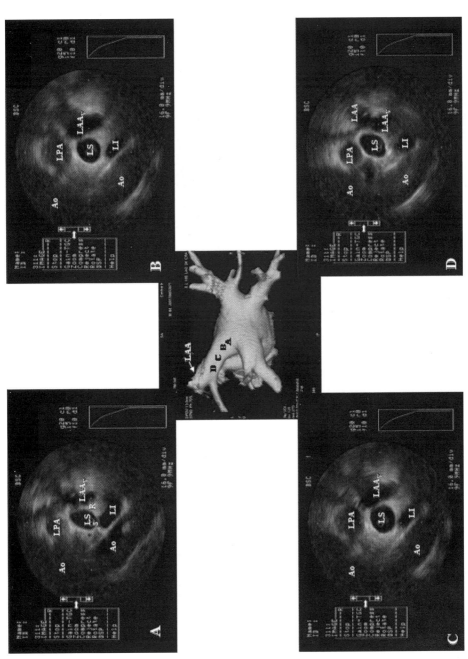

Figure 8.13 Computed tomographic image emphasizing left superior (LS) pulmonary vein (central panel). The black letters (A, B, C, D) on this CT image correspond to the approximate location of the ICE transducer in the LS pulmonary vein when the ICE images (panels A, B, C, and D) were obtained. Ao: aorta; LAA and LAAv: left atrial appendage and LAA vestibule; LI: left inferior; LPA: left pulmonary artery; P: pericardium; R: ridge; RI: right inferior; RS: right superior; S: saddle.

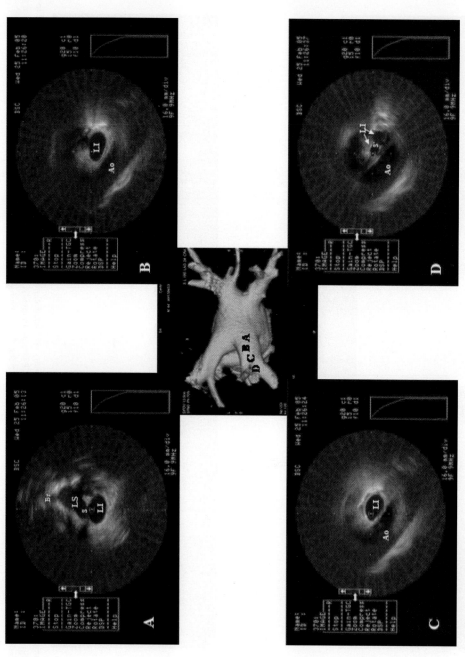

Figure 8.14 Computed tomographic image emphasizing left inferior (LI) pulmonary vein (central panel). The black letters (A, B, C, D) on this CT image correspond to the approximate location of the ICE transducer in the LI pulmonary vein when the ICE images (panels A, B, C, and D) were obtained. Ao: descending aorta; Br: branch of left superior vein; LS: left superior; S: saddle; S´: "secondary" saddle demarcating bifurcation of body of the LI pulmonary vein into branches.

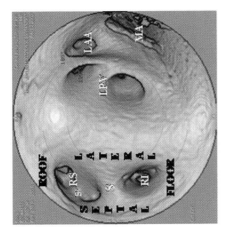

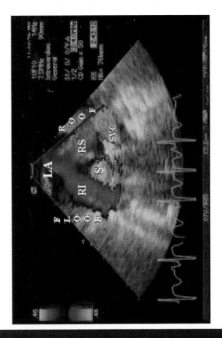

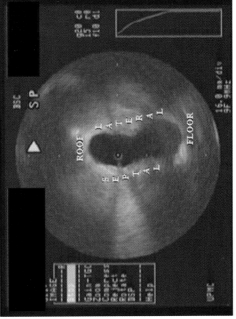

Figure 8.15 Computed tomographic (top panel), mechanical radial ICE (lower left panel, each scale = 16 mm) and AcuNav (lower right panel) images of posterior left atrium (LA) emphasizing right pulmonary venous vestibule region. Using AcuNav imaging catheter with the transducer placed in the LA through a transseptal sheath, the right superior (RS) and inferior (RI) pulmonary vein and the vestibule are imaged. SVC: superior vena cava; RPA: right pulmonary artery; S: saddle.

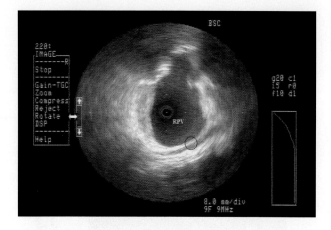

Figure 8.16 Mechanical radial ICE image of an inferior region of the right pulmonary vein (RPV) vestibule demonstrating wall thickness (2.7 mm, within the region encircled). Each scale = 8 mm.

pulmonary vein vestibule. This border has been empirically defined as 1 cm proximal to the most distal intervenous saddle. Four individual walls are identified (Figure 8.15). It is important to understand that the maximal length of the right vestibule exceeds that of the left vestibule; given the curvature of the atrial body in this region, it was not possible to demonstrate the entire structure in a single echocardiographic image. The roof wall of the vestibule abuts the superior caval vein and right pulmonary artery. The superior aspect of the septal wall abuts the superior caval vein. The vestibule has an ovoid shape; maximal dimensions are variable: roof–floor distance 3.6–7.2 cm; ridge–posterior wall distance 2.2–4.1 cm and cross-sectional area 5.9–8.1 cm^2. It is highly motile, with a maximum change in cross-sectional area of 15–30% during the cardiac mechanical cycle [3]. There is significant regional heterogeneity as to the magnitude and type of motion. For example, the lateral wall moves to a significantly greater degree than the septal wall, which appears to be relatively tethered. Wall thickness varies by region: septal wall 4–8 mm, roof wall 3–8 mm, lateral wall 2–5 mm, and floor wall 2–5 mm. However, as for the left pulmonary vein echocardiographic wall thickness does not necessarily equate with that of myocardial investiture. Although this distinction can be more difficult to make echocardiographically, our aggregate experience suggests that myocardial thickness in all regions is <5 mm (Figure 8.16).

Pulmonary veins

Pulmonary vein anatomy on the right side is more complex and variable than the left side. This fact,

combined with: (1) broader separation between veins; (2) greater angulation between veins; and (3) more difficult transducer access and stabilization, make imaging of the right veins more challenging than the left when using mechanical radial imaging catheter. As mentioned above, regardless of transducer it is not typical to be able to capture all veins in a single image plane. As we have previously noted, supernumerary right veins are common, as are proximal branches [5].

The right superior pulmonary vein orifice is apparent in approximately same imaging plane as the intervenous saddle (Figures 8.17 and 8.18). In the setting of one or more supernumerary veins, this saddle may not demarcate the junction of superior and inferior veins (Figure 8.19). Wall thickness is variable but always <3 mm. It is motile [3]. Branches are often seen proximally. It is asymmetrically invested with myocardium for a variable distance. Near the orifice, the vein is contiguous with the medial (septal) wall of the superior caval vein. This region has importance because it is occasionally contiguous to myocardial fibers which conduct directly between right and left atria (see below). The right superior pulmonary vein is also in proximity to the right pulmonary artery. More distally, the vein becomes contiguous with the posterior right atrium, from where both right atrial and pulmonary venous potentials could be recorded [6].

The right inferior vein orifice was apparent in approximately the same imaging plane as the intervenous saddle (Figures 8.20 and 8.21). In the setting of one or more supernumerary veins, this saddle may not be with the superior vein. Wall thickness is variable but measured always ≤2 mm. It is motile [3]. Branching is almost always seen proximally (Figure 8.19).

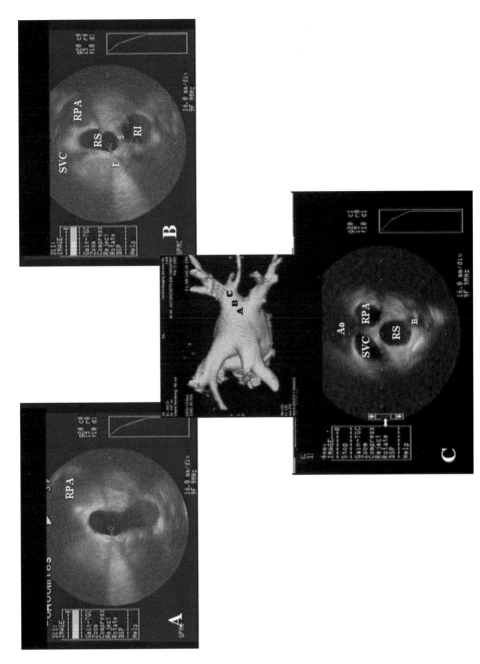

Figure 8.17 Computed tomographic image emphasizing right superior (RS) pulmonary vein (central panel). The black letters (A, B, C) on this CT image correspond to the approximate location of the ICE transducer in the RS pulmonary vein when the ICE images (panels A, B, and C) were obtained. Ao: aorta; B: vein branch; RI: right inferior pulmonary vein; RPA: right pulmonary artery; SVC: superior caval vein.

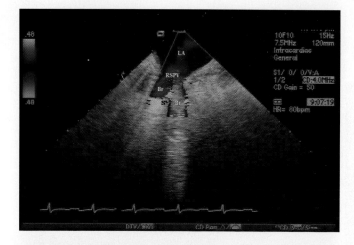

Figure 8.18 AcuNav image showing right superior pulmonary vein (RSPV) with secondary branches (Br) and saddle (S′). LA: left atrium.

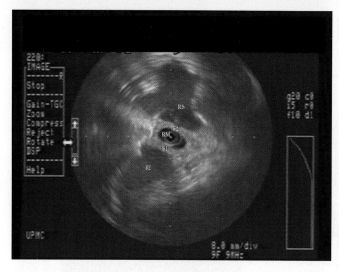

Figure 8.19 Mechanical radial ICE image with the transducer in the right middle pulmonary vein (RM) showing the middle-inferior (S1) and middle-superior (S2) saddles. Each scale = 8 mm. RI and RS: right inferior and superior pulmonary vein.

It is asymmetrically invested with myocardium for a variable distance, generally less than the superior vein. The right middle vein(s) were found small, without proximal branches, and minimally invested with myocardium (Figure 8.19).

Left atrial appendage

The left atrial appendage is very complex: (1) the orifice is asymmetric, as is the body; (2) there is marked heterogeneity in wall thickness, endocardial topography, and lobulation; (3) both orifice and body are disproportionately (e.g., relative to the left atrium body) motile; (4) blood flow is variable and non-laminar. There is much interpatient variation in each

of these features, which is poorly reported by two-dimensional ICE (Figure 8.22): this phenomenon is also true of transesophageal echocardiography. Given the stiffness, nondeflectability, and lack of control of catheter axis relative to appendage axis, using mechanical radial ICE catheter to image this structure is not recommend. Although much more reliable and clear than right atrium-based AcuNav ICE imaging, left atrium-based AcuNav ICE has not been found to provide images significantly different from those of the esophageal transducer location.

Left atrial isthmus

This region encompasses the floor of the lateral left atrium, between left venous vestibule

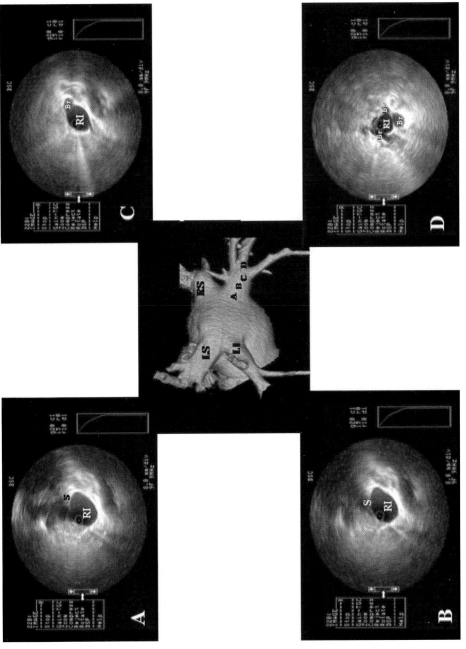

Figure 8.20 Computed tomographic image of left atrium emphasizing right inferior (RI) pulmonary vein (central panel). The black letters (A, B, C, D) on this CT image correspond to the approximate location of the ICE transducer in the right inferior pulmonary vein when the ICE images (panels A, B, C, and D) were obtained. Br: vein branch; LI and LS: left inferior and superior pulmonary vein; RS: right superior; S: saddle.

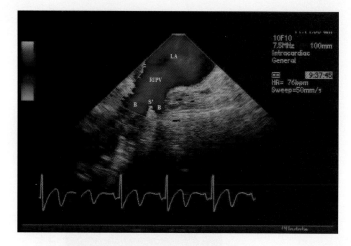

Figure 8.21 AcuNav image of the right inferior pulmonary vein (RIPV) showing secondary branches (B) and saddle (S′).

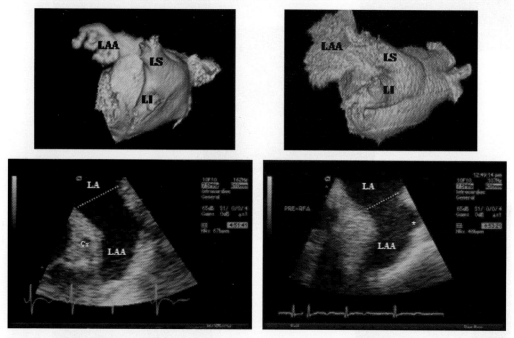

Figure 8.22 Computed tomographic (upper panels) and corresponding AcuNav ICE (lower panels) images emphasizing left atrial (LA) appendage (LAA). Marked morphologic differences apparent on CT images are not reflected by ICE. The lines demarcate orifice border. *: lobulation; Cx: circumflex coronary artery; LI and LS: left inferior and superior pulmonary vein.

and mitral annulus (Figure 8.23). Dimensions and myocardial thicknesses were quite variable within and between patients. Topographically, the endocardium may be "pitted" or trabeculated, particularly in the left atrial appendage vestibule: this has important implications for power titration during ablation.

Mitral apparatus and left ventricle

Mitral leaflets from base to apex, chordae and papillary muscles as well as left ventricular endocardium can be imaged with a high degree of resolution using the mechanical radial ICE catheter with the transducer placed in the left ventricle (Figures 8.24–8.26)

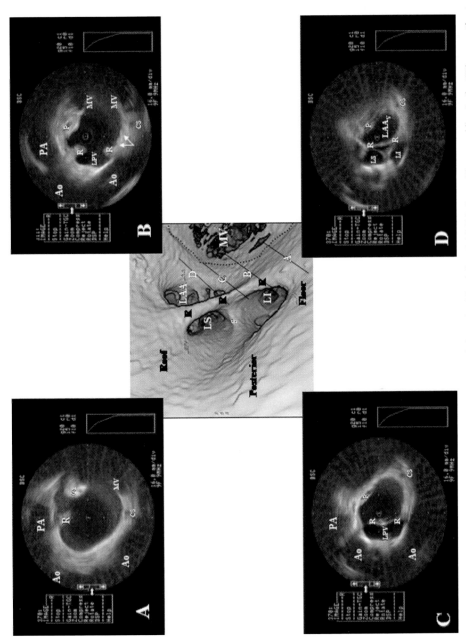

Figure 8.23 CT (central panel) and mechanical radial ICE images (panels A, B, C, and D) emphasizing left atrial (LA) isthmus. The curved line in the CT image estimates the mitral annulus; the lettered straight lines (A, B, C, D) estimate the plane of the corresponding ICE image (panels A, B, C, and D). Arrows in B emphasize the irregular endocardial contour. Ao: aorta; CS: coronary sinus; Cx: circumflex coronary artery; LAA and LAA$_V$: LA appendage and LAA vestibule; LI and LS: left inferior and superior pulmonary vein (LPV); MV: mitral valve; P: pericardium; PA: pulmonary artery; R: ridge; S: saddle.

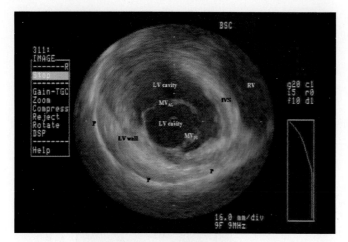

Figure 8.24 Mechanical radial ICE image with the trasducer placed approximately 1 cm distal to mitral annulus in the left ventricular (LV) inflow, showing the short-axis view of the left ventricle. "LV cavity" located anteriorly is LV outflow tract and that posteriorly is LV inflow. Each scale = 16 mm. IVS: interventricular septum; MV_{AL}: mitral valve–anterior leaflet; MV_{PS}: mitral valve–posterior leaflet; P: pericardium; RV: right ventricle.

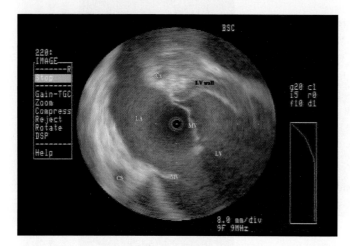

Figure 8.25 Mechanical radial ICE image with the transducer placed just below the mitral annulus in the left ventricle (LV), showing truncated long-axis of LV inflow. Each scale = 8 mm. CS: coronary sinus; C_X: circumflex coronary artery; LA: left atrium; MV: mitral valve.

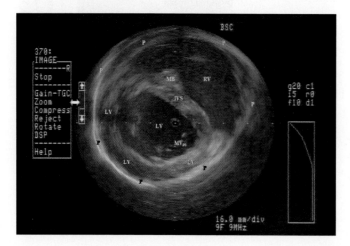

Figure 8.26 Mechanical ICE image with the transducer placed in the mid-left ventricle (LV), showing the entirety of LV endocardium in LV short-axis. Each scale = 16 mm. IVS: interventricular septum; MB: moderator band; MV_{PS}: chordae tendinae; P: pericardium; RV: right ventricle.

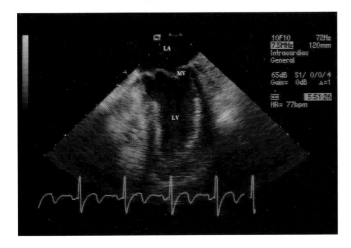

Figure 8.27 AcuNav ICE image with the transducer placed in the left atrium (LA) through a transseptal sheath, showing the left ventricle (LV) and mitral valve (MV) at end-systole.

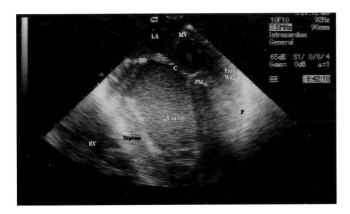

Figure 8.28 AcuNAV image with the transducer placed in the left atrium (LA) through a transseptal sheath, showing the mitral apparatus. MV: mitral valve leaflet; C: chordae tendinae; PM_{AL}: anterolateral papillary muscle; RV: right ventricle.

or AcuNav catheter (Figures 8.27 and 8.28). As detailed in Chapters 3 and 9, these regions can also be imaged with the AcuNav transducer in the right heart position.

Aorta and aortic valve

The mitral–aortic continuity region, aortic root, valves and ascending segment can be imaged using the mechanical radial catheter with the transducer placed in the left atrium near the medial atrioventricular junction (Figures 8.29 and 8.30) or the AcuNav catheter (Figure 8.31). Note also that the distal right ventricular outflow tract, pulmonic valve, and proximal main pulmonary artery are imaged. Prior images have demonstrated the mechanical radial ICE imaging of the segment of descending aorta in proximity to the posterior left atrium. As detailed in Chapters 3 and 9, these regions can also be imaged with the AcuNav transducer in the right heart position.

Esophagus

Mechanical radial ICE and AcuNav are both effective for imaging the region of contiguity between the posterior left atrium and the esophagus (Figures 8.32 and 8.33). As detailed in Chapters 7 and 11, these regions can also be imaged with the AcuNav transducer in the right heart position.

Utility of left atrial transducer position in left atrial ablation

In most patients, atrial fibrillation is primarily a disease of the left atrium. The posterior left atrium, specifically the myocardial investiture in and about the pulmonary veins, appears to play a key role in arrhythmia initiation and sustenance. The discovery of this potential Achille's heal has resulted in the rapid growth of an atrial fibrillation catheter ablation

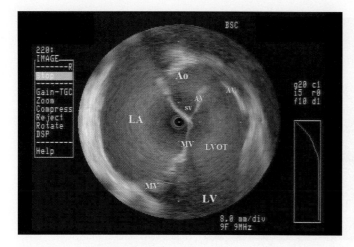

Figure 8.29 Mechanical radial ICE image with the transducer placed at the medial atrioventricular junction in the left atrium (LA), showing the mitral–aortic continuity region, aortic root (Ao), and aortic valve (AV). Each scale = 8 mm. LV and LVOT: left ventricle and LV outflow tract; MV: mitral valve; SV: aortic sinus of Valsalva.

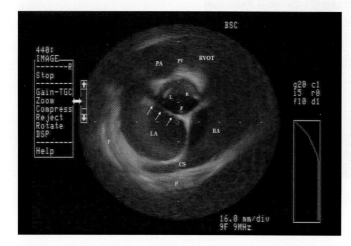

Figure 8.30 Mechanical radial ICE image with the transducer placed near the posterior wall of the aortic root (Ao) in the left atrium (LA), showing the Ao, aortic cusps (AV) and aortic wall continuity (arrows) to be projected downward to the anterior mitral valve insertion. Each scale = 16 mm. CS: coronary sinus; P: pericardium; PA: pulmonary artery; PV: pulmonic valve; RA: right atrium; RVOT: right ventricular outflow tract.

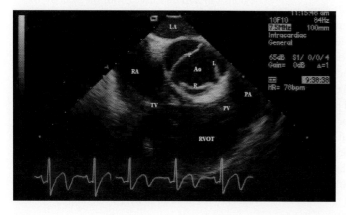

Figure 8.31 AcuNav ICE image with transducer placed in the left atrium (LA) through a transseptal sheath, showing aortic root (Ao), aortic cusps, and contiguous structures. L: left coronary cusp; P: noncoronary cusp; PA: pulmonary artery; PV: pulmonic valve; R: right coronary cusp; RA: right atrium; RVOT: right ventricular outflow tract; TV: tricuspid valve.

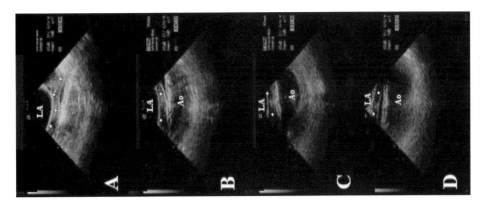

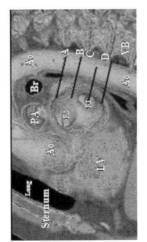

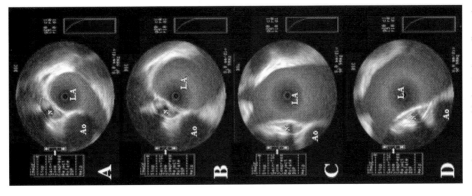

Figure 8.32 Computed tomographic (central panel), mechanical radial (left panels), and AcuNav ICE (right panels) images emphasizing the left atrial (LA) posterior wall region contiguous to the esophagus. The approximate level of the image is demarcated in the CT with letters (A, B, C, and D). In the mechanical radial ICE images, the esophagus is outlined by a white circuit. In the AcuNav images, the esophagus lumen is demarcated by asterisks. Ao: aorta; Br: bronchus; LV: left ventricle; N: nasogastric tube inserted into the esophagus; PA: pulmonary artery; RI and RS: right inferior and superior pulmonary vein; VB: vertebra.

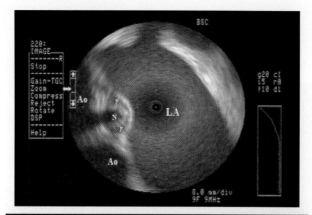

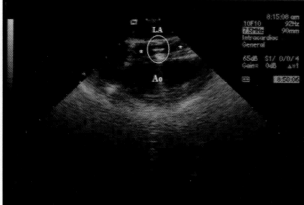

Figure 8.33 Top panel: mechanical radial ICE image recorded during manipulation of nasogastric tube (N), demonstrating protrusion of esophagus against left atrial (LA) posterior wall. The air in the nasogastric tube causes an acoustic shadow, which is apparent. P: interface between esophagus and LA posterior wall. Bottom panel: AcuNav ICE image demonstrating esophagus (asterisks) and luminal echodense object (encircled), which is a thermometric probe used during anesthesia. Ao: descending aorta.

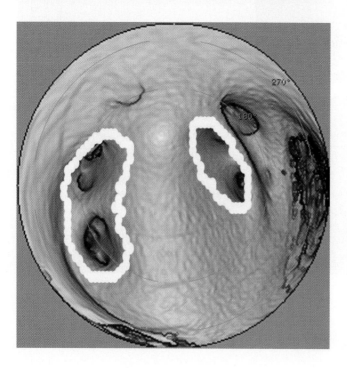

Figure 8.34 CT-derived endocardial view of posterior left atrium demonstrating approximate paths of primary ablation lesions.

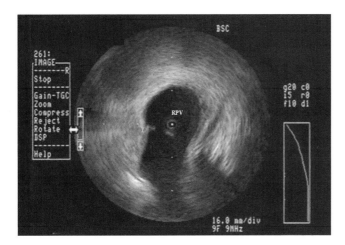

Figure 8.35 Mechanical radial ICE image of the right pulmonary venous (RPV) vestibule demonstrating standard ablation electrode (E) in contact with left atrial endocardium with distal fan-shaped shadow artifact.

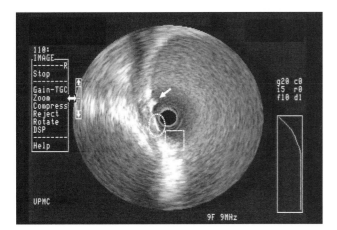

Figure 8.36 Mechanical radial ICE image demonstrating regions post-ablation where left atrial endocardial boiling occurred, evidencing hyper-echodensity of the subendocardial region (inside circle) relative to an adjacent ablated site where boiling did not occur (inside square) which is acoustically similar to unablated myocardium (region at 12 o'clock). Uncomplicated radiofrequency applications do not acutely disturb tissue architecture; applications complicated by boiling ± barotrauma destroy architecture, resulting in hyper-echodensity. The arrow points to endocardial coagulum associated with another region where boiling had occurred.

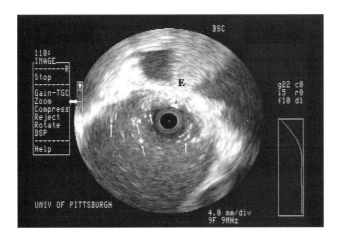

Figure 8.37 Mechanical radial ICE image showing ablation electrode (E) abutting left atrial endocardium with distal fan-shaped shadow artifact. During radiofrequency application, bubbles (arrows) eminating from the electrode–endocardial interface were observed. Bubbling denotes steam generated by myocardial boiling. Each scale = 4 mm.

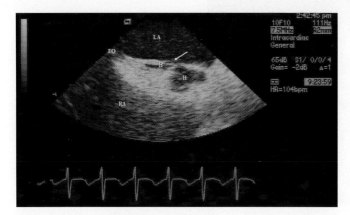

Figure 8.38 AcuNav ICE image of the right pulmonary venous vestibule, demonstrating mural tear (arrow) and subsequent intraseptal hematoma (H) resulting from barotrauma caused by explosive release of steam during interfacial boiling. The explosion was observed at an electrode temperature of approximately 48°C, radiofrequency power of 30 W, and was not associated with an impedance rise. The H was confined to the intraseptal space, and was otherwise clinically invisible except for the development of a severe form of Dressler's syndrome in this patient weeks after the procedure. FO: fossa ovalis; LA and RA: left and right atrium.

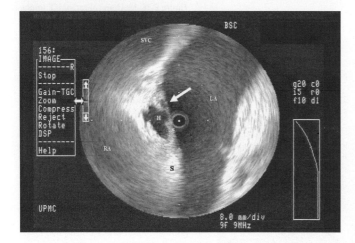

Figure 8.39 Mechanical radial ICE image of same region as in Figure 8.37. Once again, the arrow demonstrates the mural tear. Each scale = 8 mm. H: hematoma; LA and RA: left and right atrium; SVC: superior vena cava.

industry. The anatomic and biophysical complexities of the posterior left atrium have been formidable; although our ablation technique has evolved significantly, ICE has been a central component throughout. This experience serves as an excellent demonstration of the advantages and limitations of ICE, and is illustrative of how anatomic information provided by this technology can result in important electrophysiologic insight.

The past decade has witnessed impressive technological development in the field of interventional electrophysiology. However, ICE remains the only technique which provides real-time, direct imaging of the ablation electrode–endocardial interface. So-called "virtual" imaging techniques provide neither real-time nor accurate complex topographical detail. Recent publications have touted the utility of right heart-based AcuNav for facilitation of posterior left atrial ablation. Undoubtedly, this is a significant advance. However, from our vantage it does not fully utilize the capability of ICE. Specifically, direct imaging of the ablation electrode–endocardial interface before, during, and after radiofrequency energy application is usually not performed, deterred by a combination of difficult (if possible) imaging planes, plane instability, and impracticality of management of the imaging catheter by the ablationist or his/her assistant. As demonstrated above, relative to the right atrium, AcuNav imaging of the posterior left atrium is much facilitated by the left atrial transducer location. However, we have found limited utility for this, based primarily on sector orientation of the imaging

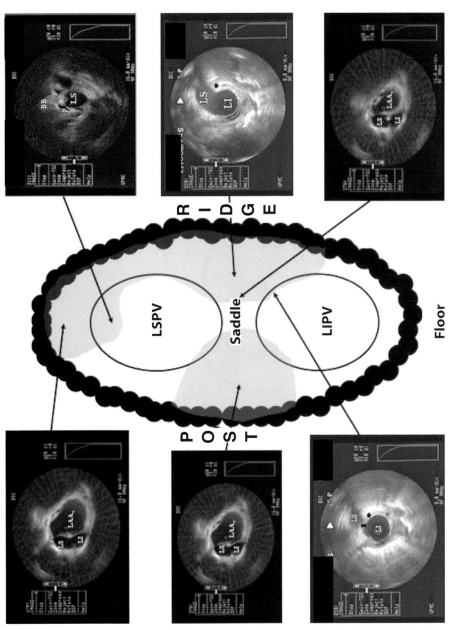

Figure 8.40 Schematic (central panel) and corresponding mechanical radial ICE images (arrows correlate with asterisks in ICE images) of left pulmonary vein vestibule myocardial territory subtended by the primary ablation lesion (collection of black circles). This figure demonstrates our aggregate experience. The red shading demarcates a region in which one or more additional radiofrequency applications were often necessary to achieve complete electrical isolation. The green shading demarcates a region where additional radiofrequency applications were less often necessary. No additional radiofrequency applications were needed in the unshaded regions. Asterisks demonstrate the specific sites to which the arrows point in the schema. BB: Bachmann's bundle; LAAv: left atrial appendage vestibule; LSPV and LIPV: left superior and inferior pulmonary vein; P: pericardium; S: saddle.

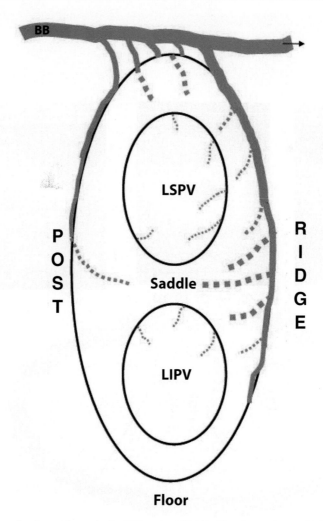

Figure 8.41 Schema, based on lessons learned using ICE as summarized in Figure 8.39, of myocardial (conduction) connections to left pulmonary vein vestibule, with thicknesses drawn to roughly parallel the girth of connection (deduced by ablation territory needed to eradicate). We believe that fibers eminating from Bachmann's bundle (BB) continue as the Marshall ridge and rain down into the vestibule, primarily via the ridge wall and roof. Connections can be seen as distal as the roof of the superior vein 2 cm distal to the venoatrial junction. Arrow: continuation of BB towards appendage; LIPV and LSPV: left inferior and superior pulmonary vein.

plane, which interfaces poorly with a circumferential ablation paradigm (below). Thus, the majority of our experience with left atrium-based ICE during atrial fibrillation ablation procedures has been with the mechanical radial ICE technology.

At present, we create circumferential lesions along the borders of the right and left pulmonary venous vestibules (Figure 8.34), with a goal of complete electrical isolation of subtended myocardium. As noted above, mechanical radial ICE is rarely capable of imaging an entire vestibule in a single frame; rather, the process is piecemeal. Also, much of the territory does not produce a unique or discrete echocardiographic signature. It is because of these issues that we have found it impossible to use ICE alone to produce these lesions. In order to maintain proper spatial orientation, we have found it essential to use ICE and virtual imaging technology (CARTO™, Biosense Webster, Diamond Bar, CA, USA) in tandem [7]. Early in our experience, we had observed using ICE that tremendous movement of the posterior left atrial endocardium correlated with the respiratory cycle, presumably due

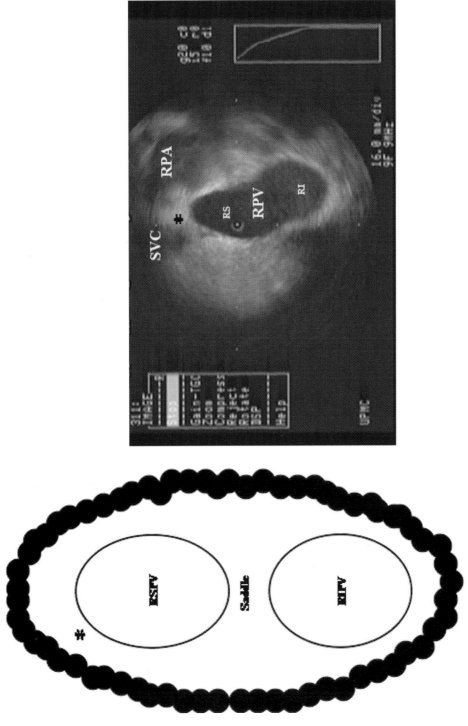

Figure 8.42 Schema of the right pulmonary vein (RPV) vestibule (left panel) demonstrating primary ablation lesion (collection of black circles) and ICE image (right panel) of RPV vestibule region. The asterisk indicates a region where in most patients with persistent conduction after the primary RPV vestibule lesion additional ablation was successful in producing complete isolation in the schema. RI and RS: inferior and superior RPV.

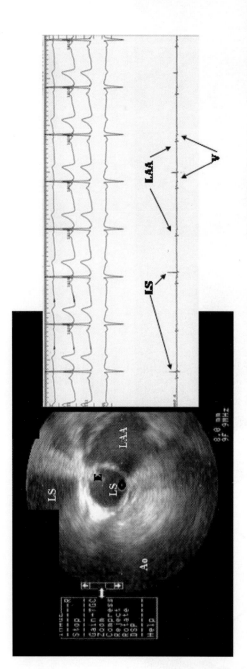

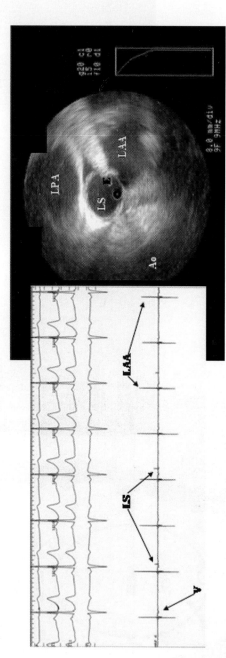

Figure 8.43 Mechanical radial ICE images and corresponding bipolar endocardial electrograms obtained after electrical isolation. On top, the ICE image demonstrates the electrode (E) abutting the roof of the left superior (LS) pulmonary vein. The electrogram at this site demonstrates a consistent appendage (LAA)-derived potential, a dissociated vein myocardium-derived potential (LS), and a ventricle-derived potential (V). On bottom, the electrode has been moved and now abuts a region of the LS vein contiguous to the LAA. In this region, large (0.3–1.2 mV) "near-field" LAA-derived potentials are recorded, as well as smaller, dissociated vein-derived potentials. Ao: aorta; LPA: left pulmonary artery.

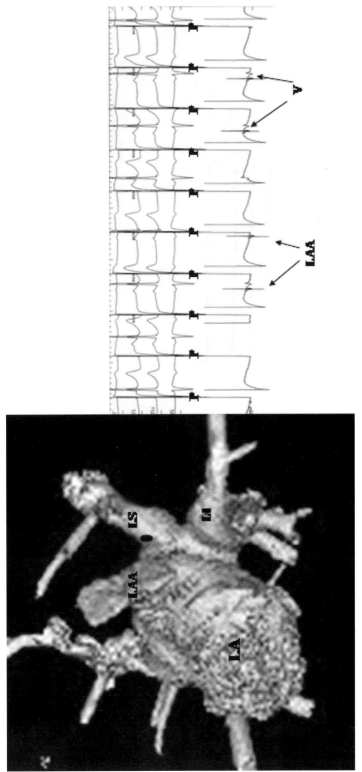

Figure 8.44 Left: Computed tomographic image estimating location of electrode shown in bottom of Figure 8.42 (black oval). To increase clarity, the image has been manipulated to enhance separation between base of appendage (LAA) and distal left vestibule/left superior (LS) vein. In reality, as can be seen from the ICE image bottom Figure 8.42, these structures are directly contiguous. Right: pacing at this site (right; P: pacing stimulus artifact) demonstrates capture of local myocardium (absence of dissociated LS potentials) and non-capture of LAA myocardium (LAA electrograms unassociated with pacing). Despite large amplitude and "near-field" properties (e.g., slow rate) of the LAA-derived potentials, and despite the close proximity of LAA myocardium to the pacing electrode, it has been our experience that the LAA myocardium cannot be captured with pacing current under 15 mA, using a standard 4 mm length ablation electrode and pacing in unipolar fashion. We presume this to be due to an insulation effect produced by the fascial plane separating the two structures.

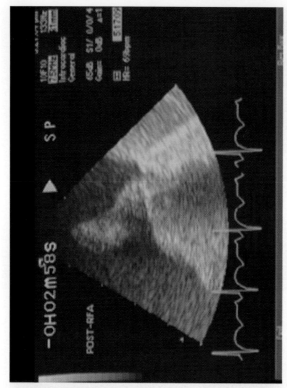

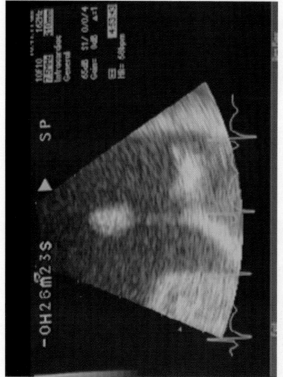

Figure 8.45 AcuNav ICE image of Marshall Ridge before (left panel) and immediately after ablation (right panel). Significant swelling is apparent after ablation. Note that swelling extended well beyond the ablation zone, which was limited in this case to the apex of the ridge. We have previously reported the phenomenon of extension of swelling beyond the ablation site [3,11].

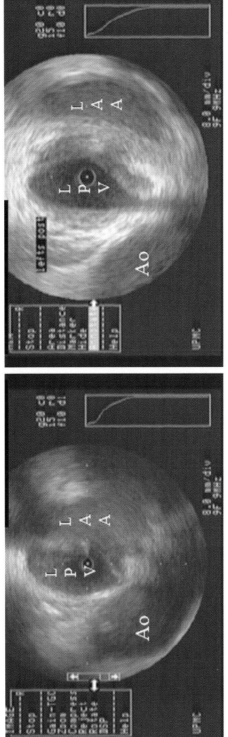

Figure 8.46 Mechanical radial ICE image of left pulmonary vein (LPV) vestibule before (left panel) and immediately after ablation (right panel). Post-ablation, circumferential myocardial swelling is apparent; this is particularly apparent in the ridge region. Each scale = 8 mm. Ao: aorta; LAA: left atrial appendage.

to its proximity to the diaphragm, which undermined ablation electrode–endocardial contact stability. In order to eliminate this motion, patients undergoing this procedure are generally anesthetized and ventilated using high frequency jet technique [8]. Prior to ablation, the lesion path for each vestibule is mapped out (Figure 8.34). On the left side, the venous vestibule edge of the Marshall ridge is traced and the path continued circumferentially in parallel orientation to the roof, floor, and posterior wall. As demonstrated above, contiguous extraatrial structures such as aorta and esophagus may be apparent, but so far we have made no effort to adjust the lesion path to avoid them. On the right side, the venoatrial junctions at the roof, mid (intervenous saddles), and floor aspects of the vestibule are located. The catheter was moved 1 cm proximally at each site, and then a path is drawn to connect these sites. Each circumferential ablation lesion was produced by applying a series of contiguous focal lesions. At each lesion site, prior to radiofrequency application, the catheter is manipulated under ICE guidance to achieve firm/stable electrode–endocardial contact (Figure 8.35). Guided by ICE, this is maintained throughout the lesion application: if it is lost the application is immediately terminated. As reported previously, stable contact is a critical element of safe and reproducible ablation [9,10]. Unfortunately, changes in tissue acoustic properties induced by ablation are not sufficiently distinct as to allow ICE to be used to guide radiofrequency power titration (Figure 8.36). Power is titrated using an electrogram amplitude reduction [10]; power requirements are consistent with regional myocardial thicknesses as assessed using ICE [11]. Although conservative, radiofrequency titration using electrogram amplitude reduction does not completely eliminate myocardial boiling [10]. Boiling and its sequelae were well reported echocardiographically but are otherwise usually invisible (Figures 8.36–8.39). They are often sudden and not heralded by ICE phenomena that could be used to avoid their occurrence.

After deployment of the initial ("primary") encircling lesions (aggregate of 91 focal lesions, on average), the myocardium subtended by the lesion was then examined under ICE guidance to confirm electrical isolation. On the left side, isolation was documented in only ≈30% of patients. One or more additional ("secondary") focal lesions within the subtended zone, deployed using ICE guidance were necessary

to produce isolation. Secondary lesion sites had a stereotypical anatomic distribution (Figure 8.40). Our experience with ablation under ICE guidance in these regions has generated a working hypothesis as to the electroanatomic logic of this region (Figure 8.41). In the right vestibule, isolation of myocardium subtended by the primary lesion was achieved in over 90% of patients. In the few patients manifesting residual conduction, most have been in a discrete anatomical region (Figure 8.42).

After successful isolation, ICE has been critical in providing insight to anatomic relationships underlying potentials which give the spurious impression of persistent conduction (Figures 8.43 and 8.44). ICE has also been instructive as to ablation-induced alterations in regional morphology and mechanical function, which were subclinical (Figures 8.45 and 8.46).

To summarize, our experience with left atrial ablation for atrial fibrillation serves to illustrate the myriad benefits of ICE using left atrial transducer technique: (1) significant insights gained as to regional electroanatomy, biophysics, and physiology; (2) real real-time endocardial imaging; (3) reliable, generally safe ablation lesion application; and (4) assurance of procedural endpoint (electrical isolation).

Conclusion

In this chapter we have reviewed imaging using the left heart ICE transducer position. Although this position provides unique windows and capabilities, as emphasized there are regions of the left heart which can be imaged from both right and left heart transducer position. In view of the potential for increased morbidity associated with left heart transducer position, the technique should be used only when it provides an important advantage. Examples would include image quality, image orientation, and image appropriateness for intervention tool guidance.

References

1 Ren J, Schwartzman D, Callans D, Marchlinski F. Intracardiac echocardiography (9 MHz) in humans: methods, imaging views and clinical utility. *Ultrasound in Med & Biol* 1999; **25**: 1077–1086.
2 Bazaz R, Schwartzman D. Site-selective atrial septal puncture. *J Cardiovasc Electrophysiol* 2003; **14**: 196–199.
3 Schwartzman D, Kanzaki H, Bazaz R, Gorcsan J. Impact of catheter ablation on pulmonary vein morphology and

mechanical function. *J Cardiovasc Electrophysiol* 2004; **15**: 161–167.

4 Schwartzman D. The common left pulmonary vein: a consistent source of arrhythmogenic atrial ectopy. *J Cardiovasc Electrophysiol* 2004; **15**: 560–566.

5 Schwartzman D, Lacomis J, Wigginton W. Characterization of left atrium and distal pulmonary vein morphology using multidimensional computed tomography. *J Am Coll Cardiol* 2003; **41**: 1349–1357.

6 Schwartzman D. Right pulmonary vein potentials recorded from the posterior right atrial endocardium. *J Cardiovasc Electrophysiol* 2000; **11**: 330–333.

7 Schwartzman D. Catheter ablation to suppress atrial fibrillation: evolution of technique at a single center. *J Intervent Cardiac Electrophysiol* 2003; **9**: 295–300.

8 Klain M, Keszler H. High-frequency jet ventilation. *Surg Clin N Am* 1985; **65**: 917–930.

9 Schwartzman D, Parizhskaya M, Devine W. Linear ablation using an irrigated electrode: electrophysiologic and histologic lesion evolution; comparison with ablation utilizing a non-irrigated electrode. *J Intervent Cardiac Electrophysiol* 2001; **5**: 17–26.

10 Schwartzman D, Michele J, Trankiem C, Ren J. Electrogram-guided radiofrequency catheter ablation of atrial tissue: comparison with thermometry-guide ablation. *J Intervent Cardiac Electrophysiol* 2001; **5**: 253–266.

11 Schwartzman D, Ren J, Devine W, Callans D. Cardiac swelling associated with linear radiofrequency ablation in the atrium. *J Intervent Cardiac Electrophysiol* 2001; **5**: 159–166.

CHAPTER 9

Intracardiac Echocardiographic Imaging in Radiofrequency Catheter Ablation for Ventricular Tachycardia

Jian-Fang Ren, MD, *& Francis E. Marchlinski,* MD

Introduction

Ventricular tachycardia may be idiopathic or caused by the presence of underlying structural heart disease. Idiopathic (repetitive monomorphic) ventricular tachycardia occurring in the absence of structural heart disease typically arises from the right ventricular outflow tract below the pulmonic valve or the left ventricular outflow tract adjacent to the mitral and aortic valves [1–10]. Verapamil sensitive ventricular tachycardia usually originates from the bottom of the left ventricular septum. The reported clinical success rate of catheter ablation of idiopathic ventricular tachycardia is 76–100% and is consistently greater than 90% for those arrhythmias arising from the right ventricular outflow tract [11–18]. Ventricular tachycardia in the setting of structural heart disease is usually caused by a reentrant mechanism in regions of patchy fibrosis which are interspersed among bundles of surviving myocardial bundles. The most common arrhythmogenic substrate among patients with reentrant ventricular tachycardia is chronic ischemic heart disease. Using traditional electrophysiologic mapping techniques, ablation of ventricular tachycardia in the setting of healed myocardial infarction is modestly successful in highly selected patients with relatively slow, well tolerated tachycardias [19,20]. The central portion of a complete transmural scar from prior infarction is commonly electrically inactive and a typical reentrant circuit uses small myocardial

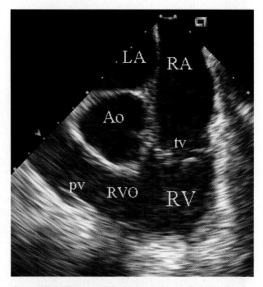

Figure 9.1 ICE image with the transducer placed in the right atrium (RA), showing the right ventricle (RV) and RV outflow tract (RVO). Ao: aorta; LA: left atrium; pv: pulmonic valve; tv: tricuspid valve.

bundles at the scar border zone as regions of slowed conduction [21,22]. In patients with posterior scar, the central conduction zone is often the isthmus between the scar and the mitral valve annulus [23]. Ablation may be accomplished at sites within the zone of slowed electrical conduction that is identified with techniques such as activation and entrainment

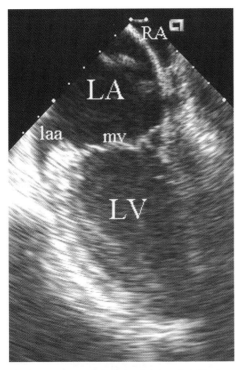

Figure 9.2 ICE image with the transducer placed in the right atrium (RA), showing the left ventricle (LV) and anterolateral and posteromedial wall. LA: left atrium; laa: LA appendage; mv: mitral valve.

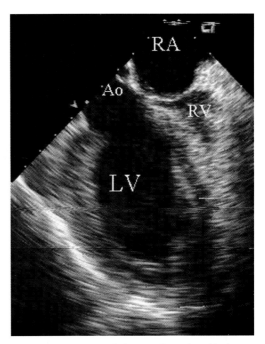

Figure 9.4 ICE image with the transducer placed in the right atrium (RA), showing the left ventricular (LV) outflow and right ventricle (RV) with the interventricular septum between them. Ao: aorta.

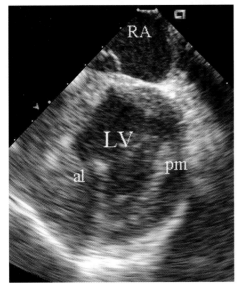

Figure 9.3 ICE image with the transducer placed in the right atrium (RA) and the tip deflected posteriorly and rotated clockwise, showing the short-axis view of the left ventricle (LV) at papillary muscle level. al and pm: anterolateral and posteromedial papillary muscles.

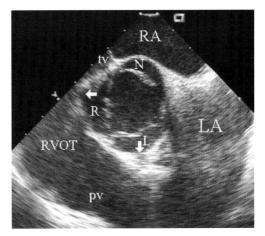

Figure 9.5 ICE image with the transducer placed in the right atrium (RA) with its tip deflected posteriorly and rotated clockwise, showing the short-axis view of the aortic root. The three aortic cusps, and left main coronary ostium (downward arrow) and right coronary arterial ostium (horizontal arrow) are identified during systole. L: left coronary aortic cusp; LA: left atrium; N: noncoronary aortic cusp; pv: pulmonic valve; R: right coronary aortic cusp; RVOT: right ventricular outflow tract; tv: tricuspid valve.

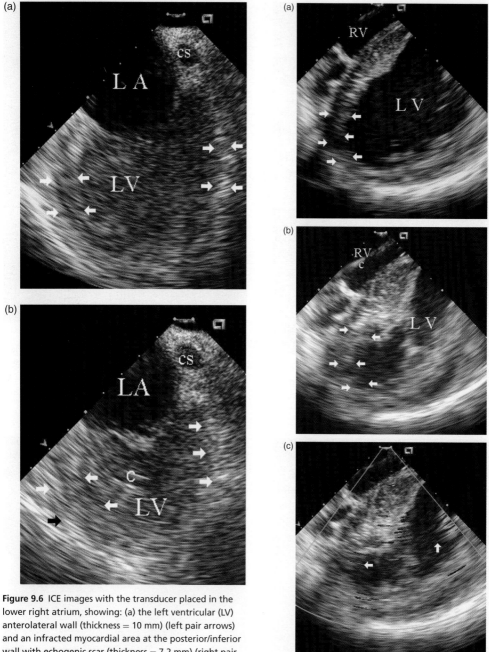

Figure 9.6 ICE images with the transducer placed in the lower right atrium, showing: (a) the left ventricular (LV) anterolateral wall (thickness = 10 mm) (left pair arrows) and an infracted myocardial area at the posterior/inferior wall with echogenic scar (thickness = 7.2 mm) (right pair arrows) during diastole (left panel); (b) as compared to the anterolateral wall (thickness = 13 mm) and the infarcted scar area without wall thickening during systole in a patient with mild LV concentric hypertrophy.

Figure 9.7 ICE images with the transducer placed in the right ventricle (RV), showing: (a) the left ventricle (LV) with an apical aneurysm (arrows) during diastole; (b) dyskinesis of wall motion (arrows) at aneurysm identified during systole; and (c) blood flow toward the mitral valvular orifice (red color, upward arrow) above the apical aneurysm in the LV but toward the dyskinetic wall (blue color, horizontal arrow) during systole in a patient with mild LV concentric hypertrophy.

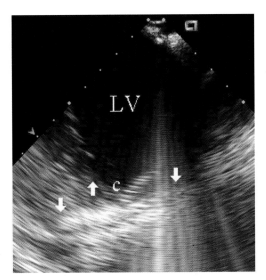

Figure 9.8 ICE image with the transducer placed near the atrioventricular junction in the right atrium, showing the development of accelerated bubbles (upward arrow) during radiofrequency energy application at the myocardial scar (between the downward arrows) at the left ventricular (LV) posteroinferior wall. c: ablation catheter.

(a)

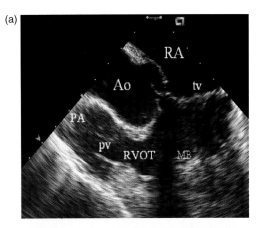

(b)

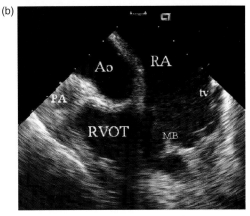

Figure 9.9 ICE images with the transducer placed in the right atrium (RA), showing: (a) the right ventricle and its outflow tract (RVOT) from the pulmonic valve (pv) to the tricuspid valve (tv); (b) the RVOT, moderator band (MB) with attached papillary muscle to the ventricular wall. Ao: aortic root; PA: pulmonary artery.

mapping [11]. Ventricular tachycardias in patients with nonischemic myopathies are typically caused by a reentrant mechanism in diffuse regions of perivalvular fibrosis mingling with normal and hypertrophied myocytes [24]. The diffuse nature of the structural abnormalities allows for dynamic changes in the reentrant circuits beat to beat and makes these patients more prone to polymorphic ventricular tachycardias [11]. Ventricular tachycardia in patients with dilated cardiomyopathy is commonly bundle branch reentrant tachycardia. Bundle branch is easily treated by ablation of the right or left bundle branch [25]. However, the majority of patients with coronary artery disease have ventricular tachycardias that are not sufficiently well tolerated to allow the prolonged mapping that is necessary for successful focal ablation. Similar limitations are frequently observed in patients with arrhythmogenic right ventricular dysplasia and ventricular tachycardia in the setting of dilated cardiomyopathy. Anatomically based ablation of the ventricular substrate obviates this difficulty by targeting lesion placement to the substrate defined by voltage mapping using three-dimensional electroanatomic mapping or abnormal myocardium

defined by intracardiac echocardiography (ICE) assistance.

ICE with catheter transducer placed in the right side heart can provide imaging of the right and left ventricular structures and identifying the ventricular tachycardia-substrate [26,27]. With optimal positioning of the ICE catheter and scanning imaging views, various regions like the right ventricular wall, tricuspid valve, right ventricular outflow tract and pulmonic valve (Figure 9.1), and left ventricular free wall and septum, the mitral valve (Figure 9.2), papillary muscles (Figure 9.3), left ventricular outflow tract (Figure 9.4), and aortic cusps are imaged (Figure 9.5). Ventricular chamber size and regional wall motion abnormalities can be qualitatively and

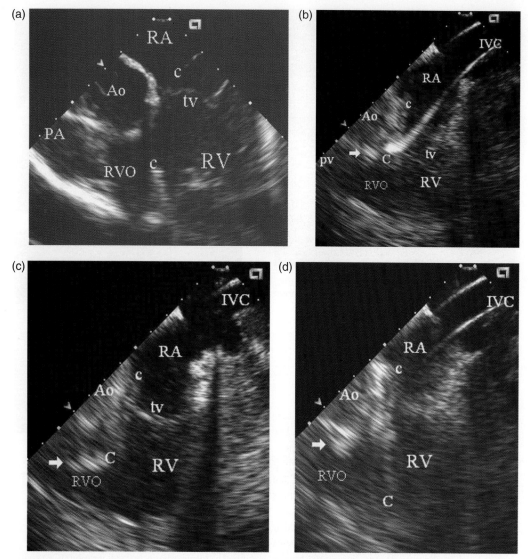

Figure 9.10 (a) ICE image with the transducer placed in the right atrium (RA), showing the right ventricle (RV) and its outflow tract (RVO) with an ablation catheter (C) positioned at the lower RVO with distal fan-shaped shadow artifact. (b–d) ICE images with the transducer just above the inferior vena cava (IVC) orifice in the RA, showing ablation catheter (C) positioned at different locations (arrow, panel b and c) of the RVO, and echogenic lesion (arrow) seen with the ablation catheter (C) and after ablation catheter moved (arrow, panel d) following radiofrequency energy application. Ao: aortic root; c: His catheter; PA: pulmonary artery; pv: pulmonic valve; tv: tricuspid valve.

quantitatively assessed. Ischemic myocardium and infarcted scar or fibrous wall can be identified by its enhanced echodensity and absence of wall thickening (Figure 9.6a,b) or dyskinesis (Figure 9.7a–c). ICE imaging can be used for assisting in positioning the mapping and ablation catheter at targeted anatomy and identifying catheter electrode–tissue contact. ICE monitoring of acute lesion morphologic changes (swelling, dimpling, crater formation and transmural echodensity) may prevent the development of significantly accelerated bubbles (Figure 9.8) followed by sudden "popping" and tissue disruption. ICE can also

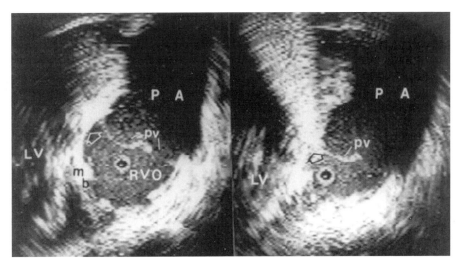

Figure 9.11 Mechanical radial ICE images with the transducer in the right ventricular outflow (RVO), showing the ablation site (arrow, left panel) and an ablation catheter electrode placed just below the pulmonic valve (pv) in the RVO with distal fan-shaped shadow artifact (arrow, right panel) guided by ICE imaging. Each scale = 5 mm. mb: moderator band; PA: pulmonary artery; LV: left ventricle.

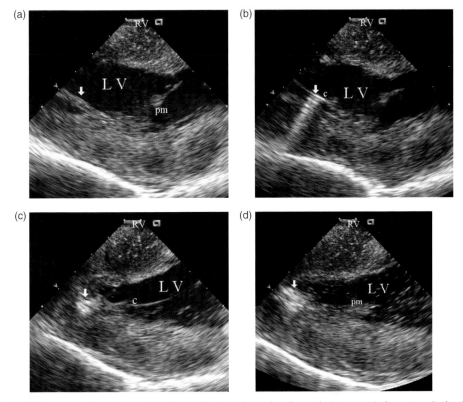

Figure 9.12 ICE images of the left ventricle (LV) with the transducer placed near the interventricular septum in the right ventricle (RV), showing: (a) a false tendon (arrow); (b) ablation catheter electrode "c" positioned at the false tendon (arrow); (c) echogenic lesion (arrow) seen following an initial radiofrequency energy application and (d) increased echogenic lesion size (arrow) following five energy applications at the false tendon in a patient with LV hypertrophy. pm: papillary muscle.

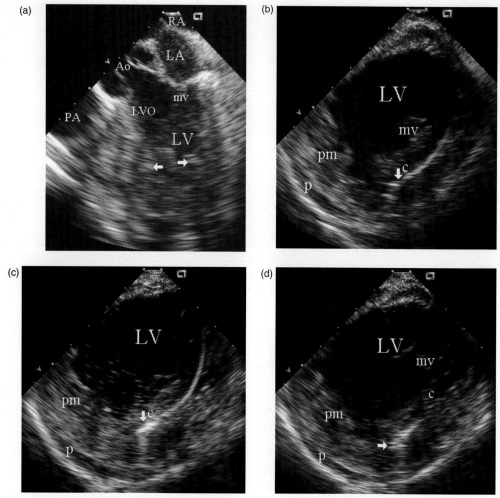

Figure 9.13 (a) ICE image with the transducer placed in the right atrium (RA), showing the left ventricle (LV) with different regions and structures, including LV inflow and outflow tract (LVO), mitral valve (mv) and papillary muscles (arrows). (b–d) Serial ICE images with the transducer placed in the right ventricle (RV), showing the ablation catheter (c) positioned at the posterolateral wall in the LV via a retrograde transaortic approach before radiofrequency ablation (arrow, panel b), accelerated bubbles seen around and echogenic change at the lesion site during ablation (arrow, panel c) and an intramural echogenic lesion development after lesion deployment (arrow, panel d). Ao: aorta; LA: left atrium; p: pericardial echo-free space, representative of epicardial fat or a small loculated anterior effusion; PA: pulmonary artery; pm: anterolateral papillary muscle.

be used to confirm stable catheter tip–endocardial contact and monitoring potential complications.

Ventricular tachycardia from right ventricular outflow tract

Localization of the catheter during activation and pacing mapping can be performed with ICE imaging. The catheter is slowly withdrawn through the pulmonic valve into the right ventricular outflow tract. Anatomic structures such as the pulmonic valve, right ventricular outflow tract, moderator band/papillary muscles, and tricuspid valve can be imaged by ICE during the procedure (Figure 9.9a,b). The ablation catheter can be advanced across the tricuspid valve into the right ventricle guided by ICE imaging or by fluoroscopy. The precise location of the ablation catheter electrode in the right ventricular outflow tract

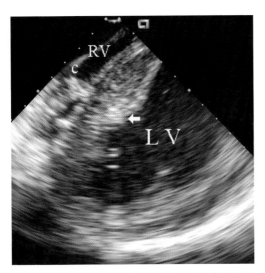

Figure 9.14 ICE image with the transducer placed in the right ventricle (RV), showing the left ventricle (LV) with the ablation catheter (arrow) positioned and energy delivered at the interventricular septum and a focal echogenic lesion identified (arrow). c: catheter.

can be identified by ICE imaging (Figures 9.10a–c and 9.11). Furthermore, ablation electrode–tissue contact, catheter movement and lesion morphology (Figure 9.10d) can be continuously monitored with ICE imaging to avoid any damage to the valvular leaflets or adjacent structures (such as aortic root) and to reduce/avoid significantly accelerated bubble formation which precedes lesion "popping" and tissue disruption.

Ventricular tachycardia from left ventricle

In patients with idiopathic left ventricular tachycardia and/or ventricular tachycardias with structural heart disease (such as ischemic or dilated cardiomyopathy), the mapping/ablation catheter is passed retrograde through the aortic valve or advanced through transseptal catheterization (see Chapter 5) with the tip of the catheter positioned in the interventricular septum and other ventricular wall regions. The relationship of left ventricular idiopathic (Belhassen) ventricular tachycardia to "false tendons" has been proposed [28]. Appropriate target sites for ablation are selected based on endocardial activation mapping [29], identification

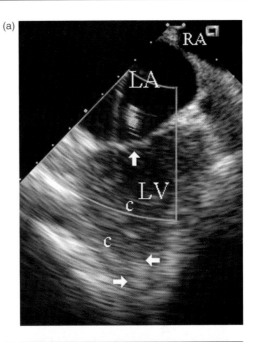

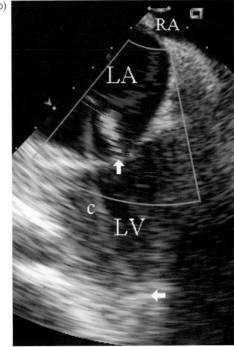

Figure 9.15 ICE images with the transducer placed in the right atrium (RA), showing: (a) the two ablation catheters (c) (one transseptum and the other retrograde) positioned in the apical region (arrows) of the left ventricle (LV); and (b) one catheter (c) moved to the posterolateral apical region (arrow). A mildly mitral regurgitant flow (red mosaic color) is imaged (upward arrow). LA: left atrium.

(a)

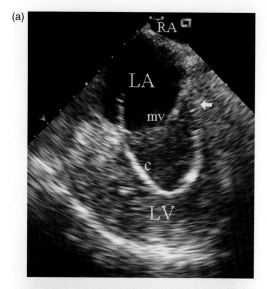

(b)

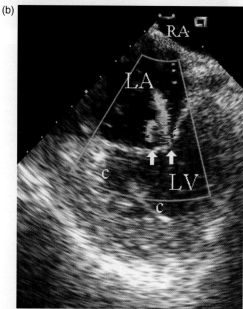

Figure 9.16 ICE images with the transducer placed in the right atrium (RA), showing: (a) the ablation catheter (c) (transseptum) positioned at the area underneath the insertion of the mitral posterior leaflet (arrow); and (b) the two jets of the mitral regurgitant flow (red mosaic color) with the two transseptal catheters (c) passed through the mitral valvular (mv) orifice into the left ventricle (LV). LA: left atrium.

of an isolated mid-diastolic potential [30], concealed entrainment [31] or pacing mapping [32,33]. Ablation is attempted at sites that demonstrate the appropriate mapping criteria [34]. ICE imaging for guiding/monitoring of ventricular tachycardia ablation in the left ventricle has the following goals: (1) track catheter location and assist precise catheter positioning at a specific structure, such as a "false tendon" (Figure 9.12a–d), papillary muscle (Figure 9.13a), or in the different regions of the left ventricle (Figure 9.13b–d), such as the outflow tract, septum (Figure 9.14), apical region (Figure 9.15a,b), and left ventricular base area underneath the insertion of the mitral valve leaflet (Figure 9.16a,b); (2) provide anatomic localization and direct tissue imaging of ischemic with regional wall motion abnormalities and/or infarcted myocardium regions with thinned akinetic/higher echogenic scar (Figure 9.17a–e); (3) monitor catheter electrode–tissue contact and stability without fluoroscopy; (4) monitor lesion morphologic changes (swelling, dimpling, or crater formation with echogenic response) (Figure 9.18a,b), especially after repeated lesions (Figure 9.19a,b), and adjust or terminate energy delivery to reduce or prevent over heating, catheter-tip coagulum or tissue disruption, especially using irrigated radiofrequency energy.

Ventricular tachycardia from the cusps of aortic valve

An unusual origin for repetitive monomorphic ventricular tachycardia in the left ventricular outflow tract region is the cusps of the aortic valve. Importantly, this site of origin may be more common than previously recognized [35–37]. The origin from aortic valve cusps is strongly suggested by the early precordial QRS transition pattern during ventricular tachycardia in lead V_1 or V_2 and broad R wave representing at least 50% of the QRS complex in these leads. A "W" pattern in lead V_1 suggests an origin from or in close proximity to the left coronary cusp [37]. Activation and pace-mapping can be used to further confirm the location. During ablation, failure to appreciate the anatomic relationship of the ablation site and proximal coronary arteries is fraught with

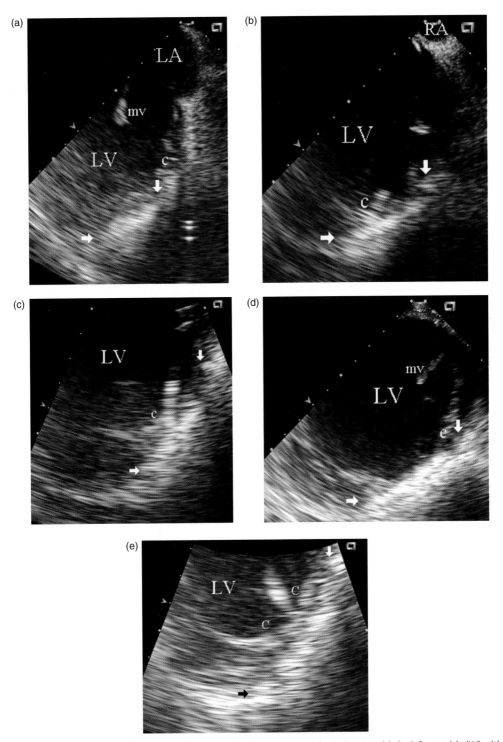

Figure 9.17 Serial ICE images with the transducer placed in the right atrium (RA), showing: (a) the left ventricle (LV) with an old myocardial infarcted region at the middle and lower posteroinferior wall (echogenic scar, between arrows); (b) radiofrequency energy delivered with the ablation catheter "c" positioned at the lower; (c) middle (zoom); and (d) upper portion of the scar region. (e) An inhomogeneous echogenic lesions along the scar (between arrows) developed with ablation (zoom). LA: left atrium; mv: mitral valve.

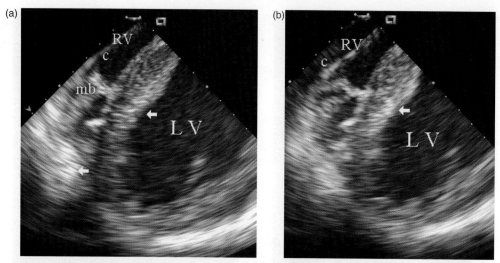

Figure 9.18 ICE images with the transducer placed in the right ventricle (RV), showing: (a) the echocardiographic characteristic changes in the lesion morphology at the left ventricular (LV) septal wall (arrow) before; and (b) after radiofrequency energy delivery. An increased echogenecity and wall thickness with a small crater (arrow) developed at the lesion site are observed after energy application. c: catheter; mb: moderator band.

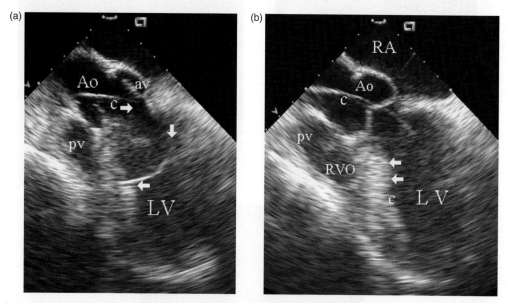

Figure 9.19 ICE images with the transducer placed in the right atrium (RA), showing: (a) left ventricle (LV) outflow with a retrograde ablation catheter (c, arrows) tip positioned at the LV anterolateral wall (leftward arrow) with a strong distal fan-shaped shadow artifact; and (b) a significantly increased wall thickness and echogenic region developed following repeated lesions and the ablation catheter tip "c" moved to the side of the lesions. Ao: aorta; av: aortic valve; pv: pulmonic valve; RVO: right ventricular outflow tract.

considerable peril [38]. Mechanical radial ICE imaging with the transducer placed at the lower anterior portion of the atrial septum adjacent to the aortic root (Figure 9.20a,b) or the base of the right ventricular outflow tract, has been used to guide positioning of the ablation catheter in the aortic root, to the coronary cusps and avoiding coronary ostia [39]. ICE imaging with AcuNav transducer placed in the right atrium

(a)

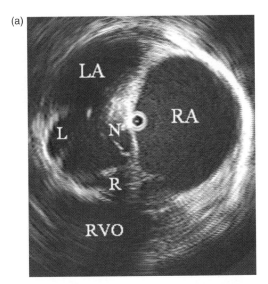

(b)

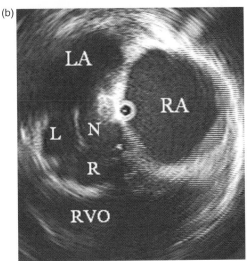

Figure 9.20 Mechanical radial ICE images with the transducer placed at the lower anterior atrial septum of the right atrium (RA) adjacent to the aortic posterior wall, showing: (a) the short-axis view of the aortic root with aortic cusps imaged during systole; and (b) diastole. L: left coronary aortic cusp; LA: left atrium; N: noncoronary aortic cusp; R: right coronary aortic cusp; RVO: right ventricular outflow tract.

(a)

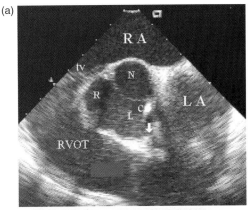

(b)

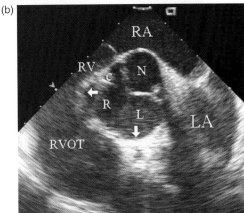

(c)

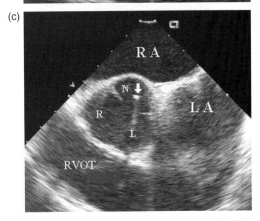

Figure 9.21 (a–c) ICE images with the transducer placed in the right atrium (RA), showing: (a) the ablation catheter electrode (c) positioned in the left coronary aortic cusp (L) area separately (13 mm) to the left main coronary aortic ostium (arrow) during diastole; (b) in the right coronary aortic cusp (R) area separately (9 mm) to the right coronary aortic ostium; and (c) in the noncoronary aortic cusp (N) area. LA: left atrium; RV: right ventricle; RVOT: RV outflow tract; tv: tricuspid valve.

and deflected anteriorly, can provide precise anatomic location of different aortic cusps and coronary arterial ostia (Figure 9.21a–c), and differentiate catheter electrode localization in the aortic sinus of Valsalva or beneath the aortic valve in the left ventricular outflow tract (Figure 9.22a–c). Despite confirmation of a safe anatomic distance, a cautious approach to

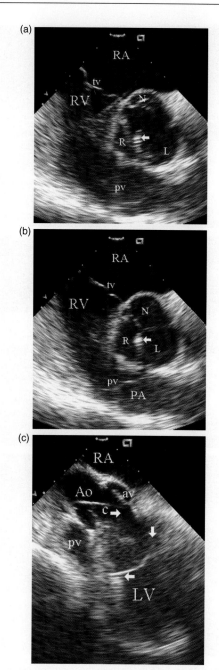

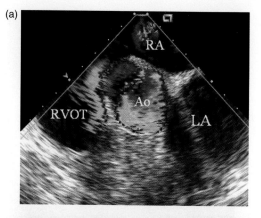

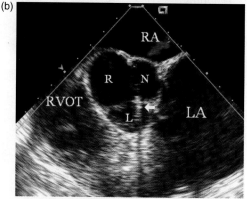

Figure 9.23 (a,b) ICE Doppler color flow images showing: (a) aortic (Ao) color flow at the aortic cusp level during systole (red color forward flow); and (b) diastole (no regurgitant flow seen). Ablation catheter electrode is positioned in the left coronary cusp area (arrow). LA: left atrium; RA and RV: right atrium and ventricle; RVOT: RV outflow tract.

Figure 9.22 ICE images with the transducer placed in the right atrium (RA), showing: (a) a retrograde ablation catheter (arrow) passing through the aortic valvular orifice during systole; and (b) diastole on a short-axis view of the aortic root; and (c) the retrograde catheter (c, arrows) finally reached the anterolateral wall (leftward arrow) in the left ventricle (LV) on the long-axis view of the LV. Ao: aorta; av: aortic valve; L: left coronary aortic cusp; N: noncoronary aortic cusp; PA: pulmonary artery; pv: pulmonic valve; R: right coronary aortic cusp; RV: right ventricle; tv: tricuspid valve.

radiofrequency energy application is required through temperature regulated energy-titrated delivery (up to maximum of 50°C, 30 W) with successful elimination of symptomatic tachycardia anticipated in most patients [37]. The experience both from our group and others [39] represents an important "proof of concept" in demonstrating how ICE imaging can assist mapping and ablation in the left ventricular outflow tract ablation procedures and potentially replace adjunctive coronary angiography in demonstrating a safe distance between the ablation target and the coronary arteries. ICE with Doppler color flow imaging can also be used to monitor and detect aortic valvular regurgitation during and following ablation at the aortic cusp region (Figure 9.23a,b).

Ventricular tachycardia from the epicardial sites of origin

The EKG pattern associated with the epicardial ventricular tachycardia sites of origin just anterior to the aortic valve may mimic the pattern associated and originating from the aortic cusp [37]. If the QRS pattern is predominantly negative in lead I and the QRS during aortic cusp pacemap has a net positive vector in lead I, then an epicardial location for the site of origin must be anticipated and epicardial mapping via pericardial puncture should be performed. Percutaneous transthoracic epicardial mapping and ablation of ventricular tachycardia is a useful ancillary approach to the management of ventricular tachycardia not amenable to ablation by conventional endocardial techniques in patients with ventricular tachycardia due to prior myocardial infarction or Chagas disease [40–45], or idiopathic nonischemic dilated cardiomyopathy [46]. Detailed endocardial and epicardial activation mapping of ventricular tachycardia in the setting of nonischemic cardiomyopathy has identified an epicardial origin in significant minority of patients [46]. ICE may be useful in guiding the subxyphoid/subcostal pericardial puncture (Figure 9.24), monitoring epicardial catheter tip positioning and lesion morphologic changes (Figure 9.25), rapidly detecting unexpected needle puncture passing through the pericardium into the right or left ventricular cavity (Figure 9.26) or identifying potential complications, such as a rapidly accumulating pericardial effusion. Of note, in patients with an increased amount of epicardial fibrous tissue undergoing epicardial ablation procedure using percutaneous pericardial approach, no evidence of bleeding into the pericardial space was noted even with activated clotting times around 200 s [45].

Potential complications

Using an ablation catheter with continuous unmodulated radiofrequency energy delivery without feedback control of catheter tip temperature for ventricular tachycardia, the first death was reported in association with radiofrequency ablation at the right ventricular outflow tract [5]. Perforation of the myocardial wall

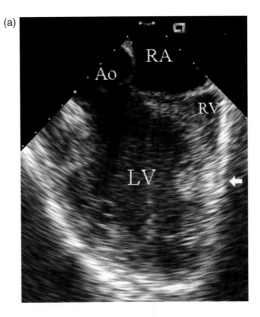

(a)

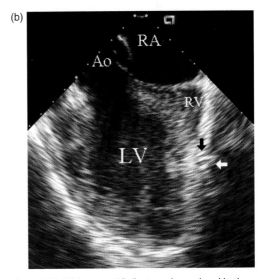

(b)

Figure 9.24 ICE images with the transducer placed in the right atrium (RA), showing: (a) the right ventricular (RV) anteroinferior wall near its apex before subcostal percutaneous pericardial puncture (arrow); and (b) after the puncture needle reached the RV epicardium with distal fan-shaped shadow artifact (arrows). Ao: aorta; LV: left ventricle.

at the lesion site was noted. Other potential complications with attempted ventricular tachycardia ablation including valvular damage resulting in valvular regurgitation, thrombus formation or thromboembolism and pericardial effusion, are presumed to be mainly

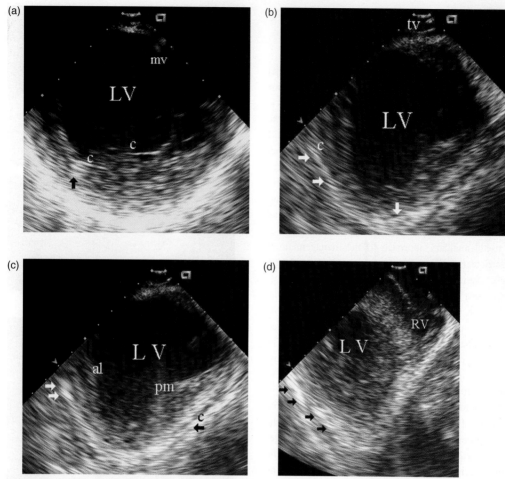

Figure 9.25 ICE images with the transducer placed in the right ventricle (RV) or atrioventricular junction, showing: (a) the left ventricular (LV) endocardial lesions (arrow) at the anterolateral papillary muscle in a patient with ventricular tachycardia due to idiopathic nonischemic dilated cardiomyopathy. (b) After an unsuccessful LV endocardial ablation, the ablation catheter (c) tip was positioned at the epicardial surface of the LV anterolateral wall within the pericardial space (arrows) using a subcostal percutaneous approach. (c) Epicardial ablation lesions developed (rightward arrows) after radiofrequency energy delivery. (d) With the ICE transducer placed in the RV showing an off-axis view of the LV, epicardial lesions (arrows) along the anterolateral wall of the left ventricle are identified. al and pm: anterolateral and posteromedial papillary muscles; tv: tricuspid valve.

related to catheter placement and manipulation. With ICE monitoring of catheter position immediate detection of catheter movement is desirable to avoid inadvertent valvular damage, perforation and pericardial effusion. A low rate of transmural injury with left ventricular lesions created by 4-mm electrode tip radiofrequency energy application eliminates the risk of free wall rupture and significant ablation-induced ventricular dysfunction [11]. However, with novel catheter designs and new energy sources, the depth

and volume of myocardial injury increases with catheter ablation. Online ICE monitoring of lesion formation and morphologic changes can document the early extent of tissue destruction. Acute monitoring of morphologic changes at the lesion site and identification of accelerating bubble formation may reduce or prevent further "popping" and abrupt tissue disruption with potential thromboembolic and hemodynamic consequences. Acute detection of thrombus formation may allow for prompt thrombus elimination

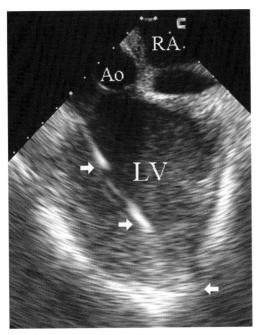

Figure 9.26 ICE image during subcostal needle puncture to access the pericardial space with the transducer placed in the right atrium (RA), showing a guide-wire (arrows) detected in the left ventricle (LV) instead of the pericardial space entering the LV apical wall (leftward arrow) by an unexpected pericardial puncture in a patient with idiopathic nonischemic dilated cardiomyopathy. The wire was safely removed and no evidence of significant bleeding into the pericardial space was found during the procedure and follow up until discharge. Repeat puncture of the pericardial space allowed access for mapping and successful ablation. Ao: aorta.

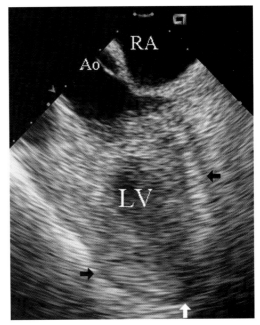

Figure 9.27 ICE image with the transducer placed in the right atrium (RA), showing a small echofree space (2–3 mm) around the left ventricle (LV) during systole representative of an acute, early developing pericardial effusion. Ao: aorta.

by withdrawal of the sheath or catheter under ICE imaging monitoring and appropriate titration of anticoagulation. Pericardial effusion can be detected at its initial stage and heparin effects can be reversed before systematic hemodynamic deterioration (Figure 9.27). With online ICE monitoring during ventricular tachycardia ablation procedures, potential complications may be prevented and/or detected and managed before any clinically serious consequence can occur [47].

References

1 Rahilly GT, Prystowsky EN, Zipes DP, Naccarelli GV, Jackman WM, Heger JJ. Clinical and electrophysiologic findings in patients with repetitive monomorphic ventricular tachycardia and otherwise normal electrocardiogram. *Am J Cardiol* 1982; **50**: 459–468.

2 Morady F, Kadish AH, DiCarlo L, *et al.* Long-term results of catheter ablation of idiopathic right ventricular tachycardia. *Circulation* 1990; **82**: 2093-2099.

3 Delacey WA, Nath S, Haines DE, Barber MJ, DiMarco JP. Adenosine and verapamil-sensitive ventricular tachycardia originating from the left ventricle: radiofrequency catheter ablation. *Pacing Clin Electrophysiol* 1992; **15**: 2240–2244.

4 Jadonath RL, Schwartzman D, Preminger MW, Gottlieb CD, Marchlinski FE. The utility of the 12-lead electrocardiogram in localizing the site of origin of right ventricular outflow tract tachycardia. *Am Heart J* 1995; **130**: 1107–1113.

5 Coggins DL, Lee RJ, Sweeney J, *et al.* Radiofrequency catheter ablation as a cure for idiopathic tachycardia of both left and right ventricular origin. *J Am Coll Cardiol* 1994; **23**: 1333–1341.

6 Movsowitz C, Schwartzman D, Callans DJ, *et al.* Idiopathic right ventricular outflow tract tachycardia: narrowing the anatomic location for successful ablation. *Am Heart J* 1996; **131**: 930–936.

7 Callans DJ, Menz V, Schwartzman D, Gottlieb CD, Marchlinski FE. Repetitive monomorphic tachycardia from the left ventricular outflow tract: electrocardiographic patterns consistent with a left ventricular site of origin. *J Am Coll Cardiol* 1997; **29**: 1023–1027.

8 Marchlinski FE, Deely MP, Zado ES. Gender specific triggers for right ventricular outflow tract tachycardia. *Am Heart J* 2000; **139**: 1009–1013.

9 Dixit S, Marchlinski FE. Clinical characteristics and catheter ablation of left ventricular tract tachycardia. *Curr Cardiol Reports* 2001; **3**: 305–313.

10 Dixit S, Gerstenfeld EP, Callans DJ, Marchlinskli FE. Electrocardiographic patterns of superior right ventricular outflow tract tachycardias: distinguishing septal and free wall sites of origin. *J Cardiovasc Electrophysiol* 2003; **14**: 1–7.

11 Haines DE. Catheter ablation therapy for arrythmias. In: Topol EJ, ed. *Textbook of Cardiovascular Medicine*, 2nd edn. Lippincott Williams & Wilkins, Philadelphia, 2002: 1547–1548, 1559–1564.

12 Wilber DJ, Baerman J Olshansky B, Kall J, Kopp D. Adenosine-sensitive ventricular tachycardia: clinical characteristics and response to catheter ablation. *Circulation* 1993; **87**: 126–134.

13 Klein LS, Shih HT, Hackett FK, Zipes DP, Miles WM. Radiofrequency catheter ablation of ventricular tachycardia in patients without structural heart disease. *Circulation* 1992; **85**: 1666–1674.

14 Calkins H, Kalbfleisch SJ, El-Atassi R, Langberg JJ, Morady F. Relation between efficacy of radiofrequency catheter ablation and site of origin of idiopathic ventricular tachycardia. *Am J Cardiol* 1993; **71**: 827–833.

15 Nakagawa H, Beckman KJ, McClelland JH, *et al.* Radiofrequency catheter ablation of idiopathic left ventricular tachycardia guided by a Purkinje potential. *Circulation* 1993; **94**: 2607–2617.

16 Wen MS, Yeh SJ, Wang CC, Lin FC, Wu D. Successful radiofrequency ablation of idiopathic left ventricular tachycardia at a site away from the tachycardia exit. *J Am Coll Cardiol* 1997; **30**: 1024–1031.

17 Peeters HA, SippensGroenewegen A, Wever EF, *et al.* Clinical application of an integrated 3-phase mapping technique for localization of the site of origin of idiopathic ventricular tachycardia. *Circulation* 1999; **99**: 1300–1311.

18 Tsuchiya T, Okumura K, Honda T, Iwasa A, Yasue H, Tabuchi T. Significance of late diastolic potential preceding Purkinje potential in verapamil-sensitive idiopathic left ventricular tachycardia. *Circulation* 1999; **99**: 2408–2413.

19 Kim YH, Sosa-Suarez G, Trouton TG, *et al.* Treatment of ventricular tachycardia by transcatheter radiofrequency ablation in patients with ischemic heart disease. *Circulation* 1994; **89**: 1094–1102.

20 Callans DJ, Zado E, Sarter BH, Schwartzman D, Gottlieb CD, Marchlinski FE. Efficacy of radiofrequency catheter ablation for ventricular tachycardia in healed myocardial infarction. *Am J Cardiol* 1998; **82**: 429–432.

21 Downar E, Kimber S, Harris L, *et al.* Endocardial mapping of ventricular tachycardia in the intact human heart. II. evidence for multiuse reentry in a functional sheet of surviving myocardium. *J Am Coll Cardiol* 1992; **20**: 869–878.

22 de Bakker JMT, Coronel R, Tasseron S, *et al.* Ventricular tachycardia in the infarcted, Langendorff-perfused human heart: role of the arrangement of surviving cardiac fibers. *J Am Coll Cardiol* 1990; **15**: 1594–1607.

23 Wilber DJ, Kopp DE, Glascock DN, Kinder CA, Kall JG. Catheter ablation of the mitral isthmus for ventricular tachycardia associated with inferior infarction. *Circulation* 1995; **92**: 3481–3489.

24 de Bakker JM, van Capelle FJ, Janse MJ, *et al.* Fractionated electrograms in dilated cardiomyopathy: origin and relation to abnormal conduction. *J Am Coll Cardiol* 1996; **27**: 1071–1078.

25 Cohen TJ, Chien WW, Lurie KG, *et al.* Radiofrequency catheter ablation for treatment of bundle branch reentrant ventricular tachycardia: results and long-term follow-up. *J Am Coll Cardiol* 1991; **18**: 1767–1773.

26 Jongbloed MRM, Bax JJ, Kies P, *et al.* Utility of intracardiac echocardiography to guide radiofrequency catheter ablation of ventricular tachycardia of different etiologies. *J Am Coll Cardiol* 2004; **43**: 359A.

27 Callans DJ, Ren J-F. Ablation of ventricular tachycardia: can the current results be improved using intracardiac echocardiography? In: Raviele A, ed. *Cardiac Arrhythmias.* Springer-Verlag Italia, Milan, 2003: 451–462.

28 Thakur RK, Klein GJ, Sivaram CA, *et al.* Anatomic substrate for idiopathic left ventricular tachycardia. *Circulation* 1996; **93**: 497–501.

29 Josephson ME, Horowitz LN, Farshidi A, Spear JE, Kastor JA, Moore EN. Recurrent sustained ventricular tachycardia II. endocardial mapping. *Circulation* 1978; **57**: 440–447.

30 Fitzgerald DM, Friday KJ, Yeung-Lai-Wah JA, Lazzara R, Jackman WM. Electrogram patterns predicting successful catheter ablation of ventricular tachycardia. *Circulation* 1988; **77**: 806–814.

31 Morady F, kadish A, Rosenheck S, *et al.* Concealed entrainment as a guide for catheter ablation of ventricular tachycardia in patients with prior myocardial infarction. *J Am Coll Cardiol* 1991; **17**: 678–689.

32 Waxman HL, Josephson ME. Ventricular activation during ventricular endocardial pacing: I. electrocardial patterns related to the site of pacing. *Am J Cardiol* 1982; **50**: 1–10.

33 Josephson ME, Waxman HL, Cain ME, Gardner MJ, Bucton AE. Ventricular activation during ventricular endocardial pacing: II. role of pace-mapping to localize origin of ventricular tachycardia. *Am J Cardiol* 1982; **50**: 11–22.

34 Morady F, Harvey M, Kalbfleisch SJ, El-Atassi R, Calkins H, Langberg JJ. Radiofrequency catheter ablation of ventricular tachycardia in patients with coronary artery disease. *Circulation* 1993; **87**: 363–372.

35 Kanagaratnum L, Tomassoni G, Scweiker R, *et al*. Ventricular tachycardia arising from the aortic sinus of valsalva: an under-recognized variant of left ventricular outflow tract tachycardia. *J Am Coll Cardiol* 2001; **37**: 1408–1414.

36 Ouyang F, Fotuhi P, Hebe J, *et al*. Repetitive monomorphic ventricular tachycardia originating from the aortic sinus cusp: electrocardiographic characterization for guiding catheter ablation. *J Am Coll Cardiol* 2002; **39**: 500–508.

37 Marchlinski FE, Lin D, Dixit S, *et al*. Ventricular Tachycardia from the aortic cusps: localization and ablation. In: Raviele A, ed. *Cardiac Arrhythmias*. Springer-Verlag Italia, Milan, 2003: 357–370.

38 Friedman PL, Stevenson WG, Bittl JA, *et al*. Left main coronary artery occlusion during radiofrequency ablation of idiopathic outflow tract ventricular tachycardia (abstr.) *PACE* 1997; **20**: 1185.

39 Lamberti F, Calo L, Pandozi C, *et al*. Radiofrequency catheter ablation of idiopathic left ventricular outflow tract tachycardia: utility of intracardiac echocardiography. *J Cardiovasc Electrophysiol* 2001; **12**: 529–535.

40 Josephson ME. Epicardial approach to the ablation of ventricular tachycardia in coronary artery disease: an alternative or ancillary approach? *J Am Coll Cardiol* 2000; **35**: 1450–1452.

41 Sosa E, Scanavacca M, D'Avila A, Pilleggi F. A new technique to perform epicardial mapping in the electrophysiology laboratory. *J Cardiovasc Electrophysiol* 1996; **7**: 531–536.

42 Sosa E, Scanavacca M, D'Avila A, *et al*. Endocardial and epicardial ablation guided by nonsurgical transthoracic epicardial mapping to treat recurrent ventricular tachycardia. *J Cardiovasc Electrophysiol* 1998; **9**: 229–239.

43 Sosa E, Scanavacca M, D'Avila A, Bellotti G, Piccioni J, Pilleggi F. Radiofrequency catheter ablation of ventricular tachycardia guided by nonsurgical epicardial mapping in chronic Chagasic heart disease. *Pacing Clin Electrophysiol* 1999; **22**: 128–130.

44 Sosa E, Scanavacca M, D'Avila A, Oliveira F, Ramires JAF. Nonsurgical transthoracic epicardial catheter ablation to treat recurrent ventricular tachycardia occurring late after myocardial infarction. *J Am Coll Cardiol* 2000; **35**: 1442–1449.

45 Sosa E, Scanavacca M, D'Avila A, Antonio J, Ramires F. Nonsurgical transthoracic epicardial approach in patients with ventricular tachycardia and previous cardiac surgery. *J Interventional Cardiac Electrophysiol* 2004; **10**: 281–288.

46 Swarup V, Morton JB, Arruda M, Wilber DJ. Ablation of epicardial macroreentrant ventricular tachycardia associated with idiopathic nonischemic dilated cardiomyopathy by a percutaneous transthoracic approach. *J Cardiovasc Electrophysiol* 2002; **13**: 1164–1168.

47 Ren JF, Marchlinski FE, Callans DJ, Herrmann HC. Clinical use of AcuNav diagnostic ultrasound catheter imaging during left heart radiofrequency ablation and transcatheter closure procedures. *J Am Soc Echocardiogr* 2002; **15**: 1301–1308.

CHAPTER 10

Intracardiac Echocardiographic Imaging in Radiofrequency Catheter Ablation in Patients with Ebstein's Anomaly

Jian-Fang Ren, MD, *& David J. Callans*, MD

Imaging the anatomic features of Ebstein's anomaly

Normally, the basal attachment of the septal tricuspid valve leaflet is positioned slightly more apically than the corresponding mitral valve leaflet; in fact, this serves as a landmark for identifying the right ventricle (Figure 10.1). Ebstein's anomaly is characterized by an excessive apical displacement of both the septal and the posterior tricuspid valve leaflets [1,2]. There is a variable degree of displacement of the proximal attachments of the tricuspid valve leaflets from the atrioventricular ring, and the distance between insertion sites of the two atrioventricular valves is diagnostic. A distance of greater than 8 mm/m^2 normalized for body surface area [3] or a maximum displacement of more than 20 mm [4] are the diagnostic criteria of Ebstein's anomaly. Just as the apical displacement may range from mild to severe, the natural history and clinical course of the syndrome are highly variable. The pathologic anatomy of Ebstein's anomaly is best demonstrated by echocardiography as well as intracardiac echocardiography (ICE) imaging [5]. An apical displacement and downward attachment of the septal leaflet is best visualized with the ICE imaging transducer placed in the right atrium during diastole and systole (Figure 10.2a,b). Typically, the leaflets are elongated and redundant with abnormal chordal attachments and the extent of leaflet tethering of the tricuspid valve can be assessed in multiple views (Figures 10.3 and 10.4). The anterior tricuspid leaflet

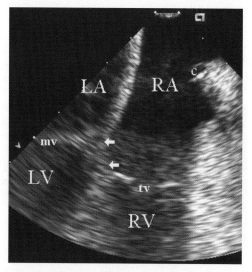

Figure 10.1 ICE image with the transducer in the high right atrium (RA) with its tip deflected slightly to the left, showing a four-chamber view of a structurally normal heart. The insertion of the septal tricuspid leaflet (tv) exhibits slight apical displacement (7 mm, between the arrows) compared to the anterior mitral leaflet (mv). c: catheter; LA and LV: left atrium and ventricle; RV: right ventricle.

is frequently larger, redundant and sail-like, and generally its basal attachment is at the atrioventricular level as compared to the tethered septal and/or posterior leaflets which are apically displaced (Figure 10.5a,b).

As a consequence of the apical displacement of the septal and posterior tricuspid leaflets, the right

(a) 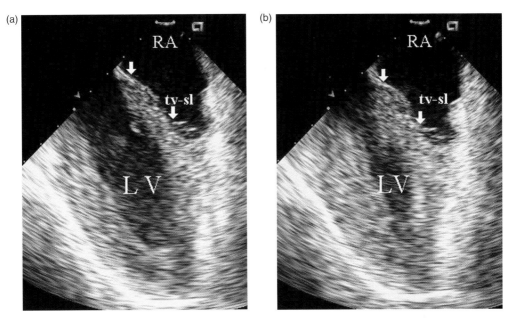 (b)

Figure 10.2 ICE images with the transducer placed in the right atrium (RA), showing apical displacement (27 mm, between the arrows) of the septal tricuspid leaflet (tv-sl) compared to the mitral valve inserted annulus: (a) during diastole; and (b) systole. LV: left ventricle.

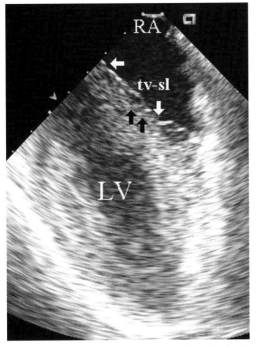

Figure 10.3 ICE image with the transducer placed in the right atrium (RA), showing tethering septal tricuspid leaflet (tv-sl, between the white arrows) to the septal wall (black arrows). LV: left ventricle.

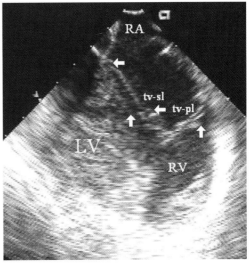

Figure 10.4 ICE image with the transducer tip deflected slightly left-anteriorly in the right atrium (RA), showing the septal (tv-sl, between the horizontal arrows) and posterior (tv-pl) tricuspid leaflets with tethering (upward arrows) to the septal and posterolateral wall, respectively. LV and RV: left and right ventricle.

(a)

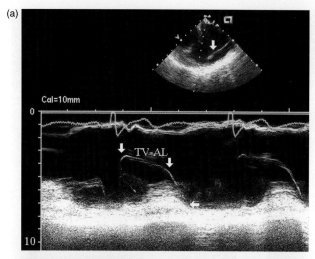

(b)

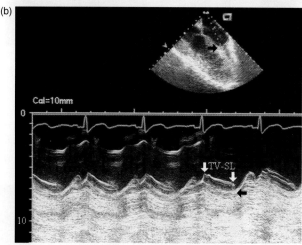

Figure 10.5 ICE M-mode recordings showing: (a) the large anterior tricuspid leaflet (TV-AL, arrow) with sail-like motion (between the arrows); (b) compared to the septal tricuspid leaflet (TV-SL, arrow) which has more limited motion during cardiac cycle.

heart consists of three portions including the true right atrium, the functional right ventricle, and an atrialized right ventricle, which is anatomically ventricular but functionally atrial tissue (Figure 10.6). This atrialized portion of the ventricle may be thinner than normal [6], frequently resulting in dilatation or even in aneurysm formation [2], located between the anatomic tricuspid annulus and the apically displaced posterior leaflet (Figure 10.6). The degree of atrialization of the right ventricle can be quantitatively evaluated by a variety of indices, such as the ratio of the area of the functional right ventricle to the total right ventricular area. If the ratio is less than 35%, the overall prognosis is poor [7,8]. In patients with Ebstein's anomaly, tricuspid regurgitation is commonly seen and can be detected using

ICE Doppler color flow imaging (Figure 10.7a,b). In adult patients with isolated Ebstein's anomaly and Wolff–Parkinson–White (WPW) syndrome, some of the pathological features are less pronounced than in children, since the malformations of the tricuspid valve associated with complex congenital malformations (such as pulmonary atresia, tetralogy of Fallot, or congenitally corrected transposition of the great arteries) are more severe.

Wolff–Parkinson–White syndrome (WPW) in Ebstein's anomaly

The anatomic substrates underlying WPW syndrome are persistent atrioventricular connections that bypass all or portions of the atrioventricular node/His bundle complex [9]. The incidence of single and multiple accessory pathways is high in Ebstein's anomaly, and many patients initially present with tachyarrhythmias. Most of these tachycardias are based on accessory pathways located along the anomalous

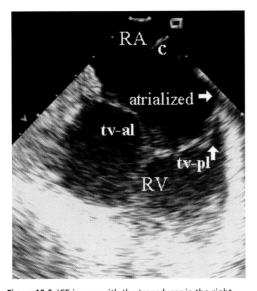

Figure 10.6 ICE image with the transducer in the right atrium (RA), showing apical displacement of the tricuspid orifice which consists of an elongated anterior tricuspid leaflet (tv-al) and a posterior leaflet (tv-pl) with tethered to the posterolateral wall (upward arrow). Aneurysmal dilation (rightward arrow) of the atrialized portion of the right ventricle (RV) between the anatomic tricuspid annulus and the apically displaced tv-pl is also seen. c: Catheter.

atrioventricular valve, found in up to 30% of this patient cohort [10]. Accessory pathways are anomalous bands of conducting tissue that form a connection between the atrium and ventricle, "bypassing" the normal atrioventricular conducting system. The majority of these accessory pathways have both antegrade and retrograde conduction properties and account for the WPW syndrome, with preexcitation during sinus rhythm in combination with paroxysmal atrioventricular reentry tachycardia. Some accessory pathways show only retrograde conduction properties, precipitating the same type of tachycardia but without preexcitation during sinus rhythm. Defects in the continuity of the annulus fibrosus may account for the subendocardial location of many right-side accessory pathyways, particularly those associated with abnormalities in the development of the atrioventricular ring, and may explain the high incidence of preexcitation syndromes in patients with Ebstein's anomaly [9,11]. Left free wall pathways usually represent residual, subepicardial, atrioventricular bridges of myocardium that fail to regress during fetal development. In congenitally corrected transposition of the great arteries, there is an increased incidence of Ebstein's anomaly of the left-sided (systemic) tricuspid valve [12–14]. Furthermore, the increased incidence of the WPW syndrome in this disorder is explained by the coexistence of Ebstein's anomaly [10]. In the case of antegrade conducting pathways, preexcitation during sinus rhythm may lead to pseudonormalization of the QRS-pattern by bridging the delayed conduction through the atrialized ventricle. Patients

(a)

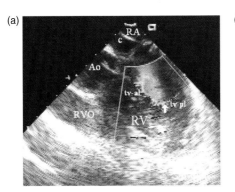

(b)

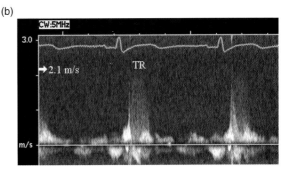

Figure 10.7 ICE images with the transducer placed in the right atrium (RA), showing: (a) Doppler color flow image of tricuspid regurgitant (TR) flow (red mosaic color, toward the RA); and (b) continuous-wave Doppler velocity spectral recording of a mildly TR jet measured at 2.1 m/s (estimated 28 mmHg of the pulmonary arterial systolic pressure gradient). Ao: aorta; c: catheter; RV: right ventricle; RVO: RV outflow tract; tv-al and tv-pl: anterior and septal tricuspid leaflets.

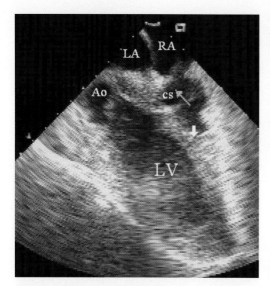

Figure 10.8 ICE image with the transducer placed in the right atrium (RA), showing the coronary sinus (cs) ostium (leftward oblique arrow) just anteromedial to the inferior vena cava orifice, and the apically displaced insertion of the septal tricuspid leaflet (downward arrow). The atrialized right ventricle is localized between the CS and the displaced leaflets. Ao: aortic root; LA and LV: left atrium and ventricle.

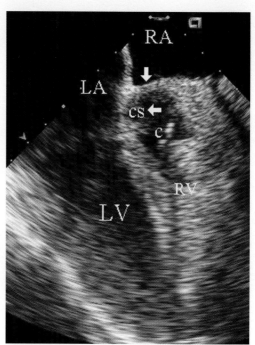

Figure 10.9 ICE image with the transducer in the right atrium (RA), showing the coronary sinus ostium (cs, leftward arrow) with Chiari network (downward arrow) extending between the inferior vena caval (eustachian) valve and the coronary sinus (thebesian) valve. The catheter (c) tip is shown in contact with the functional right ventricle (RV). LA and LV: left atrium and ventricle.

with WPW syndrome are prone to orthodromic and antidromic atrioventricular tachycardia. During orthodromic atrioventricular tachycardia, antegrade conduction to the ventricles is through the atrioventricular node/His–Purkinje system (resulting in a narrow QRS), and retrograde conduction to the atria is through the accessory pathway. As a result of the high incidence of multiple accessory pathways in patients with Ebstein's anomaly, preexcited atrioventricular tachycardia is observed using an antegrade conducting accessory pathway as the antegrade (atrioventricular) limb and either the normal conduction system or another accessory pathway as the retrograde (ventriculoatrial) one. The resulting surface ECG shows a wide QRS tachycardia with maximal preexcitation. For unclear reasons, atrioventricular reentry tachycardias may induce atrial fibrillation, which in combination to the existence of fast antegrade conducting accessory pathway may lead to death due to rapid ventricular rates and resultant ventricular fibrillation [10].

Antidromic tachycardia is also observed in patients with Mahiam fibers, a distinct rare subgroup of the preexcitation syndromes, which account for up to 13% of the patients with Ebstein's anomaly

and preexcitation [11,15]. Mahiam fibers are decrementally conducting antegrade-only accessory pathways, and have a course between the atrium or atrioventricular node and the ventricle or right bundle branch. The characteristic decremental conduction is caused by interposed atrioventricular node-like conduction tissue, either due to the atrioventricular node proper (in nodofascicular or nodoventricular pathways) or ectopic atrioventricular node tissue (in atriofascicular or atrioventricular pathways) typically located from the posterior to lateral aspect of the tricuspid valve [16–18]. Mahiam fibers conduction may mask the usual QRS morphology observed in Ebstein's anomaly by bridging the delayed antegrade conduction to the atrialized right ventricle.

Non-accessory pathway related acquired tachycardias are also observed in Ebstein's anomaly due to pathological myocardial alterations (hypertrophy, fibrosis, and chamber dilatation) and/or residual myocardial scars after surgery. Generally, these

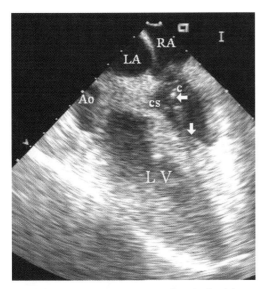

Figure 10.10 ICE image with the transducer in the right atrium (RA), showing the catheter tip (c) reaching to the level of the coronary sinus (cs) (leftward arrow) and directed 1 cm right-anteriorly to the ostium after pulling back from the functional right ventricle (below the displaced septal leaflet, downward arrow) under ICE imaging guidance. Ao: aorta; LA and LV: left atrium and ventricle.

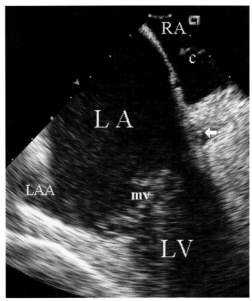

Figure 10.12 ICE image with the transducer in the right atrium (RA) and its tip rotated slightly clockwise, showing a little of the distal lumen of the coronary sinus and a catheter (arrow) inside the coronary sinus with a distal echo shadowing artifact. Successful coronary sinus entry is confirmed. c: catheter; LA and LV: left atrium and ventricle; LAA: LA appendage; mv: mitral valve.

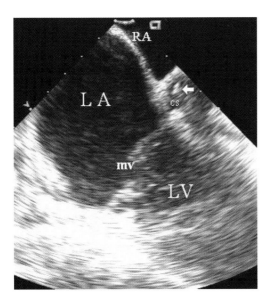

Figure 10.11 ICE image with the transducer in the right atrium (RA), showing the catheter just entering to the coronary sinus (cs) ostium (arrow) with its tip advancing left-posteriorly under ICE imaging guidance. LA and LV: left atrium and ventricle; mv: mitral valve.

acquired tachycardias include atrial fibrillation, typical atrial flutter, and incisional atrial tachycardia. Premature ventricular contractions occasionally occur, but spontaneous sustained ventricular tachycardias are rare, except in the early postoperative period. Ventricular fibrillation can be induced by catheter manipulation in the electrically sensitive atrialized right ventricle or during transvenous placement of the ventricular pacemaker leads [10,19–21].

Guiding coronary sinus catheterization in the atrialized right ventricle

Coronary sinus catheterization is routinely used during mapping and ablation procedures. The coronary sinus is located posteriorly and slightly caudal to the tricuspid annulus. In the electrophysiologic procedures coronary sinus cannulation is generally performed via the right internal jugular or femoral venous approach under fluoroscopic guidance. With the former approach [22], the catheter tip is initially pointed laterally toward the right atrial border

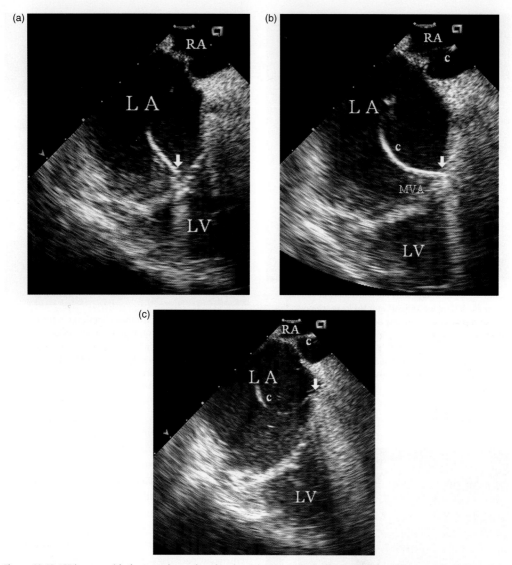

Figure 10.13 ICE images with the transducer placed in the right atrium (RA), showing a coronal cross-sectional view of the left atrium (LA) and ventricle (LV), and a mapping/ablation catheter "c" with its tip (arrow, with distal fan-shaped shadow artifact) positioned along (a) the lateral, (b) the posterolateral, and (c) the medial mitral annulus, respectively.

in the right anterior oblique projection. The catheter is then rotated counterclockwise and advanced slightly until it just enters the right ventricle. After slight additional counterclockwise rotation, the catheter is withdrawn slowly until it engages the coronary sinus ostium. Gentle readvancement of the catheter from this position leads to cannulation of the coronary sinus. Successful coronary sinus entry is confirmed by the lateral position of the catheter in the left anterior

oblique plane and by electrical recordings of sharp atrial and ventricular signals.

In patients with Ebstein's anomaly, however, the anatomic level and orientation of the coronary sinus ostium and tricuspid annulus are different from normal due to the apically displaced septal, posterior tricuspid leaflets, and the atrialized right ventricle. These morphologic and pathologic changes may prevent successful coronary sinus cannulation under

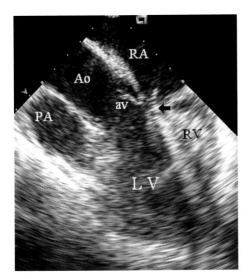

Figure 10.14 ICE image with the transducer placed in the right atrium (RA), showing the catheter tip at the His position (arrow) which is anterior to the ostium of the coronary sinus and directly above the insertion of the septal tricuspid leaflet, with a strong distal fan-shaped shadow artifact. Ao: aorta; av: aortic valve; LV and RV: left and right ventricle; PA: pulmonary artery.

fluoroscopic guidance, in which the coronary sinus ostium and anatomic structures are not visualized directly and the catheter is entirely manipulated by its position in the cardiac silhouette. ICE may provide real-time anatomic imaging and guide coronary sinus catheter manipulation by imaging the coronary sinus ostium in relationship to the displaced septal or posterior tricuspid leaflets (Figure 10.8) and the actual position of the catheter tip in relationship to the coronary sinus ostium (Figure 10.9). Under ICE imaging guidance the catheter is initially positioned at the accurate level of the coronary sinus ostium (Figure 10.10), then adjusted in terms of orientation (generally left posterior), and then advanced into the coronary sinus ostium (Figure 10.11). Successful coronary sinus entry is easily confirmed by clockwise rotation of the imaging catheter to show the distal lumen of the coronary sinus with the catheter visualized inside (Figure 10.12).

ICE guidance for accessory pathway ablation in patients with Ebstein's anomaly

The basis of arrhythmias in the WPW syndrome and its variants is the presence of accessory atrioventricular connections. These variants include the concealed (retrograde-only) bypass tracts, the permanent form of junctional reciprocating tachycardia (which is caused by a slowly conducting retrograde-only bypass tract), and Mahiam fibers [23]. In patients with symptomatic tachycardias independent of the type of pathway, catheter ablation of the accessory connections using radiofrequency energy has become the treatment of choice. The use of electrophysiologic studies for the localization of accessory atrioventricular connections in WPW syndrome requires accurate evaluation of the site of bypass tract insertion. The high success rate of radiofrequency ablation of accessory pathways is related to accurate mapping. In patients with Ebstein's anomaly, precise localization of the accessory connection may be impaired by the presence of multiple pathways and by their often complex course along the dysplastic tricuspid annulus and the atrialized right ventricle, a region where abnormal endocardial electrograms have been reported to originate [10,19]. Successful ablation is often difficult in patients with Ebstein's anomaly, especially for older patients who have large hearts with poorly defined atrioventricular grooves, leading to a lack of specificity for what appear to be excellent electrophysiologic signals in predicting a successful ablation site [24]. In addition, catheter stabilization for free wall pathways in enlarged hearts is difficult [25].

ICE is superior to angiography and X-ray modalities for defining the special orientation of anatomic structures. ICE was initially used for defining intracardiac anatomic landmarks, at first in the right heart with mechanical radial imaging [26–28] and subsequently in both the left and right heart with electronic phased-array sector imaging [29,30]. ICE can provide accurate identification of atrial and ventricular landmarks, such as an anatomic and functional tricuspid annulus with Ebstein's anomaly (Figure 10.6) and can be used to guide mapping or ablation catheter positioning at a precise location of the atrioventricular groove, such as at the tricuspid annulus [31] and along the mitral annulus (Figure 10.13a–c). Although catheter ablation has become routine for patients with symptomatic WPW syndrome because of its high efficacy (95%) and low risk [32,33], radiofrequency ablation for septal accessory pathways close to the atrioventricular node or His bundle still carries a high risk of developing complete heart block. ICE can provide accurate anatomic imaging of the His location (Figure 10.14) and

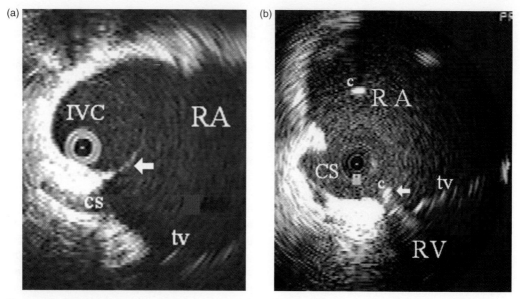

Figure 10.15 Mechanical radial ICE images with the transducer placed at the orifice of the inferior vena cava (IVC) with the eustachian valve (arrow) seen in the right atrium (RA), showing: (a) the ostium of the coronary sinus (cs) and the septal tricuspid leaflet (tv), the postero-septal aspect of the tricuspid annulus located between the insertion of tv and cs ostium; and (b) the ablation catheter (c) positioned at the tricuspid annulus (arrow). Echogenic swelling is seen at the site where radiofrequency lesions were delivered. The radius of the images = 40 mm. c: catheter; RV: right ventricle.

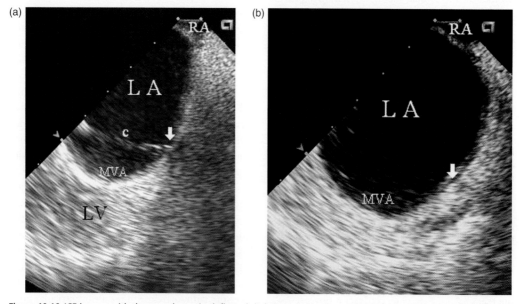

Figure 10.16 ICE images with the transducer tip deflected slightly and placed near the posterior interatrial septum in the right atrium (RA), showing: (a) a left atrial (LA) ablation catheter (c) tip (arrow) with good tissue contact, positioned at the posterolateral mitral annulus (MVA) Pre-ablation; and (b) an echogenic lesion (arrow) that developed following ablation. LV: left ventricle.

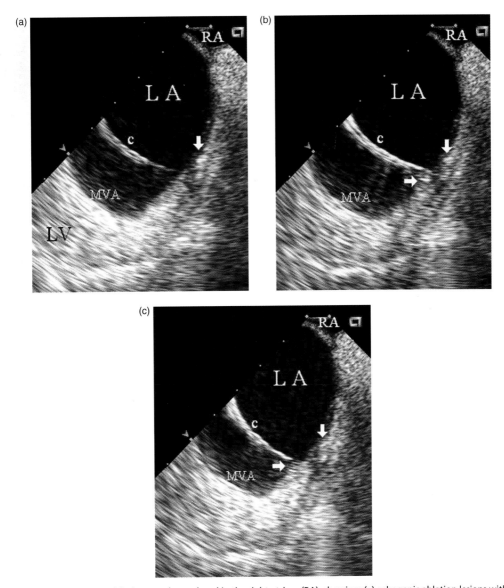

Figure 10.17 ICE images with the transducer placed in the right atrium (RA), showing: (a) echogenic ablation lesions with craters (arrow) following repeated left atrial (LA) ablation at the posterolateral mitral annulus (MVA); (b and c) serial lesions with wall swelling (rightward arrow) with ablation catheter "c" moving along the mitral annulus. LV: left ventricle.

guide power-titration of radiofrequency output [34]. The relevant anatomy surrounding the atrioventricular conduction system is defined by the triangle of Koch which is formed by the tricuspid annulus and the tendon of Todaro. The compact atrioventricular node is a superficial structure lying just beneath the right atrial endocardium, anterior to the ostium of

the coronary sinus, and directly above the insertion of the septal tricuspid leaflet [35]. According to both electrophysiologic and anatomic criteria, the slow pathway can be ablated close to the superior rim of the coronary sinus ostium at the posterior septal aspect of the tricuspid annulus. Slow pathway modification is the primary approach for cure of atrioventricular node reentry and can be accurately guided by ICE imaging [36] (Figure 10.15a,b). For ablation of left accessory atrioventricular connections, the transseptal approach to the atrial site of the mitral annulus is very safe and highly effective [37]. The atrial aspect of mitral annulus and left atrial posterolateral wall is a relatively smooth, nonobstructed surface that simplifies catheter movement, thereby permitting rapid and accurate accessory pathway location and ablation. During the ablation procedure ICE can provide real-time monitoring of catheter electrode–tissue contact and lesion morphologic changes (Figure 10.16a,b). With repeated radiofrequency ablation, serial lesions with swelling and crater development can be visualized and evaluated along the mitral annulus–left atrial posterior wall (Figure 10.17a–c). The high success rate of radiofrequency catheter ablation delivered from the endocardial approach implies that most pathways are situated closely to the endocardial surface. However, a small proportion of left free wall accessory pathways (1–4%) can only be ablated successfully from the epicardial approach via the coronary sinus and probably represent true epicardial pathways [38,39]. Transthoracic epicardial catheter ablation with ICE imaging assistance (see Chapter 9) may be effective in eliminating the rare epicardial accessory pathway which has failed attempts at conventional endocardial and coronary venous system approaches [40]. During the ablation procedure, it is possible with ICE imaging monitoring to immediately identify procedure-related complications, such as pericardial effusion, inadvertent damage to cardiac structure and thrombus formation. Immediate diagnosis can prevent more serious consequence, particularly in the setting of pericardial effusion during procedures that require high-intensity anticoagulation [30,41].

References

1 Aaron BL, Mills M, Lower RR. Congenital tricuspid insufficiency: definition and review. *Chest* 1976; **69**: 637–641.

2 Oechslin E, Buchholz S, Jenni R. Ebstein's anomaly in adults: Doppler-echocardiographic evaluation. *Thorac Cardiovasc Surg* 2000; **48**: 209–213.

3 Shiina A, Seward JB, Edwards WD, Hagler DJ, Tajik AJ. Two-dimensional echocardiographic spectrum of Ebstein's anomaly: detailed anatomic assessment. *J Am Coll Cardiol* 1984; **3**: 356–370.

4 Gussenhoven EJ, Stewart PA, Becker AE, Essed CE, Ligtovoet KM, DeVilleneuve VH. "Offsetting" of the septal tricuspid leaflet in normal hearts and in hearts with Ebstein's anomaly. *Am J Cardiol* 1984; **54**: 172–176.

5 Ren JF, Schwartzman D, Marchlinski FE, Brode SE, Lighty GW, Chaudhry FA. Intracardiac ultrasound catheter imaging in Ebstein's anomaly. *J Cardiovasc Diagnosis and Procedures* 1997; **14**: 173–176.

6 Anderson KR, Lie JT. The right ventricular myocardium in Ebstein's anomaly: a morphometric histologic study. *Mayo Clin Proc* 1979; **54**: 181–184.

7 Shiina A, Seward JB, Tajik AJ, Hagler DJ, Danielson GK. Two-dimensional echocardiographic-surgical correlation in Ebstein's anomaly: preoperative determination of patients requiring tricuspid valve plication versus replacement. *Circulation* 1983; **68**: 534–544.

8 Celermajer DS, Bull C, Till JA, *et al.* Ebstein's anomaly: presentation and outcome from fetus to adult. *J Am Coll Cardiol* 1994; **23**: 170–176.

9 Cain ME, Lindsay BD. Preexcitation syndromes: diagnostic and management strategies. In: Horowitz LN, ed. *Current Management of Arrhythmias.* B.C. Decker, Inc., Philadelphia, 1991: 91–92.

10 Hebe J. Ebstein's anomaly in adults. Arrhythmias: diagnosis and therapeutic approach. *Thorac Cardiov Surg* 2000; **48**: 214–219.

11 Smith WM, Gallagher JJ, Kerr CR, *et al.* The electrophysiologic basis and management of symptomatic recurrent tachycardia in patients with Ebstein's anomaly of the tricuspid valve. *Am J Cardiol* 1982; **49**: 1223–1234.

12 Becu LM, Swam JHJC, Du Shane JW, Edwards JE. Ebstein malformation of the left atrioventricular valve in corrected transposition of the great vessels with ventricular septal defect. *Mayo Clin Proc* 1975; **30**: 483–490.

13 Anderson KR, Danielson GK, McGoon DC, Lie JT. Ebstein's anomaly of the left-sided tricuspid valve: pathological anatomy of the valvular malformation. *Circulation* 1978; **58**(suppl. 1): 87–91.

14 Silverman NH, Gerlis LM, Horowitz ES, Ho SY, Neches WH, Anderson RH. Pathological elucidation of the echocardiographic features of Ebstein's malformation of the morphologically tricuspid valve in discordant atrioventricular connections. *Am J Cardiol* 1995; **76**: 1277–1283.

15 Ward DE, Camm J, Cory-Pearce R, Fuenmayor I, Rees GM, Spurrell RA. Ebstein's anomaly in association with anomalous nodoventricular conduction: preoperative and intraoperative electrophysiological studies. *J Electrocardiol* 1979; **12**: 227–233.

16 Anderson RH, Ho SY. Anatomy of the atrioventricular junctions with regard to ventricular preexcitation. *Pacing Clin Electrophysiol* 1997; **20**: 2072–2076.

17 Brugada J, Martinez SJ. Radiofrequency catheter ablation of atrioventricular accessory pathways guided by discrete electrical potentials recorded at the tricuspid annulus. *Pacing Clin Electrophysiol* 1995; **18**: 1388–1394.

18 Schoen WJ, Fujimura O. Variant preexcitation syndrome: a true nodoventricular Mahiam fiber or an accessory atrioventricular pathway with decremental properties? *J Cardiovasc Electrophysiol* 1995; **6**: 1117–1123.

19 Kastor JA, Goldreyer BN, Josephson ME, *et al.* Electrophysiologic characteristics of Ebstein's anomaly of the tricuspid valve. *Circulation* 1975; **52**: 987–995.

20 Oh JK, Holmers DR Jr, Porter CB, Danielson GK. Cardiac arrhythmias in patients with surgical repair of Ebstein's anomaly. *J Am Cardiol* 1985; **6**: 1351–1357.

21 Watson H. Natural history of Ebstein's anomaly of the tricuspid valve in childhood and adolescence: an international cooperative study of 505 cases. *Br Heart J* 1974; **36**: 417–427.

22 Chou TM, Zellner C, Kern MJ. Evaluation of myocardial blood flow and metabolism, chapter 18. In: Baim DS, Grossman W, eds. *Grossman's Cardiac Catheterization, Angiography, and Intervention*, 6th edn. Lippincott Williams & Wilkins, Philadelphia, 2000; 403–404.

23 Plumb VJ. Catheter ablation of the accessory pathways of the Wolff–Pakinson–White syndrome and its variants. *Progress in Cardiovasc Dis* 1995; **37**: 295–306.

24 Levine JC, Walsh EP, Saul JP. Radiofrequency ablation of accessory pathways associated with congenital heart disease including heterotaxy syndrome. *Am J Cardiol* 1993; **72**: 689–693.

25 Saul JP, Hulse JE, De W, Lock JE, Walsh EP. Catheter manipulation for ablation of accessory atrioventricular pathways in young patients: use of long vascular sheath, the transseptal approach and a retrograde left posterior parallel approach. *J Am Coll Cardiol* 1993; **21**: 571–583.

26 Schwartz SL, Gillam ID, Weintraub AR, *et al.* Intracardiac echocardiography in humans using a small-sized (6 F), low frequency (12.5 MHz) ultrasound catheter: methods, imaging planes, and clinical experience. *J Am Coll Cardiol* 1993; **21**: 189–198.

27 Chu E, Fitzpatrick AP, Chin MC, Sudhir K, Yock PG, Lesh MD. Radiofrequency catheter ablation guided by intracardiac echocardiography. *Circulation* 1994; **89**: 1301–1305.

28 Ren JF, Schwartzman D, Callans D, Marchlinski FE, Gottlieb CD, Chaudhry FA. Imaging technique and clinical utility for electrophysiologic procedures of lower frequency (9 MHz) intracardiac echocardiography. *Am J Cardiol* 1998; **82**: 1557–1560.

29 Packer DL, Stevens CL, Curley MG, *et al.* Intracardiac phased-array imaging: methods and initial clinical experience with high resolution, under blood visualization: initial experience with intracardiac phased-array ultrasound. *J Am Coll Cardiol* 2002; **39**: 509–516.

30 Ren JF, Marchlinski FE, Callans DJ, Herrmann HC. Clinical use of AcuNav diagnostic ultrasound catheter imaging during left heart radiofrequency ablation and transcatheter closure procedures. *J Am Soc Echocardiogr* 2002; **15**: 1301–1308.

31 Ren JF, Schwartzman D, Callans DJ, Marchlinski FE, Zhang LP, Chaudhry FA. Intracardiac echocardiographic imaging in guiding and monitoring radiofrequency catheter ablation at tricuspid annulus. *Echocardiography* 1998; **15**: 661–664.

32 Worley SJ. Use of a real-time three-dimensional magnetic navigation system for radiofrequency ablation of accessory pathways. *PACE* 1998; **21**: 1636–1645.

33 Ganz LI, Friedman PL. Medical progress: supraventricular tachycardia. *N Engl J Med* 1995; **332**: 162–173.

34 Lin JL, Huang SK, Lai LP, Cheng TF, Tseng YZ, Lien WP. Radiofrequency catheter ablation of septal accessory pathways within the triangle of Koch: importance of energy titration testing other than the local electrogram characteristics for identifying the successful target site. *PACE* 1998; **21**: 1909–1917.

35 Zipes DP. Genesis of cardiac arrhythmias: electrophysiological considerations. In: Braunwald E, ed. *Heart Disease – A Textbook of Cardiovascular Medicine*, 3rd edn. WB Saunders, Philadelphia, 1988: 582–583.

36 Ren JF, Marchlinski FE. Intracardiac ultrasound catheter imaging for electrophysiologic substrate of AV node reentrant tachycardia: anatomic versus electrophysiologic evidence. *J Cardiovasc Electrophysiol* 2004; **15**: 274–275.

37 Montenero AS, Crea F, Bendini MG, Bellocci F, Zecchi P. Catheter ablation of left accessory atrioventricular connections: the transseptal approach. *J Interventional Cardiol* 1995; **8**: 806–812.

38 Morady F, Strickberger A, Man KC, *et al.* Reasons for prolonged or failed attempts at radiofrequency catheter ablation of accessory pathways. *J Am Coll Cardiol* 1996; **27**: 683–689.

39 Haine DE. Catheter ablation therapy for arrhythmias. In: Topol EJ, ed. *Textbook of Cardiovascular Medicine*, 2nd edn. Lippincott Williams & Wilkins, Philadelphia, 2002; 1551–1553.

40 de Paola AA, Leite LR, Mesas CE. Nonsurgical transthoracic epicardial ablation for the treatment of a resistant posteroseptal accessory pathway. *PACE* 2004; **27**: 259–261.

41 Ren JF, Schwartzman D, Callans DJ, Brode SE, Gottlieb CD, Marchlinski FE. Intracardiac echocardiography (9 MHz) in humans: methods, imaging views, and clinical utility. *Ultrasound in Med & Biol* 1999; **25**: 1077–1086.

CHAPTER 11

Monitoring and Early Diagnosis of Procedural Complications

Jian-Fang Ren, MD, *& Francis E. Marchlinski,* MD

One of the important roles for intracardiac echocardiography (ICE) imaging is in the recognition and prevention of potential complications during interventional electrophysiologic procedures. Although various potential complications have been described in the previous individual chapters, it is important to have a dedicated focused chapter on this subject and provide a summary account with empirical emphasis and additional illustrations as a further reference for the readers.

Damage to intracardiac structures

Importantly, ICE can provide the proper imaging view of the interatrial septum (Figure 11.1a) and the structures around it to guide and facilitate safe transseptal puncture. Just as it is critical to the successful identification of the septum so is the recognition of the adjacent structures and the impact of inadvertent manipulation of the catheter during transseptal catheterization or mapping/ablation may cause damage to adjacent nonseptal structures, such as aorta, coronary sinus, left atrial appendage, valves and chordae tendineae, and atrial wall. When transseptal puncture is directed to and positioned in an anterosuperior region from the right atrium or when one mistakes a posterior wall of the aortic root for the interatrial septum (Figure 11.1b), the aortic wall may be injured or perforated. Doppler color flow imaging can easily detect the shunt flow jet from the aorta to the right atrium (Figure 11.2a,b). Inadvertent manipulation of transseptal needle or catheter into the coronary sinus or ablation directly in the coronary sinus may cause perforation and induce communication between the coronary sinus and left atrium or a

pericardial effusion. ICE can provide a longitudinal view of the coronary sinus lumen with segmental color flow imaging (Figure 11.3a–d). Parenthetically, such monitoring may also be used for real-time monitoring power titration of the radiofrequency energy within the coronary sinus to prevent intramural superheating and sudden "popping" during ablation. In patients with a dilated left atrial appendage, one can mistake the orifice of the left atrial appendage for the upper left pulmonary vein due to an anatomically posterosuperior extension of the appendage (Figure 11.4a,b). Inadvertent manipulation of the catheter when attempting to pass the catheter into the peripheral pulmonary veins may cause damage to or perforate the left atrial appendage. During the transseptal catheterization and manipulation of the catheter/sheath into the left ventricle through the mitral valve or chordae tendineae, ICE-detected mitral regurgitation that remained after withdrawal from the left ventricle not previously noted, is a sign of damage to these structures. A quantitative evaluation can identify an increase in severity of mitral regurgitation after an inadvertent manipulation of a catheter or sheath through the mitral valve in patients with known mitral regurgitation (Figure 11.5a–c). Left atrial trauma from the transseptal needle/sheath hitting against the left atrial wall immediately following puncture can be detected with ICE imaging as an increased wall thickness and echogenic changes in the local wall (Figure 11.6a–c). Radiofrequency energy delivered at the atrial wall induces focal lesions with morphologic changes. However, due to the repeated ablation or superheating, these lesions can cause severe tissue responses and imaging morphologic changes in the local as well as the whole atrial wall, including swelling, dimpling, or crater

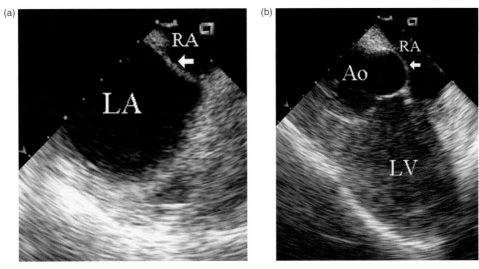

Figure 11.1 ICE images with the transducer in the high right atrium (RA), showing: (a) an interatrial septum (arrow) and the left atrium (LA); and (b) with the transducer rotated counterclockwise a prominent aortic root (Ao, diameter = 4.6 cm) with its posterior wall (arrow) which can be mistaken for the interatrial septum is identified. LV: left ventricle.

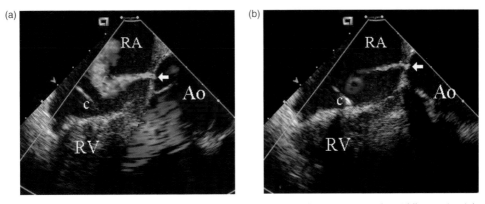

Figure 11.2 ICE Doppler color flow images with the transducer placed near the aortic root in the middle anterior right atrium (RA), showing: (a) a tiny continuous shunting flow jet (arrow) from aortic root (Ao) to RA during early systole; and (b) end-diastole. c: catheter; RV: right ventricle. (Provided by AcuNav peer training course.)

formation (Figure 11.7a–d). ICE imaging monitoring of lesion morphologic changes during energy delivery may assist power titration and prevent intramural superheating or sudden "popping" and the risk of wall perforation.

"Patent" foramen ovale and atrial septal defect

During right heart catheterization or interventional electrophysiologic study manipulation of a catheter in the right atrium (such as "crista" catheter, ultrasound imaging catheter) particularly when advancing from right atrium to superior vena cava, the catheter may inadvertently perforate and pass into the left atrium through the superoanterior limbus of the fossa ovalis. This appears to be more common in patients with a thickened or lipomatous hypertrophy of the interatrial septum (Figure 11.8a,b). With a catheter repeatedly passing through the limbus a "patent" foramen ovale with a bidirected shunting flow can be detected (Figure 11.9a,b). ICE can easily detect such an inadvertent passage and guide the catheter back to

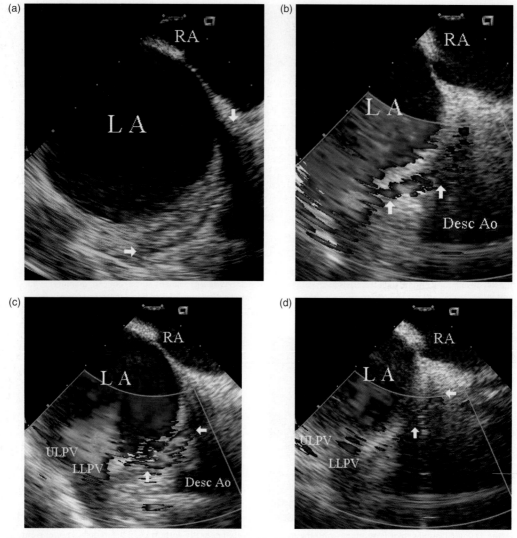

Figure 11.3 ICE images with the transducer placed in the right atrium (RA), showing: (a) a longitudinal view of the coronary sinus lumen (between the two arrows); and (b to d) the Doppler color flow imaging of the coronary sinus (red color, toward the RA) from distal to proximal segments (between the two arrows). Desc Ao: descending aorta; LA: left atrium; ULPV and LLPV: upper and lower left pulmonary vein.

the right atrium and its appropriate location to avoid further damage to the septum.

A residual atrial septal defect can be detected immediately following the removal of transseptal catheters (see Chapter 5). ICE with Doppler color flow imaging can be used to quantify the size of the residual septal defect (Figure 11.10a–c) and characterize the shunt flow (Figure 11.10d). The size of the residual septal defect changes dynamically and reduces within 10 min immediately after removal of transseptal catheters

(Figure 11.10b,c) [1,2]. The size measures generally less than 4 mm in 98% of residual atrial septal defects when transseptal catheterization involves the use of 8 Fr Mullins sheaths, and appears to be clinically insignificant. However, the size of residual septal defect may significantly increase (Figure 11.11a,b) with repeated reinsertion of the catheter/sheath passing through the defect during the ablation procedure due to inadvertent return of the left atrial catheter to the right atrium. Importantly, we have noted at follow-up study

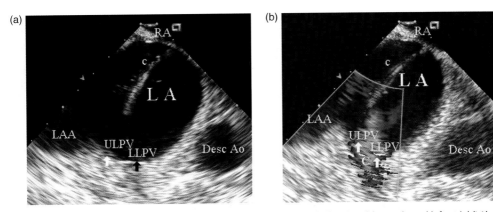

Figure 11.4 ICE images with the transducer placed in the right atrium (RA), showing: (a) an enlarged left atrial (LA) appendage (LAA) and a shared ostium (arrows) of the upper (ULPV) and lower left pulmonary vein (LLPV); and (b) Doppler color flow from the LPVs toward the LA (red color) different from that toward the LAA (blue color) during systole; a Lasso catheter (c) positioned at the shared LPV ostium in both panels. Desc Ao: descending aorta.

in patients with repeated left atrial ablation procedures that the residual atrial septal defects created by individual puncture and passage of an 8 Fr sheath typically resolves completely within 6 months [2]. A persistent defect may be present after catheterization with larger sized catheters and sheaths.

Right and left atrial thrombus formation

Atrial thrombus formation has been recognized as one of the major complications during catheter ablation procedures for tachyarrhythmias. Using continuous ICE imaging monitoring, the incidence of detected right atrial thrombus formation has been reported to be as high as 32% during right atrial ablation when long sheaths are used and anticoagulation is minimized [3]. The incidence of left atrial thrombus formation during left atrial ablation procedure when anticoagulation is maintained after dual transseptal catheterization targeting an activated clotting time (ACT) >250–300 s has been reported as high as 10.3% [4]. These thrombi are usually single, linear, and mobile and of relatively small size, and are typically attached firmly to a catheter or sheath (Figure 11.12). Occasionally the thrombus can be identified attached to the interatrial septal wall at the transseptal punctural point (Figure 11.13) or to the atrial wall at the lesion site (see Chapter 6). The thrombus attached to the catheter can also be seen in the right atrial

appendage (Figure 11.14) and the coronary sinus (Figure 11.15).

Careful management of the left atrial thrombus is important since it may have serious systemic embolic consequences. A tubular type of left atrial thrombus may rarely occur when the left atrial sheath is flushed with aspirated blood during transseptal catheterization by an inexperienced operator (Figure 11.16). The majority of the left atrial thrombi appear to be firmly attached to the catheter or sheath in patients with online ICE imaging monitoring during the ablation procedure. In 90% patients with online imaging detected left atrial thrombus, successful withdrawal of the thrombus-attached catheter/sheath from the left atrium (Figure 11.17a–d) into the right atrium has been reported to prevent any serious systemic embolic consequences [4]. In attempting to pull back into the right atrium, the left atrial thrombi may rarely become wedged into the interatrial septal puncture site (Figure 11.18) and incompletely withdrawn into the right atrium. Reinsertion of the catheters through the interatrial septum into the left atrium is avoided since it can easily cause dislodgement of a wedged thrombus. In our experience in two patients in whom this was observed aggressive anticoagulation for 24–48 h led to gradual diminution and/or dissolution of thrombus without evidence of clinical embolic phenomenon [4]. Importantly, an increased left atrial size and the presence of spontaneous echo contrast appear

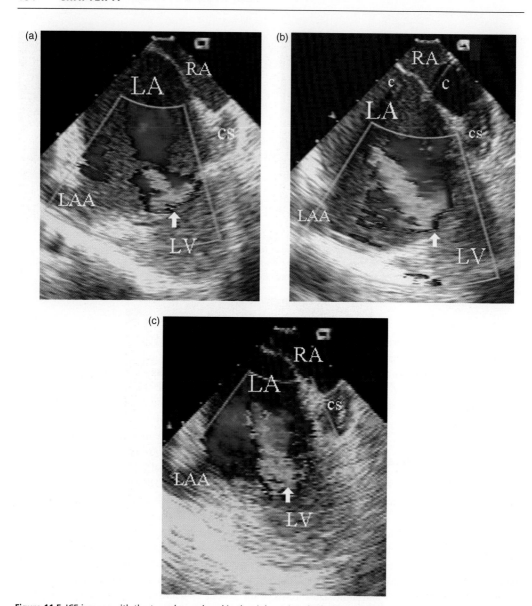

Figure 11.5 ICE images with the transducer placed in the right atrium (RA), showing changes in the severity of the mitral regurgitation (arrow) during/after ablation procedure: (a) mild regurgitation prior to dual transseptal catheterization; (b) moderate immediately with manipulation of the catheters placed in the left ventricle (LV); and (c) moderate mitral regurgitation remained after ablation procedure. c: catheter; cs: coronary sinus; LA: left atrium; LAA: LA appendage.

to be significant risk factors for the development of left atrial thrombi. When spontaneous echocardiographic contrast is detected before transseptal catheterization and left heart ablation procedure (Figure 11.19), increased anticoagulation to maintain ACT >325–350 s reduces the risk of left atrial thrombus formation [5].

Pulmonary vein ostial stenosis and its management with balloon angioplasty and stent placement

Pulmonary vein ostial stenosis
Pulmonary vein stenosis is one of the serious complications associated with pulmonary vein ostial

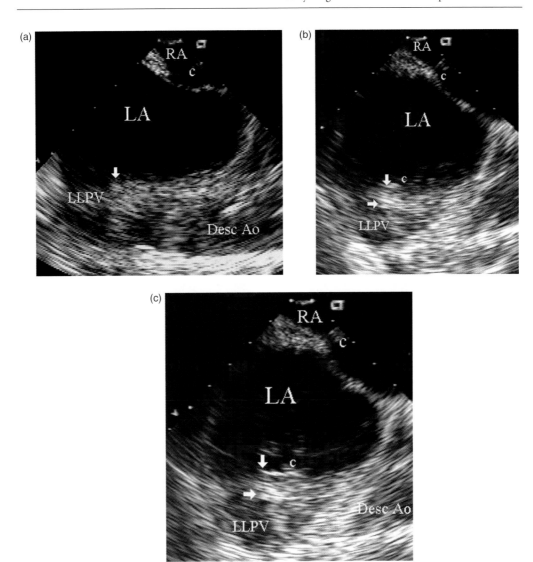

Figure 11.6 ICE images with the transducer placed in the higher right atrium (RA), showing: (a) the left atrial (LA) wall (arrows) at the lower edge of the lower left pulmonary vein (LLPV) ostium before; and (b) with increase of echogenic density and wall thickness (changing from 8 to 11 mm) immediately following the punctural sheath "c" hitting against it; and (c) the sheath "c" moved aside.

isolation/ablation. Any effective ablation lesion deployed inside or at the inner edge of the pulmonary vein ostium may cause narrowing (with tissue swelling/necrosis), which can be detected by an increased ostial peak flow velocity (Figure 11.20) [6].

When a circular multipolar mapping catheter (Lasso) is used at the ostium of the upper left pulmonary vein, one has to recognize that the superior portion of the Lasso is always wedged into the ostium as shown by ICE imaging (Figure 11.21). Therefore, ablation lesions have to be deployed proximal to the Lasso poles with documentation of ablation catheter tip location just outside the ostium identified with ICE imaging. The narrowing effect of acute lesion deployment becomes significant if radiofrequency lesions are deployed just distal or even proximal to the Lasso poles but within the ostium (Figure 11.22).

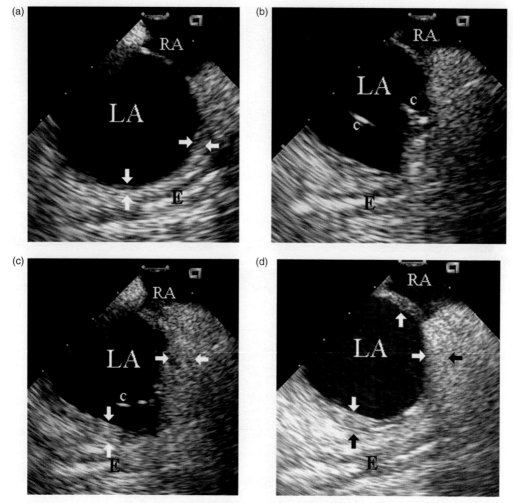

Figure 11.7 ICE images with the transducer placed in the right atrium (RA), showing morphologic changes in the imaging features and the thickness of the atrial wall with lesion formation (between the two arrows): (a) a 3 mm atrial wall thickness noted pre-ablation; (b) the ablation/mapping catheters "c" positioned at the atrial wall during; and (c) with significant swelling (7–8 mm), dimpling, and multiple small surface craters; (d) swelling in the atrial septum (a white upward arrow) is also identified after radiofrequency lesions are delivered to the middle and lower right pulmonary vein ostial region. Esophagus (E) contiguous to the atrial posterior wall is imaged in its longitudinal cross-sectional view.

The ligament of Marshall region always requires repeat radiofrequency lesion application (see Chapter 7), especially at the carina between the left pulmonary vein ostia and the left atrial appendage (Figure 11.23a–c). Radiofrequency lesions delivered in this region cause a certain degree of narrowing in the upper and lower left pulmonary vein ostia with significant swelling and echogenic morphologic changes (Figure 11.23c). In addition to a quantitative evaluation for an increase in flow velocity, Doppler color flow imaging can provide a qualitative evaluation for the presence of narrowing. With marked narrowing a homogeneous color flow becomes mosaic (Figure 11.24a). The qualitative changes should accompany an increased peak flow velocity as determined by the pulsed- or continuous-wave Doppler velocity spectral recording (Figure 11.24b).

Online ICE monitoring of pulmonary vein ostial flow with combined color flow imaging and velocity spectral recording provides a powerful tool to

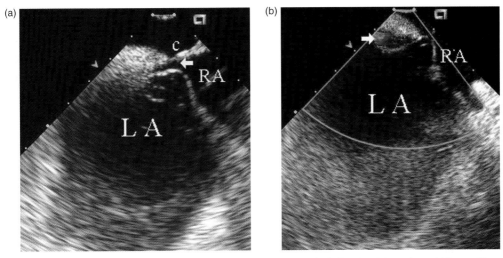

Figure 11.8 ICE images with the transducer placed in the high right atrium (RA), showing: (a) a catheter (c) inserted into the superoanterior limbus of the fossa ovalis (arrow) with an aneurysmatic and mild lipomatous hypertrophic interatrial septum. (b) After the catheter is pulled back, a residual "patent" foramen ovale with a red color flow (arrow) directing from the left atrium (LA) to the RA is identified.

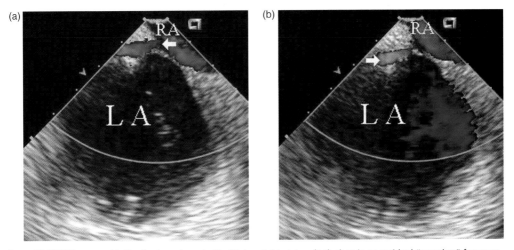

Figure 11.9 ICE images with the the transducer in the higher right atrium (RA), showing a residual "opening" foramen ovale with a bi-directional flow (arrow) through it between the left atrium (LA) and the RA during a cardiac cycle in a patient with lipomatous hypertrophy of the interatrial septum: (a) the blue color indicates the flow (arrow) directing from RA to LA and (b) the red color flow (arrow), from LA to RA.

prevent pulmonary vein ostial narrowing in patients undergoing pulmonary vein ostial ablation for atrial fibrillation. Of note, when isoproterenol is used as a provocative maneuver during mapping of pulmonary vein triggers for atrial fibrillation, it may increase ostial peak flow velocity [7]. Therefore, one should not misinterpret as clinically significant increase in pulmonary vein flow velocity consistent with pathologic narrowing if an isoproterenol-increased pulmonary vein ostial flow velocity is noted.

We remain consistent in our attempt to confirm that pulmonary vein flow velocity remains less than 100 cm/s after radiofrequency lesion placement. Values above 100 cm/s warrant a reassessment of

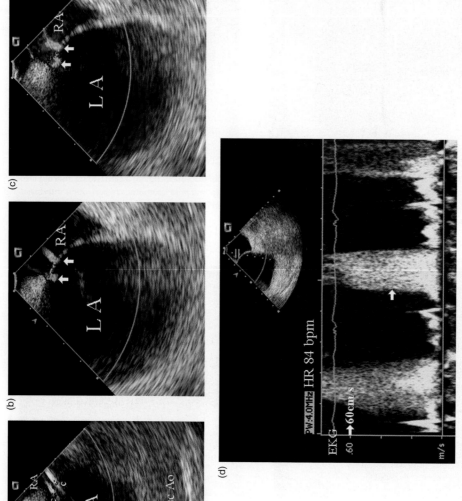

Figure 11.10 ICE images with the transducer placed in the high right atrium (RA), showing: (a) dual transseptal catheterization with two 8 Fr Mullins sheaths "c" in a patient with lipomatous hypertrophy of interatrial septum; and (b) the residual atrial septal defects (arrows, the red mosaic color flow/left-to-right shunting jet) with an acute change in the diameters from 4.9 and 4.4 mm immediately; (c) to 3.8 and 3.4 mm at 3 min after withdrawal of the catheters/sheaths. (d) Pulsed-wave Doppler spectral recording reveals mildly turbulent shunting flow velocity especially during late systole and early diastole (arrow). bpm: beats per min; Desc Ao: descending aorta; EKG: electrocardiogram; HR: heart rate; LA: left atrium.

(a)

(b)

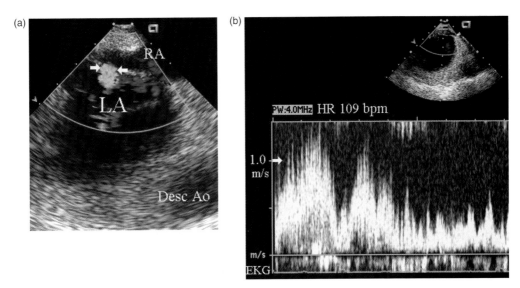

Figure 11.11 Doppler color flow ICE image with the transducer placed in the high right atrium (RA), showing: (a) the residual interatrial septal defect (between the two arrows, diameter = 7.9 mm) with blue mosaic color flow; and (b) pulsed-wave Doppler spectral recording of the bi-directional turbulent shunt flow with significant continuous left-to-right shunting (arrow) identified. Desc Ao: descending aorta; EKG: electrocardiogram; LA: left atrium.

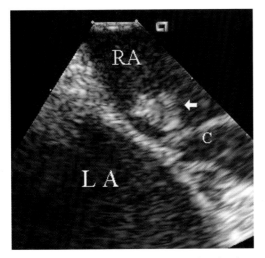

Figure 11.12 ICE image with the transducer placed in the right atrium (RA), showing a twisted thrombus (arrow) attached firmly at the catheter sheath (c) in the RA. LA: left atrium.

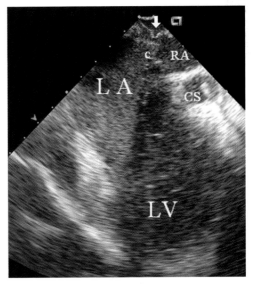

Figure 11.13 ICE image with the transducer in the right atrium (RA), showing the thrombus attached to the atrial septum (arrow) at the transseptal catheter (c) punctural site on the RA side. CS: coronary sinus; LA and LV: left atrium and ventricle.

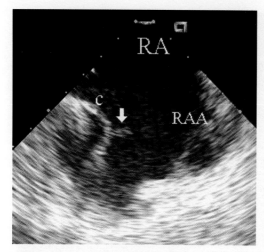

Figure 11.14 ICE image with the transducer in the right atrium (RA), showing the RA appendage (RAA) and a thrombus (arrow) attached the catheter (c).

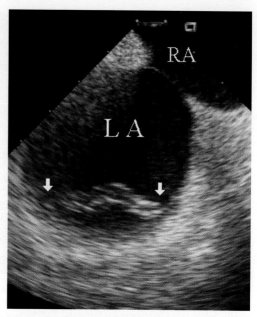

Figure 11.16 ICE image with the transducer placed in the right atrium (RA), showing a tubular thrombus (between the two arrows) immediately following flushing of the left atrial (LA) sheath with aspirated blood during transseptal catheterization.

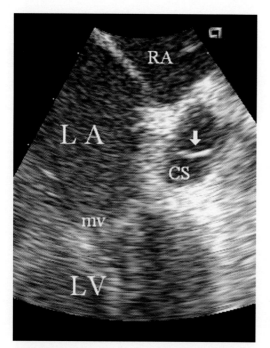

Figure 11.15 Magnified ICE image with the transducer placed in the right atrium (RA), showing left ventricular inflow view and a thrombus (arrow) attached at the catheter in the coronary sinus (CS). mv: mitral valve; LA and LV: left atrium and ventricle.

optimal lesion placement to avoid further increases. An increase to a level above 128 cm/s will result in our terminating any additional attempts at a specific pulmonary vein isolation unless lesion placement is so proximal, confirmed by ICE, as to pose no threat for producing a further increase in flow velocity.

Pulmonary vein balloon angioplasty and stent implantation

Percutaneous balloon angioplasty and stent placement have been used successfully in patients with severe pulmonary vein stenosis [8–10]. ICE with Doppler color flow imaging can be used to quantify pulmonary vein ostial velocity and to estimate a pressure gradient that indexes the severity of stenosis before and after balloon angioplasty (Figure 11.25) or stent placement (Figure 11.26). It can be used for determination of the diameter (Figure 11.25B,E,F, and K) of the ostium/lumen and guide balloon or stent (Figure 11.26B) placement at a stenotic region during the dilatation procedure. ICE Doppler color flow imaging provides a reliable sign for balloon positioned at a stenotic region when ostial flow reduces and

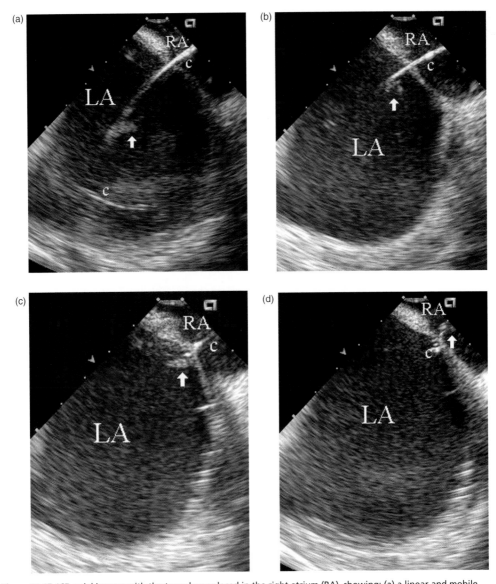

Figure 11.17 ICE serial images with the transducer placed in the right atrium (RA), showing: (a) a linear and mobile thrombus (arrow, size 10.0×4.7 mm^2) attached at distal shaft of Lasso; (b and c) the sheath/Lasso "c" with the thrombus pulled back; and (d) withdrawal of the thrombus from the left atrium (LA) into the RA.

finally disappears when the balloon gradually inflated (Figure 11.25E,J).

Esophageal injury

The esophagus is immediately contiguous to the left atrial posterior wall. Esophageal injury with the development of atrio-esophageal fistula has been reported with delivery of radiofrequency lesions at the left atrial posterior wall contiguous to the esophagus during left atrial intraoperative or percutaneous transcatheter ablation for atrial fibrillation [11–15]. The risk appears greatest especially in very thin patients or those with a small left atria. Although

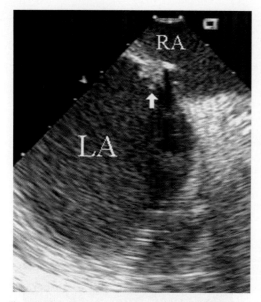

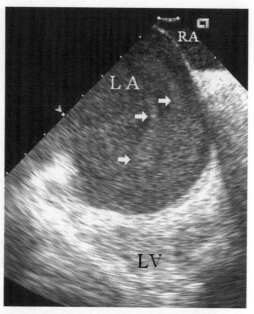

Figure 11.18 ICE images with the transducer placed in the right atrium (RA), showing a thrombus (arrow) wedged in the interatrial septum during pulling back from the left atrium (LA).

Figure 11.19 ICE image with the transducer (at ultrasound frequency 7.5 MHz) placed in the right atrium (RA), showing spontaneous echocardiographic contrast in the left atrium (LA) as a swirling, "smoke-like" cloud (arrows). LV: left ventricle.

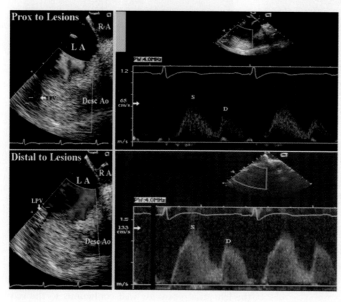

Figure 11.20 ICE images with the transducer placed in the right atrium (RA) and sampling volume in the lumen of the left pulmonary vein (LPV) (proximal to lesions) (upper panels) and outside the ostium (distal to lesions) (lower panels), showing the peak flow velocity increased from 65 cm/s to 133 cm/s with turbulent features across the ostial region of the lesions.
D and S: peak flow velocity at diastole and systole; LA: left atrium; Desc Ao: descending aorta.

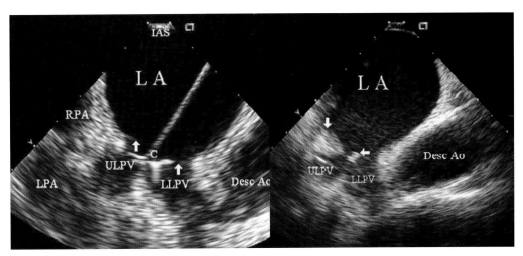

Figure 11.21 ICE images with the transducer placed in the right atrium (RA), showing the Lasso catheter (c) positioned at the shared common ostium (arrows) of the upper (ULPV) and lower left pulmonary vein (LLPV) (left panel), and the superior portion of the Lasso wedged into the ULPV ostium when positioning at its ostium (directed by leftward arrow) with ostial tissue swelling (downward arrow) following development of lesions proximal to the Lasso (right panel). Desc Ao: descending aorta; IAS: interatrial septum; LA: left atrium; LPA and RPA: left and right pulmonary artery.

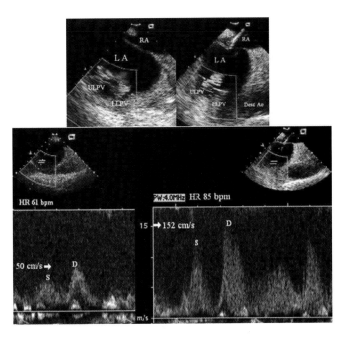

Figure 11.22 ICE images with the transducer placed in the right atrium (RA) and sampling volume at the upper left pulmonary vein (ULPV) ostium, showing the pulsed-wave Doppler spectral recording of the ULPV ostial flow velocity before (left upper and lower panels) and after lesions deployed just proximal to the superior Lasso poles within the ostium (right upper and lower panels), with a significant increased peak flow velocity from 50 cm/s (baseline) to 152 cm/s with turbulent features identified.
bpm: beats per min; D and S: peak velocity at diastole and systole; Desc Ao: descending aorta; HR: heart rate; LA: left atrium.

atrio-esophageal fistulas following left atrial ablation procedure have been rarely reported with an incidence of 0.05–1.3% [12,15], this risk may be underestimated [12]. Atrio-esophageal fistula/perforation may initially create clinical symptoms compatible with endocarditis and subsequently cause multiple gaseous and/or septic embolic events including cerebral, myocardial, and extensive systemic embolization. The high mortality rate associated with such esophageal injury mandates all possible effort to protect the

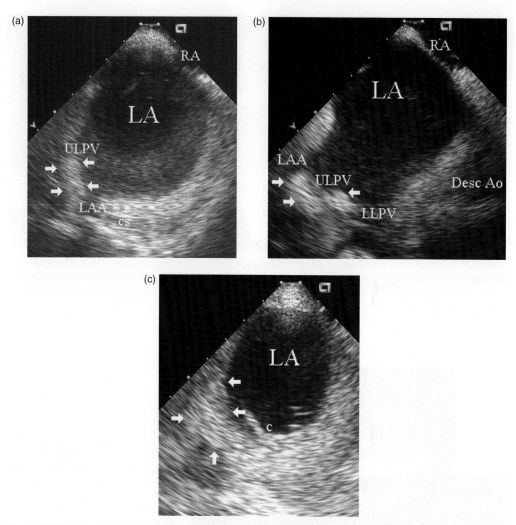

Figure 11.23 ICE images with the transducer placed in the right atrium (RA), showing: (a) the ligament of Marshall tissue region (arrows) above distal coronary sinus (cs) between the upper left pulmonary vein (ULPV) and left atrial appendage (LAA); (b) and the carina between the ULPV and lower LPV (LLPV) (leftward arrow) and the LAA (rightward arrows); (c) the ligament of Marshall tissue region thickened significantly (between arrows) after lesions were deployed. c: Lasso catheter; Desc Ao: descending aorta; LA: left atrium.

esophagus and avoid this deleterious complication. To avoid potential injury of the esophagus, ICE can provide real-time imaging of the esophagus and monitoring of lesion location and development during left atrial ablation.

Imaging characteristics of the atrio-esophageal anatomic region

With the ICE transducer placed in the right atrium and scanning between the lower right and left pulmonary vein ostia, a longitudinal view of the esophagus and atrio-esophageal region (Figure 11.27) is obtained. The ultrasound appearance of the esophagus depends on whether the esophagus is collapsed or distended. A variety of esophageal imaging features including whether filled with gas (Figure 11.28a,b), fluid (Figure 11.29), or both (Figure 11.30), movement within its segments, or variably collapsed lumen (Figure 11.31) may identify the esophagus with real-time ICE imaging monitoring during left atrial ablation procedure. Movement of fluid (salivation) within its segments or by requesting active swallowing

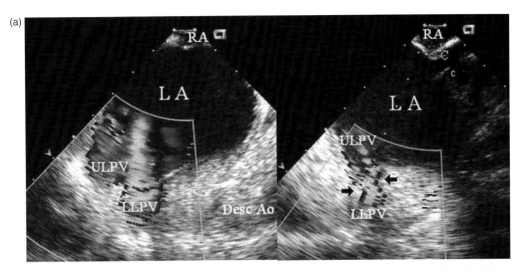

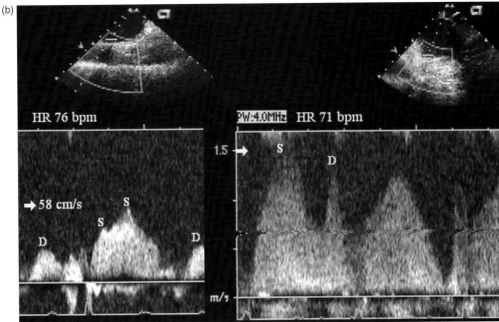

Figure 11.24 (a) Doppler color flow images of the upper (ULPV) and lower left pulmonary vein (LLPV) ostial flow, showing homogeneous red color flow from ostial lumens toward the left atrium (LA) and the diameter of LLPV ostium measured 15 mm before ablation lesions at the ostia (left panel), and the mosaic greenish color flow passing through the narrowing (diameter = 7.5 mm) region (arrows) after lesions at the ostium of LLPV (right panel); (b) pulsed-wave Doppler velocity spectra recorded from the lower left pulmonary vein ostium, showing the peak flow velocity which measured 58 cm/s before ablation lesions (left panel), and 150 cm/s (estimated pressure gradient = 9 mmHg) after lesions (right panel) indicating flow acceleration through the ostial narrowing of 50%. c: catheter; Desc Ao: descending aorta; RA: right atrium; bpm: beats per min; D and S: peak velocity at diastole and systole; HR: heart rate.

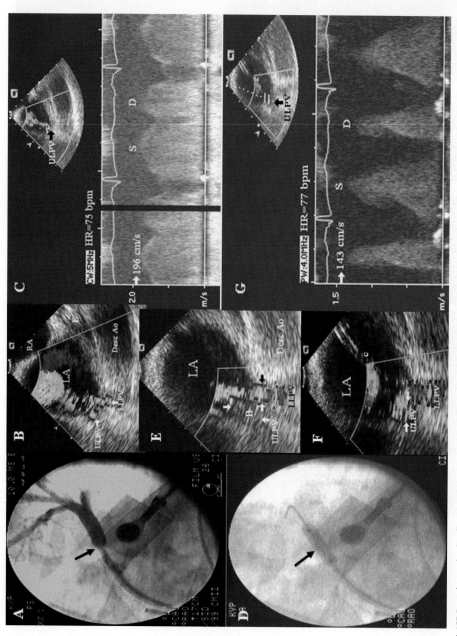

Figure 11.25(A–G) ICE Doppler and color flow images and angiograms of the upper left pulmonary vein (ULPV, panels A–G), showing the ULPV ostial stenosis (arrow, panel A) with the diameter of 3.5 mm (mosaic color flow, panel B) and ostial flow velocity of 196 cm/s (an estimated pressure gradient 15.4 mmHg, panel C) before balloon angioplasty, and the balloon inflated (arrow, panel D) at ostial narrowing region without color flow from ULPV (panel E) during balloon dilatation, and increased ostial diameter (at 7.5 mm, arrows, panel F) and reduced ostial flow velocity (at 143 cm/s, pressure gradient 6.8 mmHg, panel G) after balloon angioplasty. B: balloon; bpm: beats per min; c: catheter; HR: heart rate; LA: left atrium; LLPV: left lower pulmonary vein.

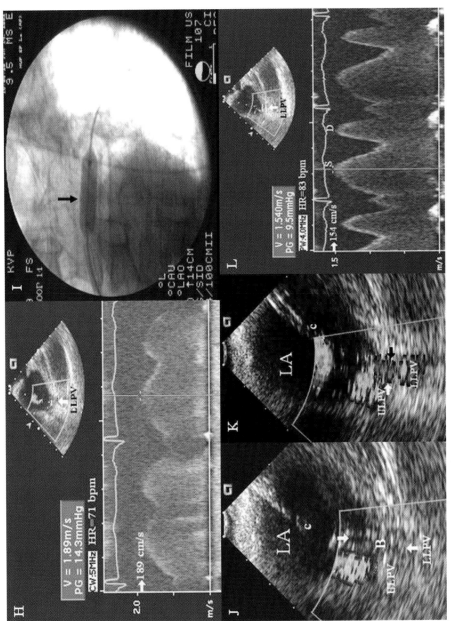

Figure 11.25(H–L) ICE Doppler and color flow images and angiogram of the lower left pulmonary vein (LLPV) showing the LLPV ostial stenosis with the diameter of 3.6 mm (see panel B) and ostial flow velocity of 189 cm/s (pressure gradient 14.3 mmHg, panel H) before balloon angioplasty, and the balloon inflated (arrow, panel I) at region of ostial narrowing obliterating the color flow from LLPV (panel J) during balloon dilatation, and increased ostial diameter (at 7 mm, arrows, panel K) and reduced ostial flow velocity (at 154 cm/s, pressure gradient 9.5 mmHg, panel L) after balloon angioplasty. B: balloon; bpm: beats per min; c: catheter; HR: heart rate; LA: left atrium.

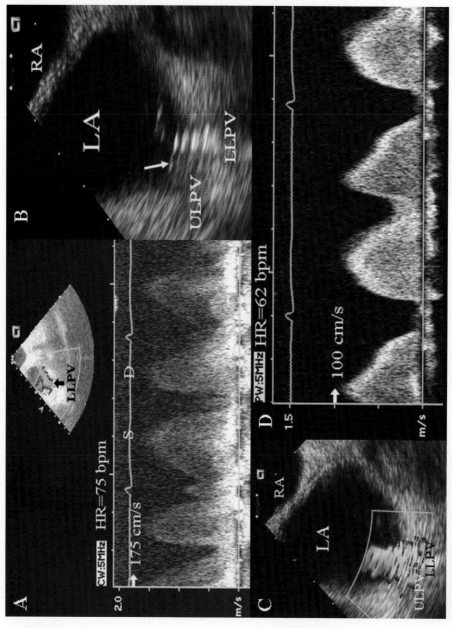

Figure 11.26 ICE Doppler and color flow images of stent placement, showing the continuous-wave Doppler spectrum with the peak flow velocity of 175 cm/s (pressure gradient 12.2 mmHg) recorded from the lower left pulmonary vein (LLPV) ostium before stent placement (panel A), a stent with echogenic acoustic artifact positioned optimally at the ostial narrowing of the LLPV (panel B), significant ostial color (red) flow toward the left atrium (LA) (panel C) and reduced ostial peak flow velocity (at 100 cm/s, pressure gradient 4 mmHg) of the LLPV after stent placement (panel D). bpm: beats per min; HR: heart rate; RA: right atrium; ULPV: upper left pulmonary vein.

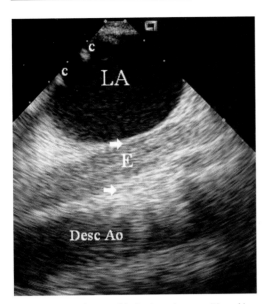

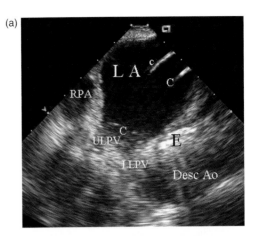

(a)

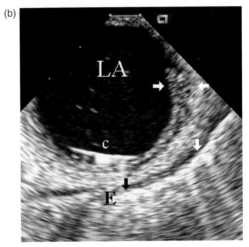

(b)

Figure 11.27 ICE image with the transducer positioned in the high right atrium while scanning between the left and right lower pulmonary vein ostia illustrates a longitudinal view of the esophagus (E) located between the left atrial (LA) posterior wall and descending aorta (Desc Ao) (between the two arrows). The esophageal lumen filled with digestive fluid is imaged just following suction of extra secretion and saliva from the mouth. c: catheter.

enhances esophageal imaging. The anterior wall of the esophagus contiguous to the left atrial posterior wall can always be imaged. However, esophageal gas can cause significant scattering of the ultrasound beam, thus temporarily/partially obscuring deeper structures including the esophageal posterior wall. The esophageal diameter can be determined by imaging its posterior border along the descending aorta (Figure 11.32). The contiguous left atrio-esophageal length, esophageal diameter and anterior wall, and contiguous left atrial posterior wall thickness have been measured using ICE (Figure 11.33) in 42 patients (age 56 ± 12 years, 33 men) with atrial fibrillation undergoing left atrial ablation (Table 11.1) [16]. The contiguous atrio-esophageal length is longer in patients with dilated than normal left atrium since the length in continuity is correlated to the left atrial diameter ($r = 0.78, p < 0.01$).

Monitoring lesion morphologic changes with radiofrequency power titration

As previously described with ICE imaging the radiofrequency lesion morphologic changes in the atrial

Figure 11.28 (a) ICE image with the transducer placed in the high right atrium shows a cross-sectional view of esophageal segment (E) filled with echogenic gas (accompanying distal ultrasonic scattering artifact), located adjacent to the lower left pulmonary vein (LLPV) ostium between the left atrial (LA) posterior wall and the descending aorta (Desc Ao). C: catheter; ULPV: upper LPV; RPV: right pulmonary artery. (b) ICE image with the transducer placed in the middle right atrium, showing the left atrial (LA) posterior wall contiguous to the esophagus (E) filled with gas (downward arrows) with distal scattered ultrasonic artifact, which obscures imaging of the deeper structures. LA inferoposterior wall is significantly thickened (7.5 mm, between the two horizontal arrows) after radiofrequency lesions delivered around the orifice of the lower right pulmonary vein. c: catheter.

wall can be identified with creation of wall swelling, dimpling, crater formation, or echogenic enhancement (see Chapters 6 and 7). In patients with atrial fibrillation undergoing radiofrequency left atrial pulmonary vein isolation using an 8 mm electrode

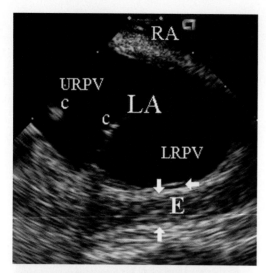

Figure 11.29 ICE image with the transducer placed in the high right atrium (RA), showing the left atrial (LA) posterior wall (leftward arrow) contiguous to the esophagus (E, between the two arrows) filled with digestive fluid. c: catheter; LRPV and URPV: lower and upper right pulmonary vein.

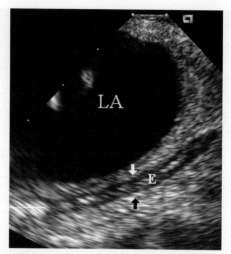

Figure 11.31 ICE image with the transducer placed in the lower right atrium, showing a longitudinal segmental view of a flat "collapsed" esophagus (E, between the two arrows, diameter = 5.2 mm) posterior to the left atrium (LA); the central linear hyper-echoic structure in the E represents mucus and trapped air, and the anechoic structures on both sides of the central line, mainly the muscular wall.

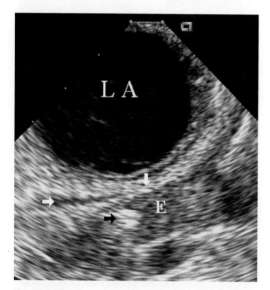

Figure 11.30 ICE image with the transducer placed in the middle right atrium, showing the left atrial (LA) posterior wall contiguous (downward arrow) to the esophagus (E) filled with fluid in which a floating gas "mass" (black rightward arrow) is seen. The oblique sinus (white rightward arrow) is partially opened between the LA posterior wall and E.

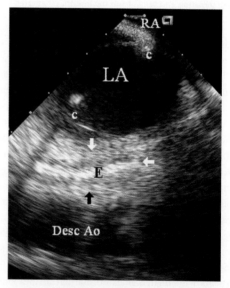

Figure 11.32 ICE image with the transducer placed in the middle right atrium (RA), showing a longitudinal segmental view of the esophagus (E, between the two arrows) posterior to the left atrium (LA), and the central linear hyper-echoic area (leftward arrow) in the E representing mucus and trapped air with distal scattered artifact. The posterior wall of the E (black upward arrow) is identified based on its bordering with the descending aorta (Desc Ao). c: catheter.

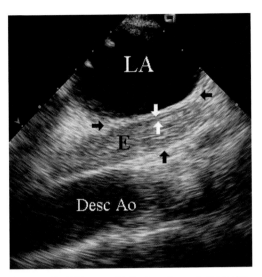

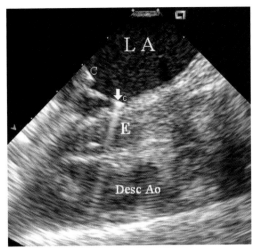

Figure 11.34 ICE image showing ablation catheter (c) tip (arrow, with distal fan-shaped artifact) positioned at the left atrial (LA) posterior wall contiguous to the esophageal (E) anterior wall, identification of this position allows for monitoring lesions during LA ablation procedure and power titration. Desc Ao: descending aorta.

Figure 11.33 ICE image with the transducer placed in the higher right atrium while scanning left atrial (LA) posterior wall between the lower left and right pulmonary vein ostia, showing a longitudinal segmental view of the esophagus (E). The measured length of the region over which the atrium is continuous with the esophagus is 32 mm (between the two black horizontal arrows). E diameter (14 mm between the white downward and black upward arrows), anterior E wall thickness (3 mm between the two white arrows) and LA posterior wall (2.5 mm) are identified. Desc Ao: descending aorta.

Table 11.2 Changes in echogenic wall thickness of contiguous left atrial posterior wall and esophageal wall post-routine versus power titrating radiofrequency ablation.

	LAPW–esophagus wall (mm)	Echogenic wall	
		Post-RF (mm)	Post-power titration RF (mm)
Mean ± SD	6.1 ± 0.9	10.8 ± 2.2	4.8 ± 1.5*
Range	5.0–8.5	7.0–15.0	3.0–8.3

* $p < 0.01$ versus post-RF.

Table 11.1 Anatomic measurements for contiguous length and wall thickness of left atrium and esophagus.

	LAPW–esophagus length	Esophagus diameter	Esophagus anterior wall	LAPW	LA diameter
	(mm)				
Mean ± SD	26.5 ± 6.5	16.6 ± 3.2	3.4 ± 0.5	2.7 ± 0.5	48 ± 5
Range	15.0–47.0	9.0–22.0	2.5–4.5	2.0–4.0	38–63

LA: left atrium; PW: posterior wall

(70 W, up to 50–52°C, 60 s) or Chilli catheter (up to 40°C, 60 s), the lesion morphologic changes at the contiguous atrio-esophageal region has been reported under routine circumstance ($n = 44$) and during power titration ($n = 29$) using ICE imaging monitoring (Figure 11.34) [17]. There were 4.3 ± 3.2 lesions/patient delivered to this atrio-esophageal region during radiofrequency ablation at the left atrial posterior wall around the lower/middle

right and lower left pulmonary vein ostia. The left atrio-esophageal wall thickness and changes in echogenic lesion thickness were measured pre- and post-radiofrequency lesions (Table 11.2). The findings indicate that radiofrequency lesions with 8 mm electrode or Chilli catheter delivered at the contiguous left atrio-esophageal wall induce echogenic lesion morphologic changes including crater formation (Figure 11.35a–c) and could involve the esophageal anterior wall (Figure 11.36). Echogenic lesion morphologic changes can be controlled and limited to the left atrial posterior wall (Figure 11.37) with power titration guided by ICE lesion monitoring [17].

These results demonstrate that ICE imaging can provide real-time imaging monitoring of the lesion

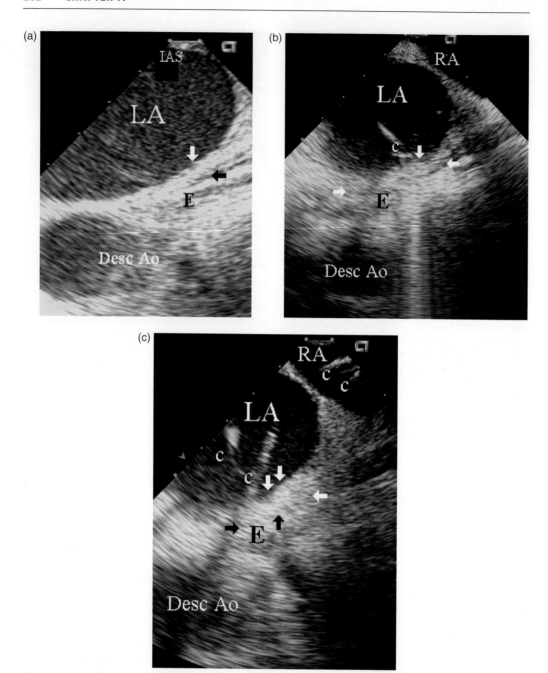

Figure 11.35 ICE images with the transducer placed in the higher right atrium (RA), showing the left atrium (LA) and LA posterior wall (downward arrow, thickness = 3.0 mm) contiguous to the esophageal (E) anterior wall (horizontal arrows, linear anechoic/hypoechoic structure, thickness = 2.5 mm): (a) pre-ablation; (b) with ablation catheter (c) tip positioned at the LA posterior wall (downward arrow, thickness = 3.0 mm) with distal fan-shaped artifact during; and (c) crater/lesion formation (downward and upward arrows) with increase in echogenic wall thickness to 8.5 mm and extending to the E anterior wall with catheter moved aside immediately following radiofrequency lesion application. c: catheter; Desc Ao: ascending aorta.

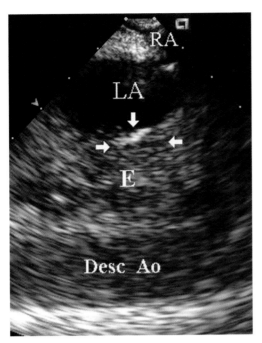

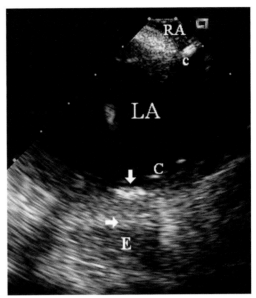

Figure 11.37 ICE image with the transducer placed in the middle right atrium (RA), showing radiofrequency lesion morphologic changes with swelling and thickening (8 mm) of the left atrial (LA) posterior wall contiguous to the esophagus (E), and an echogenic lesion depth (downward arrow) controlled at 5 mm before reaching to the anterior wall of the E (rightward arrow) during power titration under ICE monitoring. C: catheter.

Figure 11.36 ICE image with the transducer placed in the high right atrium (RA), showing radiofrequency-induced echogenic lesions (downward arrow) at left atrial (LA) posterior wall partially extending to the esophageal (E) anterior wall (horizontal arrows). Desc Ao: descending aorta.

morphologic changes at the atrio-esophageal wall, and esophageal injury can be limited and possibly completely avoided with radiofrequency power titration during a left atrial ablation procedure while carefully monitoring lesion formation.

Pericardial effusion

Pericardial effusion is one of common serious complications associated with catheter/needle manipulation during transseptal catheterization and interventional electrophysiologic procedures. It may occur immediately following catheter perforation of cardiac structures, such as coronary sinus, atrial appendage, and cardiac wall, during transseptal puncture (see Chapter 5) or catheter manipulation for mapping and ablation (see Chapter 7). ICE imaging monitoring may provide early detection and accurate diagnosis of pericardial effusion prior to arterial blood pressure and hemodynamic changes during transseptal puncture and catheter ablation procedure. Where the fluid

collects probably depends on how the pericardium can expand and where the perforation/damage is located. The posterior cul-de-sac and lateral walls are more expandable. These areas offer less resistance to stretching of the pericardium, providing an area where fluid initially collects (Figure 11.38a). Later, the pericardial effusion increases posteriorly (Figure 11.38b). In a moderately large effusion, the echo-free fluid primarily collects posteriorly with a smaller apical fluid anteriorly (Figure 11.38c). In patients with large effusion, fluid totally surrounds the heart (Figure 11.38d) and the heart seems to settle or drop posteriorly within the fluid and the accumulation of pericardial fluid becomes primarily anterior (Figure 11.38e) [18]. A pericardial effusion that increases to a moderately large amount can be detected anterolateral to the right ventricle (Figure 11.39a,b). However, the usual ICE diagnosis of pericardial effusion has emphasized the detection of pericardial fluid posterior to the left ventricle, because anterior fluid may be negligible with small effusions and relatively echo-free spaces anteriorly may represent epicardial fat (Figure 11.40), which

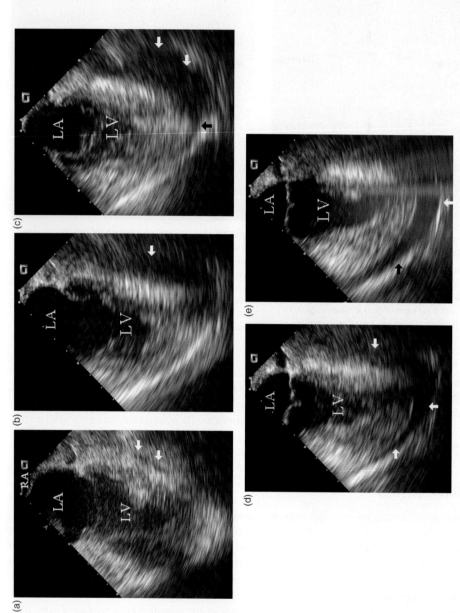

Figure 11.38 ICE serial images of a left ventricular (LV) inflow view, showing changes in anatomic distribution progressing pericardial effusion (arrows): (a) initially small pericardial effusion (echo-free space = 2.5 mm) accumulated in the posterior region; (b) effusion increased in the posterior region (echo-free space = 12 mm) and did not extend to anterior and apical regions; (c) further increased in the posterior region (echo-free space = 23 mm) expanding to the apical region (black upward arrow) with a moderately large effusion; (d) further expansion to the apical and anterior regions; and (e) heart moving freely to settle more posteriorly in a large effusion. LA: left atrium; RA: right atrium.

(a)

(b)

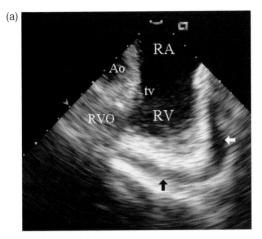
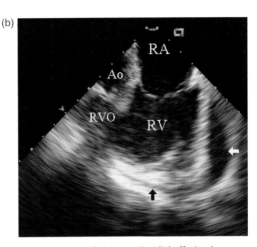

Figure 11.39 ICE images of a right ventricular (RV) inflow view, showing a moderately large pericardial effusion (arrows, echo-free space): (a) during diastole; (b) systole. Ao: aorta; RA: right atrium; RVO: RV outflow tract; tv: tricuspid valve.

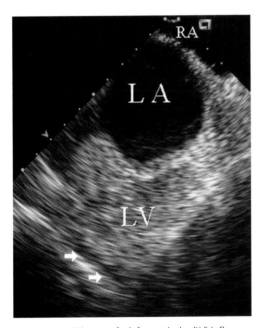

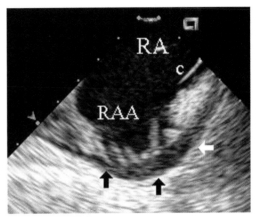

Figure 11.41 ICE image with the transducer placed in the higher right atrium (RA) while scanning the posterolateral RA, showing the pericardial echo-free fluid (arrows) surrounding the RA appendage (RAA) with pectinate muscles seen inside this structure. c: catheter.

Figure 11.40 ICE image of a left ventricular (LV) inflow view, showing an echofree space (arrows) only in pericardial anterior region and not the posterior region. This space represented epicardial fat in a patient with obesity and body weight of 302 lb. LA: left atrium; RA: right atrium.

can be mistaken for pericardial effusion. Pericardial fluid may not always collect uniformly around the heart and it may collect relatively more anteriorly or posteriorly, or even in the posterior cardiac base surrounding the right atrial appendage (Figure 11.41).

In patients with previous cardiac surgery, loculated pericardial effusion may be present due to adhesions in certain areas of the pericardium. Based on our clinical observation using ICE imaging, a semiquantitative evaluation of pericardial effusion can be made according to the size of the echo-free pericardial fluid space at its greatest width surrounding the heart, as a mild moderate (<8 mm), moderately large (8–12 mm), or large (>12 mm) amount. A small effusion is one that is only detected posteriorly.

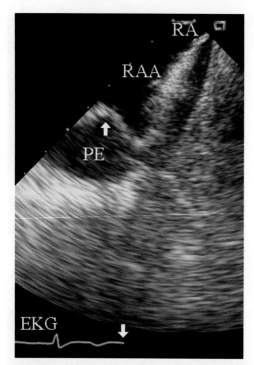

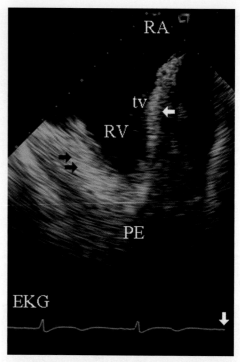

Figure 11.42 ICE image of a large pericardial effusion (PE) surrounding the right atrial (RA) appendage (RAA) with invagination (arrow) during diastole (arrow on EKG recording) in a patient with cardiac tamponade.

Figure 11.43 ICE image of a large pericardial effusion (PE) surrounding the right ventricular (RV) wall with invagination (arrows) at end-diastole (arrow on EKG recording) indicated by a complete opening of the tricuspid valve (tv) in a patient with cardiac tamponade. RA: right atrium.

In patients with cardiac tamponade the most popular and reliable echocardiographic sign is collapse of the cardiac chambers in diastole, especially with diastolic invagination of the right ventricular and/or right atrial wall during diastole [19–23]. The dynamic wall motion of the right atrium and its appendage (Figure 11.42) and the right ventricle (Figure 11.43) can be evaluated with ICE imaging and its invagination during diastole may be easily detected when cardiac tamponade occurs. Timing of the collapse is more apparent on the M-mode recording or can be made by correlating it with the tricuspid valve opening (Figure 11.43).

References

1 Ren JF, Marchlinski FE, Callans DJ. Quantitative evaluation of atrial septal defect resulting from dual transseptal catheterization for ablation of atrial fibrillation: a Doppler color flow imaging study (abstr). *PACE* 2002; **24**: 559.

2 Ren JF, Marchlinski FE, Callans DJ. Residual atrial septal defect following dual transseptal catheterization: a Doppler color flow imaging follow-up (abstr). *J Am Coll Cardiol* 2003; **41**: 95A.

3 Ren JF, Callans DJ, Schwartzman D, Marchlinski FE. Significant incidence of right atrial thrombus associated with long catheter sheath during ablation procedures (abstr). *PACE* 2001; **24**: 603.

4 Ren JF, Marchlinski FE, Callans DJ. Left atrial thrombus associated with ablation for atrial fibrillation: identification with intracardiac echocardiography. *J Am Coll Cardiol* 2004; **43**: 1861–1867.

5 Ren JF, Marchlinski FE, Callans DJ, *et al.* Increased intensity of anticoagulation may reduce risk of thrombus during atrial fibrillation ablation procedure in patients with spontaneous echo contrast. *J Cardiovasc Electrophysiol* 2005; **16**: 474–477.

6 Ren JF, Marchlinski FE, Callans DJ, Zado ES. Intracardiac Doppler echocardiographic quantification of pulmonary vein flow velocity: an effective technique for monitoring pulmonary vein ostia narrowing during focal atrial fibrillation ablation. *J Cardiovasc Electrophysiol* 2002; **13**: 1076–1081.

7 Ren JF, Marchlinski FE, Callans DJ. Effect of heart rate and isoproterenol on pulmonary vein flow velocity following radiofrequency ablation: a Doppler color flow imaging study. *J Interventional Cardiac Electrophysiol* 2004; **10**: 265–269.

8 Coulson JD, Bullaboy CA. Concentric placement of stents to relieve an obstructed anomalous pulmonary venous connection. *Catheterization & Cardiovasc Diagnosis* 1997; **42**: 201–204.

9 Hyde JA, Stumper O, Barth MJ, *et al*. Total anomalous pulmonary venous connection: outcome of surgical correction and management of recurrent venous obstruction. *Eur J Cardio-Thoracic Surg* 1999; **15**: 735–740.

10 Ussia GP, Marasini M, Rimini A, Pongiglione G. Atresia of right pulmonary veins with intact atrial septum and major aorto-pulmonary collateral treated with percutaneous stent implantation and embolization. *J Interventional Cardiol* 2004; **17**: 183–187.

11 Gillinov AM, Pettersson G, Rice TW. Esophageal injury during radiofrequency ablation for atrial fibrillation. *J Thorac Cardiovasc Surg* 2001; **122**: 1239–1240.

12 Mohr FW, Fabicius AM, Falk V, *et al*. Curative treatment of atrial fibrillation with intraoperative radiofrequency ablation: short-term and mid-term results. *J Thorac Cardiovasc Surg* 2002; **123**: 919–927.

13 Kottkamp H, Hindricks G, Autschbach R, *et al*. Specific linear left atrial lesions in atrial fibrillation: intraoperative radiofrequency ablation using minimally invasive surgical techniques. *J Am Coll Cardiol* 2002; **40**: 475–480.

14 Sonmez B, Demirsoy E, Yagan N, *et al*. Fatal complication due to radiofrequency ablation for atrial fibrillation: atrio-esophageal fistula. *Ann Thorac Surg* 2003; **76**: 281–283.

15 Pappone C, Oral H, Santinelli V, *et al*. Atrio-esophageal fistula as a complication of percutaneous transcatheter ablation of atrial fibrillation. *Circulation* 2004; **109**: 2724–2726.

16 Ren JF, Marchlinski FE, Callans DJ. Esophageal imaging characteristics and structural measurement during left atrial ablation for atrial fibrillation: an intracardiac echocardiographic study (abstr). *J Am Coll Cardiol* 2005; **45**: 114A.

17 Ren JF, Callans DJ, Marchlinski FE, Nayak H, Lin D, Gerstenfeld EP. Avoiding esophageal injury with power titrating during left atrial ablation for atrial fibrillation: an intracardiac echocardiographic imaging study (abstr). *J Am Coll Cardiol* 2005; **45**: 114A.

18 Feigenbaum H. *Echocardiography*. Lea & Febiger, Philadelphia, 1994: 556–557.

19 Armstrong WF, Schilt BF, Helper DJ, Dillon JC, Feigenbaum H. Diastolic collapse of the right ventricle with tamponade: an echocardiographic study. *Circulation* 1982; **65**: 1491–1496.

20 Gillam LD, Guyer DE, Gibson TC, King ME, Marshall JE, Weyman AE. Hydrodynamic compression of the right atrium: a new echocardiographic sign of cardiac tamponade. *Circulation* 1983; **68**: 294–301.

21 Kronzon I, Cohen ML, Winer HE. Diastolic atrial compression: a sensitive echocardiographic sign of cardiac tamponade. *J Am Coll Cardiol* 1983; **2**: 770–775.

22 Singh S, Wann LS, Schuchard GH, *et al*. Right ventricular and right atrial collapse in patients with cardiac tamponade – a combined echocardiographic and hemodynamic study. *Circulation* 1984; **70**: 966–971.

23 Singh S, Wann LS, Klopfenstein HS, Hartz A, Brooks HL. Usefulness of right ventricular diastolic collapse in diagnosing cardiac tamponade and comparison to pulsus paradoxus. *Am J Cardiol* 1986; **57**: 652–656.

CHAPTER 12

Utility for Experimental Electrophysiological Procedures in Swine

Jian-Fang Ren, MD, *David J. Callans,* MD, *&*
David Schwartzman, MD

Introduction

Swine have become an animal model of choice in experimental cardiovascular studies since there are many similarities between the human and swine cardiovascular systems. The large swine model with body weight ranging 50–114 kg may provide comparable transesophageal echocardiographic values to those found in human adults (Tables 12.1 and 12.2) [1]. However, it is difficult to obtain high-quality echocardiographic images from a transthoracic approach due to the swine's chest configuration. With multiplane transesophageal echocardiography, complete imaging of the short-axis view of the left ventricle and right heart structures in swine is frequently more difficult than in humans, due to the location of the cardiac apex in a more anterior transverse plane and interference by air in the trachea and lungs [1]. Intracardiac echocardiography (ICE) was initially performed by placing a lower frequency (5 or 7 MHz) probe in the right atrium and/or superior vena cava and right ventricle through a venous approach in an experimental animal (dog or swine), which provided imaging that was superior to transthoracic examinations and comparable with transesophageal approach [2–6]. Recently, catheter-based ICE with mechanical (9 Fr, 9 MHz) ultrasonic imaging [7,8], and electronic phased-array (10 Fr, 5.5–10 MHz) ultrasound and Doppler velocity and color flow imaging [9,10] have been developed for clinical cardiovascular diagnosis and functional evaluation. The latter imaging catheter also provides a novel

Table 12.1 Normal values (mean ± SD) of swine cardiac chamber dimensions and great vessel diameters determined by transesophageal echocardiography (TEE).

		Human adults	
	Swine	TEE	TTE
LV inner dimension (d)	48 ± 3	47 ± 5	48 ± 6
LV inner dimension (s)	33 ± 3	33 ± 4	31 ± 5
IVS thickness (d)	7 ± 2	—	—
IVS thickness (s)	12 ± 2	—	—
LV PW thickness (d)	7 ± 1	—	—
LV PW thickness (s)	12 ± 2	—	—
RV inner dimension (d)	23 ± 4	28 ± 5	28 ± 4
RV inner dimension (s)	16 ± 3	19 ± 3	—
RV wall thickness (d)	4 ± 2	—	4 ± 1
RV wall thickness (s)	8 ± 2	—	—
LA dimension (s)	48 ± 6	44 ± 6	36 ± 4
Ao diameter (s)	26 ± 3	—	29 ± 3
Descending Ao diameter	16 ± 2	—	—
PA diameter (s)	26 ± 3	20 ± 2	22 ± 4
Right upper PV diameter	12 ± 2	—	—

—: no report or not available; Ao: aorta; d: at end-diastole; LA: left atrium; LV: left ventricle; PV: pulmonary vein; PW: posterior wall; RV: right ventricle; s: at end-systole; TTE: transthoracic two-dimensional echocardiography. Reproduced with permission [1].

imaging modality with high resolution images of the cardiac structures for experimental research applications [1]. This chapter describes these catheter-based ICE techniques, imaging views, and some applications in experimental catheter ablation procedures in a large swine model.

Table 12.2 Left ventricular volumes and function measurements by transesophageal (TEE, $n = 24$) and intracardiac echocardiography (ICE, $n = 10$).

	EDV (ml)	ESV (ml)	EF (%)	SV (ml)	HR (bpm)	CI (ml/min/kg)
Swine						
TEE	156 ± 48	57 ± 22	64 ± 6	98 ± 29	93 ± 19	111 ± 22
Doppler	—	—	—	86 ± 14	100 ± 20	107 ± 20
ICE	100 ± 28	36 ± 14	64 ± 7	—	—	—
Human						
TTE	96 ± 19	39 ± 10	60 ± 6	—	—	—

—: No report or not available; CI: cardiac index; EDV and ESV: left ventricular end-diastolic and end-systolic volume; EF: ejection fraction; HR: heart rate (beats per min); SV: stroke volume; TTE: transthoracic two-dimensional echocardiography. Reproduced with permission [1].

The imaging orientation and transducer manipulation have been described earlier (see Chapter 3). For the mechanical radial imaging catheter the orientation of the image can change with the inferior or superior vena cava approach (see Chapter 3). In addition, the imaging views are a little different from those in man due to the orientation of the swine heart which has a more anterior and transverse apex and a relatively cephalad right ventricular apex compared to the left ventricle. These anatomic features make imaging of the pulmonary artery and its bifurcation easier, but detection of the right pulmonary vein ostia is more difficult in swine than in man. In addition, transseptal catheterization is more difficult in the swine model.

ICE imaging technique and normal cardiac structural views in swine

AcuNav phased-array ultrasound catheter imaging

From the right atrium

With the transducer placed in the right atrium just above the inferior vena cava orifice, the eustachian valve, coronary sinus orifice, aortic root, left ventricle, and right ventricular outflow are imaged (Figure 12.1). With the transducer placed near the coronary sinus orifice, rotated counterclockwise and facing posteriorly to the interventricular septum and the septal leaflet of the tricuspid valve, the subeustachian isthmus region (useful for ablation of atrial flutter) including the "posterior" (or inferior) and the septal (superior) isthmus can be imaged in a

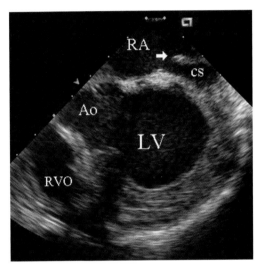

Figure 12.1 ICE image with the transducer placed in the right atrium (RA) just above the inferior vena cava orifice in a swine, showing the eustachian valve (arrow), coronary sinus (CS) ostium, aortic root (Ao), right ventricular outflow (RVO), and a truncated left ventricle (LV).

cross-sectional view (Figure 12.2). With the transducer rotated further clockwise and advanced, the left ventricular outflow is imaged as well as a better view of the aortic root is imaged (Figure 12.3). With the transducer advanced and the tip deflected a little anteriorly, the pulmonary artery and the pulmonic valve are imaged (Figure 12.4). When the transducer is rotated clockwise, the left atrium with its appendage is imaged (Figure 12.5). This is the optimal view of the interatrial septum (fossa ovalis) for guiding transseptal punctures. With the transducer slightly

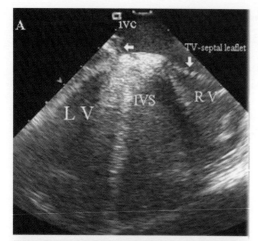

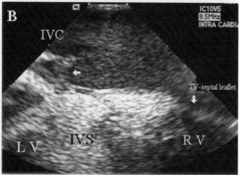

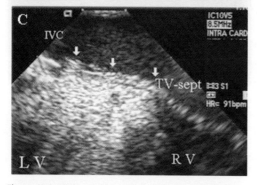

Figure 12.2 ICE images in a swine, with the transducer placed just above the orifice of inferior vena cava (IVC), showing IVC-tricuspid valve (TV) isthmus region. The septal isthmus (A) with its amplified image (B) shows the area between the margin of the coronary sinus (a horizontal arrow) and the septal leaflet of the TV (a downward arrow). The "central" (inferior) isthmus image (C) with the transducer oriented a little posteriorly, shows the area (arrows) between the eustachian valve (ridge) posteriorly and the hinge of the TV anteriorly. The anterior section close to the hinge of the TV septal leaflet consists of the myocardium that formed the full thickness of the atrial wall as seen with thickened echogenicity images in these figures. IVS: interventricular septum; LV and RV: left and right ventricle.

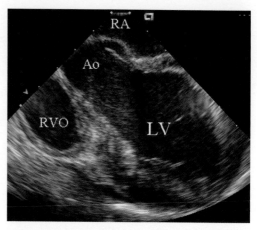

Figure 12.3 ICE image with the transducer advanced and rotated slightly clockwise in the right atrium (RA) in a swine; left ventricular (LV) outflow and aortic root (Ao) are imaged. RVO: right ventricular outflow.

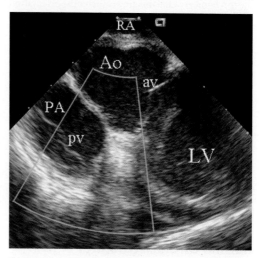

Figure 12.4 ICE images with the transducer advanced and deflected a little anteriorly in the right atrium (RA) in a swine, showing pulmonary artery (PA) and pulmonic valve (pv), aortic root and its cusps (av), and truncated left ventricle (LV).

advanced and further rotated, the pulmonary artery and its bifurcation are imaged (Figure 12.6). The upper left pulmonary vein can be identified when scanning near to the distal end of the left pulmonary artery. With a minor adjustment of the transducer level and subtle rotation clockwise or counterclockwise, both the upper and lower left pulmonary vein ostia are imaged (Figure 12.7a). When the transducer is just rotated clockwise or advanced a little, the lower and upper right pulmonary vein ostia

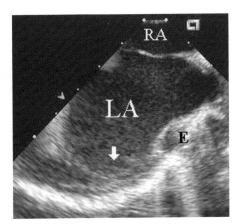

Figure 12.5 ICE image with the transducer placed in the middle right atrium (RA) in a swine, showing the left atrium (LA), interatrial septum, and LA appendage with pectinate muscles (arrow). The esophagus (E) in its short-axis view contiguous to the LA posterior wall is imaged with gas-induced distal scattering of the ultrasound beam.

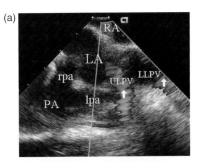

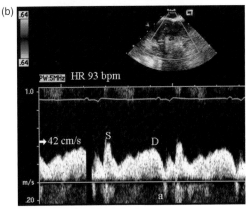

Figure 12.7 ICE Doppler color flow imaging with the transducer placed in the right atrium (RA) in a swine, showing: (a) the left atrium (LA) and the upper (ULPV) and lower left pulmonary vein (LLPV) (arrows) with red color flow toward the LA; and (b) Doppler velocity spectrum recorded with sampling volume at ostium of the ULPV. a: late reversal wave due to atrial contraction. bpm: beats per min; D and S: peak diastolic and systolic flow velocity; HR: heart rate; lpa and rpa: left and right pulmonary artery (PA).

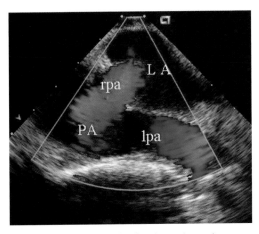

Figure 12.6 ICE Doppler color flow image in a swine, showing the left atrium (LA) and the pulmonary artery (PA) and its bifurcation – the right (rpa) and left PA (lpa).

can be imaged (Figure 12.8a) if an imaging overlap of the right pulmonary artery is avoided. Pulmonary vein ostial flow velocity can be determined with pulsed/continuous-wave Doppler spectral and color flow imaging (Figure 12.7b and 12.8b,c). With the transducer advanced and deflected anteriorly, the aortic root and the aortic cusps in the short-axis view are imaged (Figure 12.9). When the transducer is advanced and rotated counterclockwise the inflow portion of the right ventricle is imaged (Figure 12.10). When the transducer is advanced to the junction of the

superior vena cava and right atrium, the right atrial appendage and the superolateral crista terminalis are imaged (Figure 12.11).

From the tricuspid annulus and right ventricle

With the transducer advanced and just passing over the aortic root, the right ventricle and its outflow tract are imaged (Figure 12.12). When the transducer is placed near the tricuspid orifice, the moderator band in the right ventricle is imaged (Figure 12.13). The catheter can be directed through the tricuspid valve into the right ventricle using ICE imaging guidance. This is helpful in imaging the left ventricle in its long-axis (Figure 12.14) and short-axis views (Figure 12.15a,b).

(a)

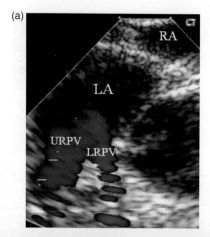

(b)

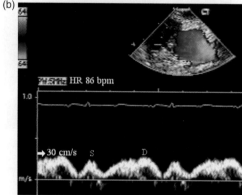

(c)

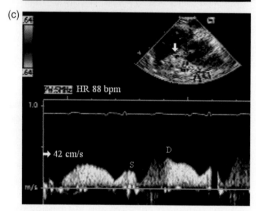

Figure 12.8 ICE Doppler color flow imaging with the transducer placed in the junction of the right atrium (RA) and superior vena cava in a swine, showing: (a) the upper (URPV) and lower right pulmonary vein (LRPV) with red color flow toward the left atrium (LA); and (b) Doppler velocity spectra recorded with sampling volume placed at the ostium of the URPV; and (c) LRPV. bpm: beats per min; D and S: peak diastolic and systolic flow velocity; HR: heart rate.

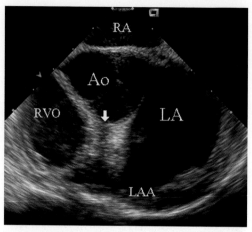

Figure 12.9 ICE image with the transducer in the anterior right atrium (RA) in a swine, showing the short-axis view of the aortic root (Ao) with aortic cusps imaged during diastole. The left main coronary artery is visualized with its ostium in the left aortic sinus of Valsalva (arrow). LA and LAA: left atrium and LA appendage; RVO: right ventricular outflow.

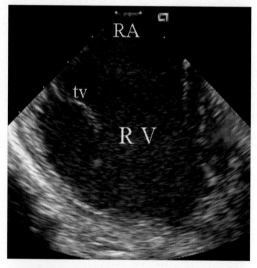

Figure 12.10 ICE image with the transducer in the anterior right atrium (RA) in a swine, showing the right ventricular (RV) inflow tract and the tricuspid valve (tv).

Mechanical radial ultrasound catheter imaging

From the right atrium

With the transducer placed just above the inferior vena cava orifice in the lower right atrium, the eustachian valve, coronary sinus ostium, right atrium and left atrium, right pulmonary vein and artery, and left and right ventricle are imaged (Figure 12.16a–c).

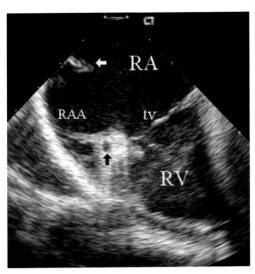

Figure 12.11 ICE image with the transducer placed in the junction of the right atrium (RA) and superior vena cava in a swine, showing the superolateral crista terminalis (arrow) which is the most prominent ridge between the superior vena cava orifice and the RA appendage (RAA), and the right ventricular (RV) inflow. The right coronary artery passing behind the anterolateral tricuspid annulus (black upward arrow) is clearly imaged. tv: tricuspid valve.

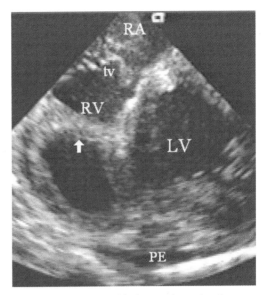

Figure 12.13 ICE image with the transducer placed near the tricuspid orifice in a swine, showing the moderator band (arrow) in the right ventricle (RV), left ventricle (LV), and small pericardial effusion (PE). tv: tricuspid valve.

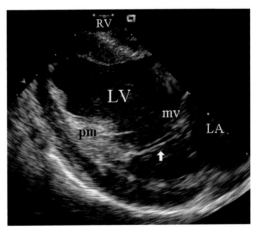

Figure 12.14 ICE image with the transducer placed in the right ventricle (RV) in a swine, showing the left ventricle (LV) in its long-axis view with the anterolateral papillary muscle (pm), mitral valve (mv), and chordae tendineae (arrow). LA: left atrium.

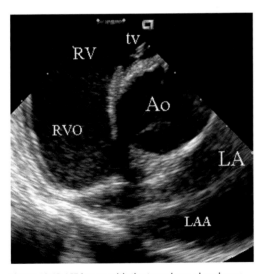

Figure 12.12 ICE image with the transducer placed near the tricuspid valvular (tv) annulus in a swine, showing the right ventricle (RV) and its outflow tract (RVO), aortic root (Ao) and a portion of the left atrium (LA). LAA: LA appendage.

With the transducer placed at the level of the fossa ovalis, the upper left and right pulmonary vein ostia can be imaged (Figure 12.17). When the transducer is advanced into the middle right atrium, the posterolateral crista terminalis at middle level, aortic root, left atrium, and right ventricle are imaged

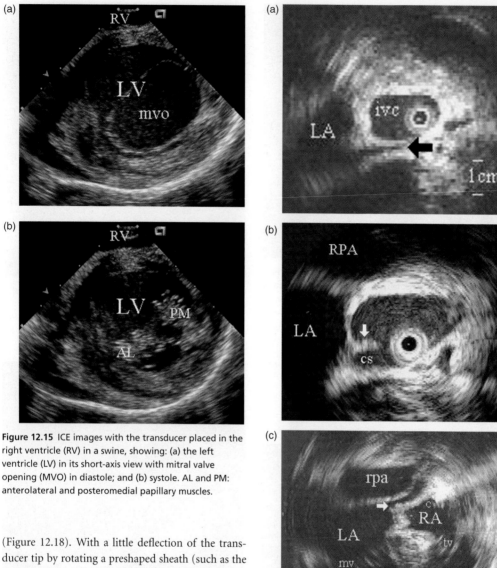

Figure 12.15 ICE images with the transducer placed in the right ventricle (RV) in a swine, showing: (a) the left ventricle (LV) in its short-axis view with mitral valve opening (MVO) in diastole; and (b) systole. AL and PM: anterolateral and posteromedial papillary muscles.

(Figure 12.18). With a little deflection of the transducer tip by rotating a preshaped sheath (such as the tip with 15 or 30° angling) (see Chapter 3), a short-axis view of the aortic root at the aortic cusp level is imaged (Figure 12.19). With the transducer advanced to the high right atrium, the ascending aorta and the junction of the right atrium and superior vena cava at the superior posterolateral crista terminalis are imaged (Figure 12.20).

From the superior vena cava

With the transducer placed just above the orifice in the superior vena cava, the right atrial appendage and ascending aorta surrounding it are imaged (Figure 12.21a) and the superior posterolateral

Figure 12.16 Mechanical radial ICE images with the transducer placed in the low right atrium (RA) in a swine, showing: (a) inferior vena cava orifice (ivc), and coronary sinus (arrow) and left atrium (LA) around it just above the ivc; (b) eustachian valve (arrow), coronary sinus ostium (CS), LA and right pulmonary artery (RPA) with transducer advanced slightly higher (the radius of the image = 3 cm); (c) the left (LV) and right ventricular (RV) inflow, right pulmonary vein (arrow) and artery (rpa) are imaged with transducer positioned close to the interatrial septum (the radius of the image = 6 cm).

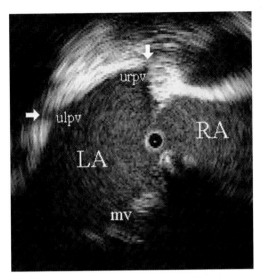

Figure 12.17 Mechanical radial ICE image with the transducer placed at the fossa ovalis in the right atrium (RA) in a swine, showing the left atrium (LA) with the upper left (ulpv) and right pulmonary vein (urpv) ostia (the radius of the image = 4 cm). mv: mitral valve.

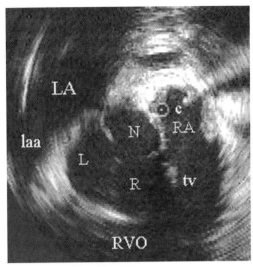

Figure 12.19 Mechanical radial ICE image of a short-axis view of the aortic root in a swine, showing the aortic cusps during diastole (the radius of the image = 6 cm). c: catheter; L: left coronary aortic cusp; LA: left atrium; laa: LA appendage; N: noncoronary aortic cusp; R: right coronary aortic cusp; RA: right atrium; RVO: right ventricular outflow; tv: tricuspid valve.

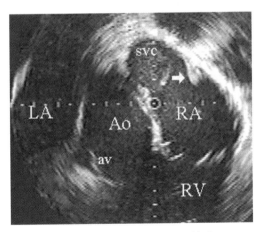

Figure 12.18 Mechanical radial ICE image with the transducer placed anteriorly in the mid-right atrium (RA) in a swine, showing the posterolateral crista terminalis (arrow), aortic root (Ao), left atrium (LA) and the posterior wall of the superior vena cava (svc) (the radius of the image = 6 cm). av: aortic valve; RV: right ventricle.

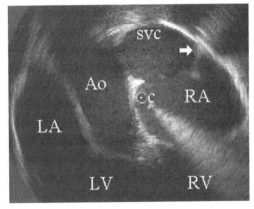

Figure 12.20 Mechanical radial ICE image with the transducer placed in the medial high right atrium (RA) in a swine, showing ascending aorta (Ao) and the superior posterolateral crista terminalis (arrow) at the junction of RA and the superior vena cava (svc) orifice (the radius of the image = 6 cm). c: catheter; LA and LV: left atrium and ventricle; RV: right ventricle.

crista terminalis is visualized during a cardiac cycle (Figure 12.21b). The pulmonary artery may be imaged distal to the ascending aorta (Figure 12.22). With transducer placed further cephalad, the azygos vein orifice is imaged (Figure 12.23).

From the tricuspid annulus and right ventricle

With the transducer placed in the atrioventricular junction, a four-chamber view with both ventricular inflows is imaged (Figure 12.24). With the transducer placed at different levels of the right

(a)

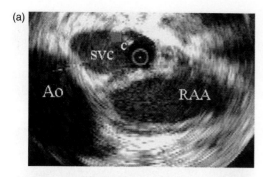

(b)

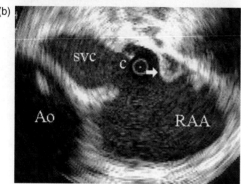

Figure 12.21 Mechanical radial ICE images with the transducer placed in the superior vena cava (svc) in a swine, showing: (a) right atrial appendage (RAA) and ascending aorta (Ao); (b) and the superior posterolateral crista terminalis (arrow) during a cardiac cycle (the radius of the image = 4 cm).

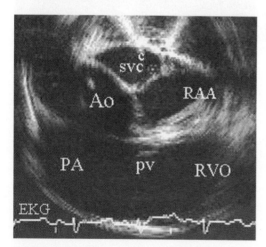

Figure 12.22 Mechanical radial ICE image with the transducer placed in the superior vena cava (SVC) in a swine, showing pulmonary artery (PA) in its long-axis view distal to the ascending aorta (Ao) (the radius of the image = 8 cm). c: catheter; EKG: electrocardiogram; pv: pulmonic valve; RAA: right atrial appendage; RVO: right ventricular outflow.

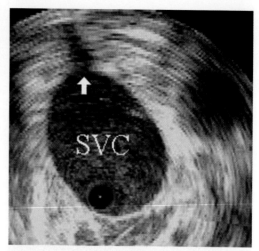

Figure 12.23 Mechanical radial ICE image with the transducer placed in the superior vena cava (SVC) from a right jugular vein approach in the swine model, showing the azygos vein and its orifice (arrow) (the radius of the image = 3 cm).

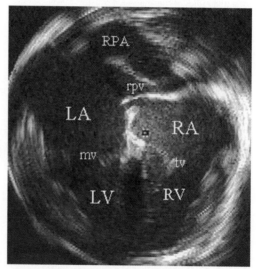

Figure 12.24 Mechanical radial ICE image with the transducer placed in the right side of the cardiac crux in a swine, showing a four-chamber view of the left and right atria (LA and RA) and ventricles (LV and RV) (the radius of the image = 8 cm). mv: mitral valve; RPA and rpv: right pulmonary artery and vein; tv: tricuspid valve.

ventricle, left ventricular short-axis views are imaged, and the left ventricular regional wall motion and global systolic function can be evaluated from its linear dimension, area or volumetric changes during diastole and systole (Figure 12.25a,b).

(a)

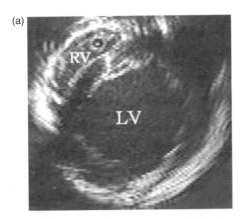

(b)

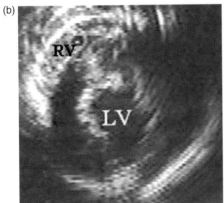

Figure 12.25 Mechanical radial ICE image with the transducer placed in the right ventricle (RV) in a swine, showing: (a) left ventricle (LV) in its short-axis view at end-diastole; and (b) end-systole (the radius of the image = 6 cm).

From the aortic root and left ventricle

From a retrograde femoral artery approach or transseptal catheterization near-field images of left heart structures can be obtained. When the transducer is advanced retrograde to the aortic root, the left main coronary artery ostium and it proximal segment and the anatomic structures around the aortic root can be imaged (Figure 12.26). Positioning the transducer within the left ventricle yields a short-axis view at each level of the imaging catheter, allowing evaluation of left ventricular regional wall thickness, motion, chamber dimension and area, and volume (Figure 12.27).

Transseptal catheterization guided by ICE

ICE imaging has been helpful in guiding transseptal catheterization, improving both the efficacy and safety

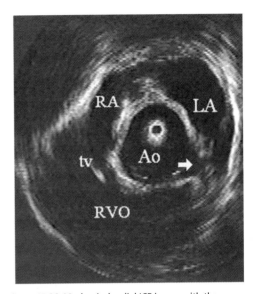

Figure 12.26 Mechanical radial ICE image with the transducer placed retrograde in the aortic root (Ao) in a swine, showing the left main coronary artery and its proximal branches (arrow), and the left atrium (LA), right atrium (RA) and right ventricular outflow tract (RVO) around Ao (the radius of the image = 8 cm).

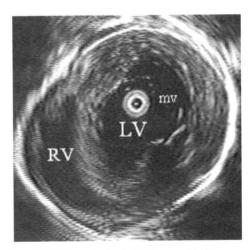

Figure 12.27 Mechanical radial ICE image with the transducer placed retrograde in the left ventricle (LV) in a swine, showing LV and right ventricle (RV) in their short-axis views. The ventricular wall thickness, chamber dimension and area can be evaluated (the radius of the image = 6 cm). mv: mitral valve.

of transseptal procedures. ICE can provide real-time imaging assistance and guidance by imaging the position of puncture needle related to the interatrial septum and its adjacent cardiac structures. Transseptal catheterization in a swine model is technically

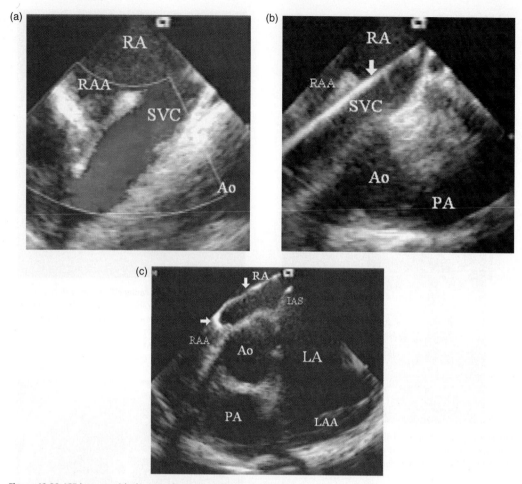

Figure 12.28 ICE images with the transducer placed in the high right atrium (RA) in a swine, showing: (a) the superior vena cava (SVC, red color flow toward the RA) adjacent to the RA appendage (RAA); (b) a guide wire (arrow) positioning in the SVC; or (c) at the orifice of RAA during transseptal catheterization. Ao: aorta; IAS: interatrial septum; LA and LAA: left atrium and LA appendage; PA: pulmonary artery.

more difficult than in man; frequent procedural failure and significant complications have been observed using fluoroscopic guidance alone, including damage to pulmonary artery, coronary sinus and left ventricle, and pericardial effusion. This may be secondary to the parallel orientation of the interatrial septum relative to transseptal catheter as delivered from an inferior vena cava approach in swine. These anatomic structural relationships are not apparent with real-time fluoroscopic imaging guided entirely by catheter position in cardiac silhouette. Transseptal catheterization is performed with a Brockenbrough needle in conjunction with Mullins sheath/dilator unit from an inferior vena cava approach (see Chapter 5).

Transseptal catheterization guided by AcuNav ICE imaging without fluoroscopic imaging *in vivo* is possible and safe since the relationship of the transseptal catheter tip and adjacent structures can be clearly imaged [11]. ICE imaging guidance for transseptal catheterization without fluoroscopy, allows adequate visualization of each procedural step: (1) positioning of the guide wire within the superior vena cava (Figure 12.28a,b) or near the orifice of the right atrial appendage (Figure 12.28c); (2) positioning of the Brockenbrough needle at the fossa ovalis with tenting of the atrial septum (Figure 12.29a,b); (3) ensuring optimal left atrial "target" positioning after puncture (Figure 12.29c).

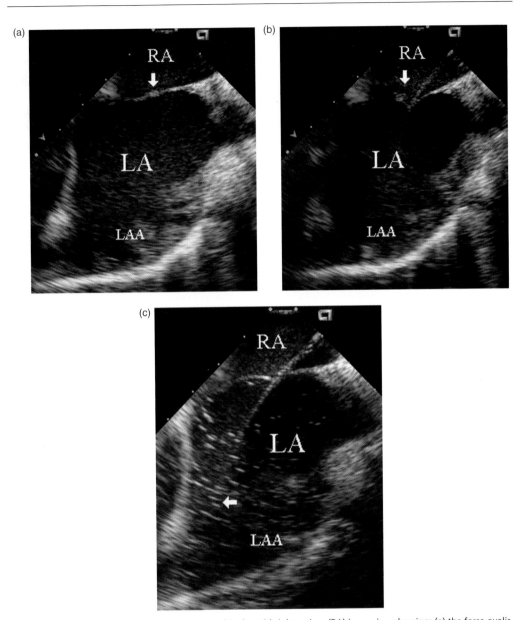

Figure 12.29 ICE images with the transducer placed in the mid-right atrium (RA) in a swine, showing: (a) the fossa ovalis (arrow) before puncture; (b) needle tenting (arrow) during; and (c) optimal "target" positioning (arrow) after puncture. Flushing of the catheter with saline results in characteristic bubbles seen in the left atrium (LA), verifying LA position of the sheath. LAA: LA appendage.

Mechanical radial ICE, even with its relatively high (9 MHz) ultrasound frequency transducer and limited imaging depth for the left heart structures, can be used properly for guiding transseptal needle positioning at the fossa ovalis and tenting with an optimal direction into the left atrium (Figure 12.30a,b) during transseptal catheterization.

Radiofrequency energy ablation in the atria and left ventricle

Swine model, normal and post anterior myocardial infarction

Normal swine model

Domestic healthy swine weighing between 35–130 kg are kept on a minimum 12 h fast prior to the

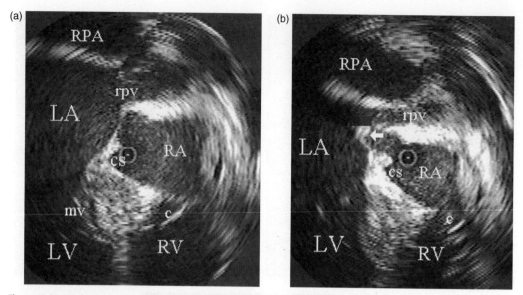

Figure 12.30 Mechanical radial ICE images with the transducer placed near the fossa ovalis of the interatrial septum in the right atrium (RA) in a swine, showing: (a) the fossa ovalis just above the coronary sinus (CS) ostium before puncture; and (b) needle tenting with an optimal direction (arrow) into the left atrium (LA) during the transseptal puncture (the radius of the image = 4 cm). c: catheter; LV and RV: left and right ventricle; mv: mitral valve; RPA and rpv: right pulmonary artery and vein.

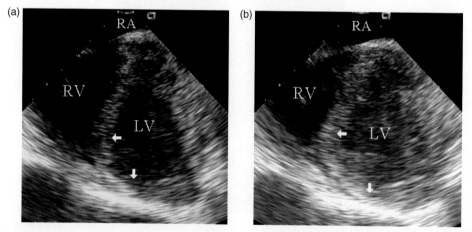

Figure 12.31 ICE images with the transducer placed near the atrioventricular junction in the right atrium (RA) in a swine model of healed myocardial infarction, showing: left ventricular regional wall thinning, increased echogenicity (scar), and akinesis (between the two arrows) in the anteroseptal region: (a) at diastole; and (b) systole.

procedure and given drinking water *ad libitum*. Swine are premedicated with an intramuscular injection of droperidol (0.1 mg/kg) and pethidine HCl (2 mg/kg) 20 min before anesthesia and the ECG is monitored. An intravenous catheter (auricular marginal vein) is used to administer fluids (0.9% saline, 10 mg per h) or drugs. Premedication is intravenous thiopental sodium (10–12 mg/kg). Endotracheal intubation is performed after inducement of hypnotic state and anesthesia maintained with forane (2–4%) in oxygen (Ohio, 30/70 proportioner anesthesia machine) [1,12]. Swine are subjected to atrial and ventricular endocardial mapping and ablation.

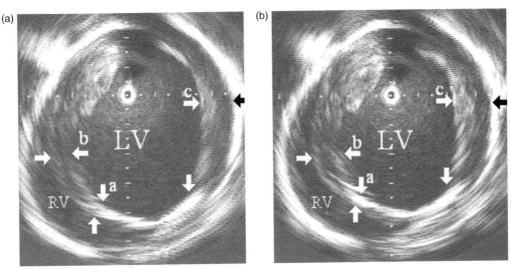

Figure 12.32 Mechanical radial ICE images with the transducer placed in the left ventricle (LV) via retrograde transaortic approach in a swine model of healed myocardial infarction, showing a LV short-axis view with changes in LV regional wall thickness: (a) at end-diastole; and (b) end-systole 45 days after myocardial infarction. LV wall thinning (3 mm), akinesis, and increased echogenicity (scar) is seen in the anteroseptal region between the two downward arrows. LV wall thickening is preserved, but reduced in the other septal (b, thickness 7.5–10 mm) and posterolateral wall region (c, 10–13 mm) (each scale = 5 mm).

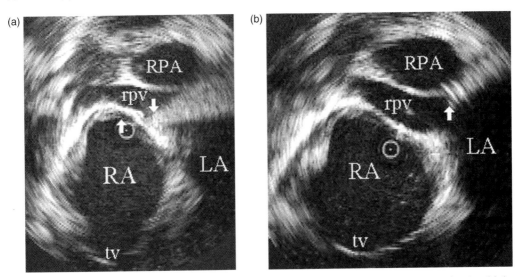

Figure 12.33 Mechanical radial ICE images with the transducer placed in the right atrium (RA) in a swine, showing: (a) the RA posterior smooth wall region (upward arrow), and the ablation catheter positioned at the lower edge (downward arrow); and (b) the upper edge (upward arrow) of the right pulmonary vein (rpv) ostium with distal fan-shaped shadow artifact in the left atrium (LA) (the radius of the image = 4 cm). RPA: right pulmonary artery; tv: tricuspid valve.

Swine model of anterior myocardial infarction

Swine are warmed with a water-circulating heating pad. The closed-chest infarction procedure [13,14] is performed in swine under endotracheal intubation and general anesthesia with inhaled forane in oxygen (60%) and N_2O (40%) after an overnight fast and premedication with ketamine 22 mg/kg, acetylpromazine 1.1 mg/kg, and atropine 0.05 mg/kg IM. Arterial blood gas measurements

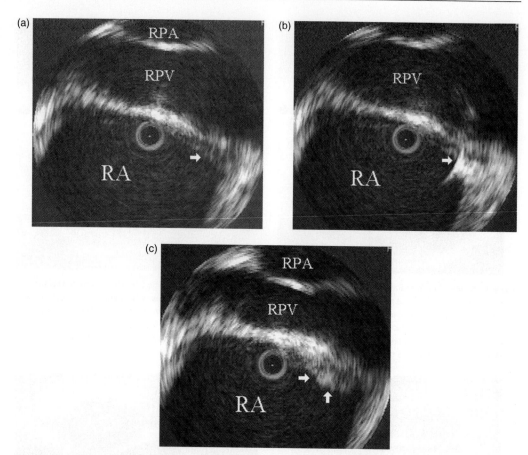

Figure 12.34 Mechanical radial ICE images of the right atrium (RA) in a swine, showing: (a) the posterior wall thickness at baseline (arrow, thickness = 2.2 mm); (b) an ablation catheter electrode positioned during ablation; and (c) increased wall thickness (5.5 mm) and echogenicity with dimpling and craters (arrows) immediately after radiofrequency lesion application (the radius of the image = 2 cm). RPA and RPV: right pulmonary artery and vein.

are performed throughout the procedure (when clinically indicated) and intravenous fluids are administered. A 9 F sheath is placed percutaneously in the left femoral artery by the Seldinger technique to monitor blood pressure and to allow arterial access. An 8 F AL 1 or 2 guide catheter was placed at the ostium of the left anterior descending coronary artery (LAD), and a 2- to 2.5-mm angioplasty balloon is advanced to the distal LAD at the site of the second diagonal branch. Thirty seconds after balloon inflation (6 atm), 300 μL of agarose gel beads (diameter of 75–150 μm; Bio-Rad Laboratories) diluted in 1.5 ml saline is injected through the balloon lumen. The balloon is deflated and the catheter withdrawn. The evolving anterior infarction is assessed by continuous ECG and hemodynamic monitoring. The swine is maintained

under general anesthesia until the arterial sheath is removed 30 min after the infarction procedure, and buprenorphine 0.3 mg IM was given to alleviate discomfort on awakening. After extubation, the swine is observed until it is able to walk without assistance. After 6–10 weeks of infarct healing, swine are subjected to left ventricular endocardial mapping and ablation. A typical healed myocardial infarction involving left ventricular anterior-septal regions can be revealed with wall thinning, increased echogenicity (scar) and akinesis or dyskinesis by AcuNav (Figure 12.31a,b) or mechanical radial ICE imaging (Figure 12.32a,b).

Ablation procedure

Arterial and venous access is obtained to the carotid artery and the femoral vessels under general

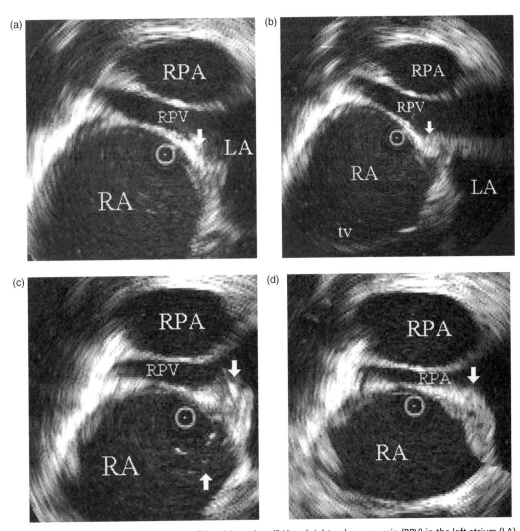

Figure 12.35 Mechanical radial ICE images of the right atrium (RA) and right pulmonary vein (RPV) in the left atrium (LA) in a swine, showing: (a) the lower edge of the RPV ostium (arrow, wall thickness = 4 mm) before; (b) a LA ablation catheter electrode (arrow); (c) wall swelling (downward arrow), bubbles (upward arrow) on the opposite RA side during; and (d) increased wall thickness (arrow, 6 mm) after lesion application (the radius of the image = 4cm). RPA: right pulmonary artery; tv: tricuspid valve.

anesthesia. Heparin is given intravenously at initial dose of 10 000 units with repeated dose every 90 min. Discrete and/or linear radiofrequency lesions are made in the right atrium posterior smooth wall (Figure 12.33a) and in the left atrial medial posterior wall adjacent to the orifice of the upper right pulmonary vein (Figure 12.33a,b) with a transseptal catheterization using a standard 4.5-mm length ablation electrode (Navistar, CARTO system, Biosense Ltd., Israel) under ICE imaging guidance [12,15]. A prototype 3.5-mm, 7-Fr irrigated-tip thermocouple catheter (with room temperature saline at 30–40 ml/min using a Rolerflex pump) or a standard radiofrequency ablation catheter is introduced to the left ventricle using a retrograde transaortic approach via the femoral and/or carotid artery. ICE-guided radiofrequency applications (30–50 W, up to 120 s) are used to deploy discrete and/or linear lesions at the border of the infarct region or the normal left ventricular posterior/lateral wall [15–17]. Catheter contact with atrial and left ventricular endocardium and its stability are continuously assessed and

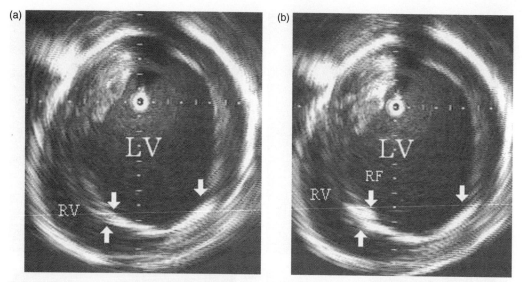

Figure 12.36 Mechanical radial ICE images of the left ventricle (LV) short-axis view with the transducer advanced to the LV via a retrograde transaortic approach in a swine model, showing: (a) an infarcted anteroseptal wall with thinning (thickness = 3 mm between the two downward arrows) with akinesis and increased echogenicity before; and (b) increased wall thickness (from 5–9 mm) and echogenicity at the infarcted border (between the two opposite arrows) after lesion application (RF).

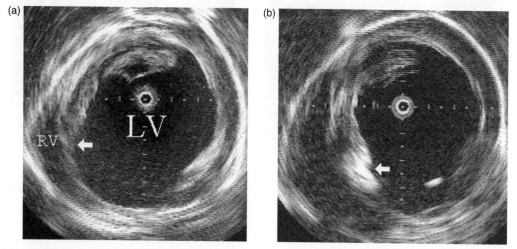

Figure 12.37 Mechanical radial ICE images of the left ventricular (LV) short-axis view in a swine model of anteroseptal myocardial infarction, showing: (a) the anteroseptal thickness (5 mm, arrow) at the border of an infarcted zone before; and (b) increased wall thickness (9 mm) and echogenicity with crater formation (arrow) after lesion deployment. Each scale = 5 mm. RV: right ventricle.

monitored with ICE imaging, and radiofrequency energy is delivered only when adequate electrode–tissue contact is assured using ICE monitoring. During the ablation, fluoroscopy is occasionally used for catheter positioning as reference and comparison.

Lesion morphologic changes in atrial and ventricular tissue

The ability to evaluate lesion creation *in vivo* may have important clinical and experimental applications for ablation therapy [12,18,19]. At present, when radiofrequency energy delivery does not result

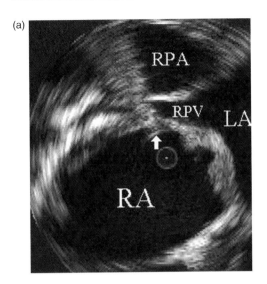
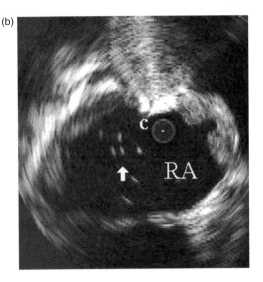
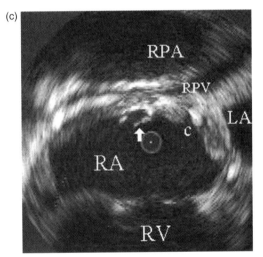

Figure 12.38 Mechanical radial ICE images of right atrium (RA) in a swine model, showing: (a) an ablation catheter positioned (arrow) at the RA posterior wall (thickness = 2.5 mm) before; (b) bubbles (arrow) in the RA during; and (c) increased wall thickness (4 mm) with echogenic crater formation and thrombus attached (arrow) following lesion application (the radius of the image = 3 cm). c: catheter; LA: left atrium; RPA and RPV: right pulmonary artery and vein.

in arrhythmia termination, it is difficult to distinguish ineffective lesion delivery from insufficient accuracy in mapping. ICE imaging provides online verification that the intended radiofrequency lesion actually affects the underlying tissue with serial morphologic changes. Based on findings of ICE guided right atrial radiofrequency ablations (25–50 W, or 70°C, up to 120 s) creating 423 intercaval linear and 47 special separation lesions in 12 large swine (117–127 kg), with serial radiofrequency energy

applications, morphologic evolution of local right atrial wall with three phases [18] are: (1) Phase I, increased wall thickness to 120% relative to baseline, increased or mixed with unchanged echogenicity, consistent with swelling and edema; (2) Phase II, dimpling, increased wall thickness to 150% relative to baseline, increased and inhomogeneous echogenicity, consistent with edema and ischemic to resistive heating; (3) Phase III, crater formation, increased, unchanged or reduced (relative to phase II) wall

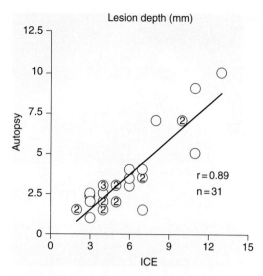

Figure 12.39 Correlation between intracardiac echocardiography (ICE) imaging local atrial and left ventricular wall thickness following radiofrequency deployment and pathologic lesion depth ($p < 0.01$) in a swine model. Reproduced with permission [15].

Table 12.3 ICE imaging wall thickness at the lesion site pre- and post-radiofrequency deployment and pathologic lesion size.

	ICE wall thickness (mm)			Pathologic lesion depth (mm)
	Pre-	Post-RF*	Change	
Atria (n = 24)	2.3 ± 1.0	4.5 ± 1.5	2.2 ± 1.2	2.4 ± 0.8
LV (n = 7)	6.8 ± 2.2	9.8 ± 2.3	3.0 ± 1.4	7.0 ± 2.1

*$p < 0.01$: post- versus pre-RF. ICE: intracardiac echocardiography; LV: left ventricle; RF: radiofrequency. Reproduced with permission [15].

thickness, shaggy appearance of the endocardium with occasional thrombus formation, reduced central and strongly increased lesion surface/peripheral echogenicity, consistent with findings of coagulative necrosis, and edema at pathologic analysis. It has been well established that therapeutic radiofrequency ablation causes right (Figure 12.34a–c), left atrial (Figure 12.35a–d), and ventricular lesions (Figure 12.36a,b) with mixed mural swelling, dimpling, and crater formation (Figure 12.37a,b) associated with echogenicity changes or occasional thrombus formation (Figure 12.38a–c) detected by ICE imaging [8,12,15–20]. Radiofrequency ablation-induced changes in wall thickness determined by ICE imaging are correlated with pathologic lesion depth at autopsy (Table 12.3, Figure 12.39) in the atria ($r = 0.82, p < 0.01$) and the left ventricle ($r = 0.85, p < 0.05$) [15]. ICE quantification of atrial wall thickness changes, following radiofrequency ablation has been studied at different atrial sites including the high, middle, and lower right atrium, superior vena cava, and left atrium (Table 12.4) [19]. Important features of atrial wall response to lesion application include increased wall thickness relative to baseline with distortion of endocardial contour at the point of electrode–endocardial contact within 1 min post-lesion, gradually tapering on either side. At 30 and 150 min post-lesion wall thickening is progressive and more diffuse [19]. Similar morphologic findings have been revealed on left ventricular mural swelling from radiofrequency ablation using irrigated-tip and standard catheter in a swine model of healed anterior myocardial infarction [16,17]. Furthermore, as demonstrated by ICE imaging, irrigated radiofrequency ablation produces quantitatively greater changes in wall thickness and tissue echogenicity than standard radiofrequency

Table 12.4 ICE quantification of atrial and superior vena cava wall thickness following radiofrequency ablation in swine (n = 7, 80–120 kg).

	High RA	Middle RA	Low RA	SVC	LA
Baseline (mm)	3.0 ± 1.2	2.8 ± 1.0	1.8 ± 0.8	2.9 ± 1.3	3.2 ± 1.5
1' Post- (mm)	5.0 ± 1.5	5.2 ± 1.4	3.9 ± 1.3	4.4 ± 1.6	5.8 ± 2.0
30' Post- (mm)	6.4 ± 2.3	7.0 ± 1.4	5.0 ± 1.1	7.2 ± 2.3	6.7 ± 1.5
150' Post- (mm)	6.8 ± 1.9	10.1 ± 3.1	—	8.5 ± 3.5	11.0 ± 5.6

$p < 0.01$: all Post- versus Baseline. ICE: intracardiac echocardiography; LA: left atrial wall thickness; Post-: post-radiofrequency ablation; RA: right atrial wall thickness; SVC: superior vena cava wall thickness.

Table 12.5 Left ventricular wall measurements at lesion site pre- and post-radiofrequency ablation using irrigated and standard catheter.

Wall thickness (mm)	Irrigated		Standard	
	Septal/Anterior	Infarcted*	Septal/Anterior	Infarcted
Pre-	8.5 ± 1.4	5.9 ± 1.8	8.6 ± 2.8	5.0 ± 1.0
1′ Post-	10.3 ± 1.8	8.3 ± 2.3	9.9 ± 2.7	5.6 ± 1.1
Difference	1.8 ± 1.4	2.4 ± 1.6	1.3 ± 0.7	0.6 ± 0.2
Δ% (versus Pre-)	21.2	40.7	15.1	12.0

*$p < 0.0007$: versus Infarcted using standard catheter. Reproduced with permission [16].

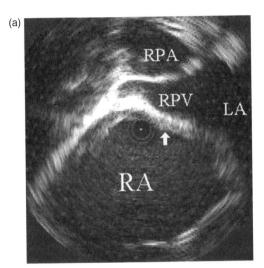 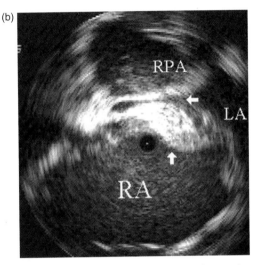

Figure 12.40 Mechanical radial ICE images of right atrium (RA) and adjacent upper right pulmonary vein (RPV) in a swine model, showing: (a) RA posterior wall (arrow, thickness = 3 mm) before; and (b) increased wall thickness (11 mm, upward arrow) and echogenicity with adjacent RPV luminal narrowing (leftward arrow) after radiofrequency lesions deployed (the radius of the image = 3 cm). LA: left atrium; RPA: right pulmonary artery.

Table 12.6 Evolution of right atrial wall thickness and adjacent right pulmonary vein luminal diameter after right atrial linear radiofrequency ablation in 12 swines.

(mm)	Pre-	Post-	1 week	1 month	2 months	3 months
Wall thickness	1.8 ± 0.6	6.1 ± 1.1*	4.2 ± 0.5*	1.8 ± 0.2	2.5 ± 0.7	2.7 ± 0.6
Lumen diameter	7.5 ± 1.7	5.0 ± 1.5*	4.5 ± 0.7*	6.3 ± 1.0	5.8 ± 2.5	8.1 ± 3.6

*$p < 0.05$: versus Pre-. Pre- and Post-: Pre- and Post-radiofrequency ablation.

ablation (Table 12.5) [16]. Because changes in tissue parameters that can be quantified by ICE imaging directly reflect lesion size, ICE imaging may be helpful for "dosing" energy delivery using irrigated radiofrequency energy delivery.

Narrowing effect of right atrial mural swelling on adjacent pulmonary vein lumen and its regression

Right atrial linear radiofrequency ablation consistently causes mural swelling and produces adjacent

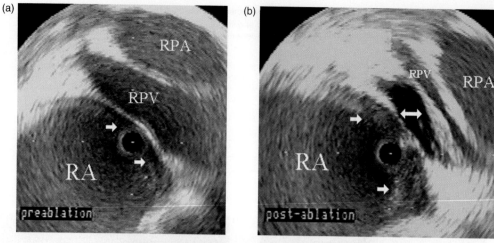

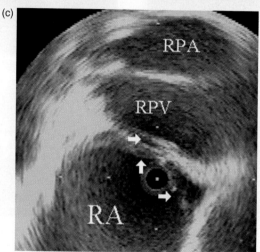

Figure 12.41 Mechanical radial ICE images of the right atrium (RA) and adjacent upper right pulmonary vein (RPV) in a healthy swine model, showing: (a) the RA posterior wall thickness (2.2 and 2.6 mm, at the arrows) and RPV luminal diameter (6.2–9.0 mm) at baseline; and (b) increased wall thickness (4.8 and 6.9 mm) and diminished RPV luminal diameter (1.8–1.7 mm) with the development of an echo-free interstitial space (5 mm, bi-directional arrow) immediately post-ablation. (c) At 1 week post-ablation, the RA posterior wall thickness (3.2 and 7.0 mm) decreases, but is still significantly greater than baseline and the RPV luminal diameter (8.0–9.0 mm) returns to baseline with a trivial interstitial space left between them (higher rightward arrow). Each scale = 8 mm. RPA: right pulmonary artery.

Table 12.7 Changes in left ventricular wall thickness and regional fractional shortening associated with radiofrequency ablation (85 lesions) in swine myocardial infarcted model ($n = 8$).

	Interventricular septum		Anterior		Lateral/Posterior	
	THK (mm)	FS (%)	THK (mm)	FS (%)	THK (mm)	FS (%)
Pre-	9.2 ± 3.0	32 ± 25	6.8 ± 1.9	40 ± 24	10.7 ± 2.0	49 ± 29
1'Post–*	11.6 ± 3.8	14 ± 12	8.5 ± 2.2	29 ± 26	11.9 ± 2.4	25 ± 20
*p: versus Pre-	< 0.003	$=0.06$	< 0.001	< 0.003	< 0.0001	< 0.02

THK: thickness; FS: fractional shortening.

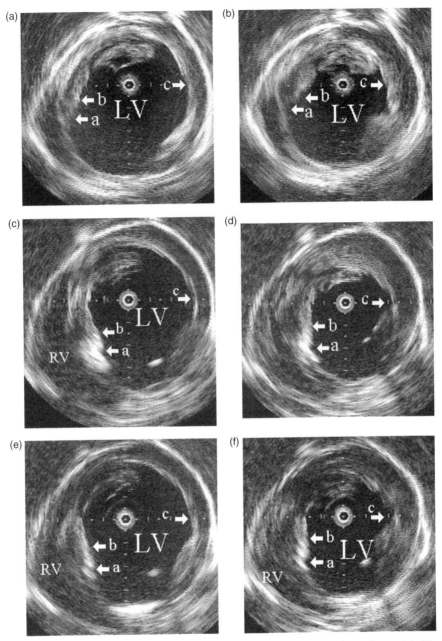

Figure 12.42 Mechanical radial ICE images of the left ventricle (LV) in the short-axis view in a swine model of the anteroseptal myocardial infarction, showing the wall thickness at the ablated site of the infarcted border zone (a, arrow), 1 cm adjacent to the ablated site (b, arrow) and the normal wall on the opposite site (c, arrow): (a) at end-diastole (thickness at "a" = 5 mm; "b" = 11 mm; "c" = 10 mm); and (b) end-systole ("a" = 5 mm; "b" = 12.5 mm; "c" = 17 mm) before; and (c) changes in wall thickness associated with ablation-increased wall thickness and echogenicity with crater formation at "a" at end-diastole ("a" = 9 mm; "b" = 14.5 mm; "c" = 7.5 mm); and (d) end-systole ("a" = 9 mm; "b" = 15 mm; "c" = 14 mm); immediately after; and those (e) at end-diastole ("a" = 9 mm; "b" = 14 mm; "c" = 9 mm); and (f) end-systole ("a" = 9 mm; "b" = 17.5 mm; "c" = 15 mm) at 30 min after lesion deployment. The regional wall fractional shortening decreases from 13.6% to 3.4% at the adjacent wall "b" and increases from 70% to 86.7% at the distal normal wall associated with morphologic changes at the ablated site "a" immediately after lesion application, and its returning to preablation values (25% at "b" and 66.6% at "c") observed at 30 min following lesion deployment.

Table 12.8 Radiofrequency-induced changes in left ventricular wall thickness and regional wall motion function in the swine model of myocardial infarction.

		Post-radiofrequency lesion			
	Pre-	1 min	30 min	60 min	90 min
Wall thickness (mm)	7.7 ± 1.8	$9.6 \pm 2.0^*$	$11.0 \pm 2.0^*$	$12.2 \pm 2.0^*$	$12.3 \pm 2.1^*$
Fractional shortening (%)	29 ± 13	$16 \pm 10^*$	27 ± 11	27 ± 12	27 ± 12

$^*p < 0.05$: versus Pre-(radiofrequency lesion) values. Reproduced with permission [17].

(a)
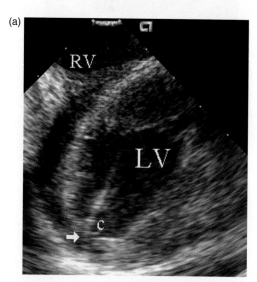

(b)
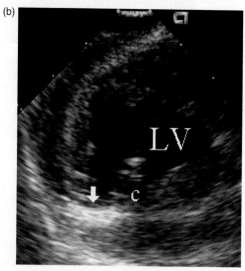

Figure 12.43 ICE images of the left ventricle (LV) in the short-axis view with the transducer placed in a swine right ventricle (RV), showing: (a) the catheter (c) needle (arrow) positioned just beneath the endocardium before ablation; and (b) an intramural lesion (arrow) development with increased echogenicity and wall thickness immediately after alcohol injection and the catheter (c) withdrawn.

Table 12.9 Morphologic characteristics of left ventricular myocardial ethanol lesion in swine.

Needle type	Lesion volume (mm³)	Lesion depth (mm)	Depth from endocardium (mm)
Single port	$1910 \pm 1066^*$	$8.9 \pm 3.3^*$	$1.8 \pm 1.2^{**}$
Multiport	825 ± 753	4.9 ± 2.5	0.3 ± 0.7

$^*p < 0.05$ and $^{**}p < 0.01$: versus multiport. Reproduced with permission [32].

pulmonary vein and aortic wall edema that is observed both in a large swine model and man [21]. Linear radiofrequency ablation in the posterior right atrium causes immediate swelling of the walls of contiguous right upper pulmonary vein, resulting in a decrease in the pulmonary vein luminal diameter

(Figure 12.40a,b) as observed with ICE imaging in 12 healthy swine [22]. The right atrial posterior wall thickness and adjacent right pulmonary vein luminal diameter are measured pre-, immediately post-lesion deployment and subsequently at intervals of 1 week, and 1, 2, and 3 months (Table 12.6). The findings indicate that the magnitude of right atrial wall thickness increase and adjacent right pulmonary vein luminal diameter decrease is maximal early, and importantly, these lesion morphologic changes can resolve (Figure 12.41a–c) by 1 month [22].

Left ventricular regional wall motion associated with lesion morphologic changes

ICE imaging provides capability of evaluating regional wall motion function expressed as the fractional shortening (%) which is (the difference of wall thickness

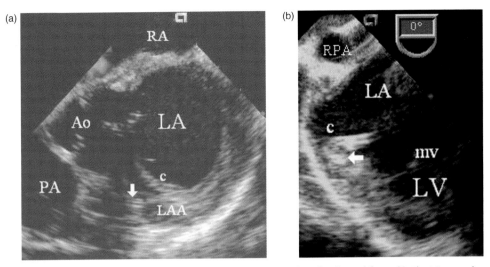

Figure 12.44 ICE image of the left atrium (LA) in a swine, showing: (a) a thrombus (arrow) formed in the LA appendage (LAA) after injection of thrombin through a catheter (c) which is withdrawn aside; and (b) the thrombus (arrow) and catheter (c) also imaged in the LA appendage by transesophageal echocardiography. Ao: aortic root; LV: left ventricle; mv: mitral valve; PA: pulmonary artery; RA: right atrium; RPA: right pulmonary artery.

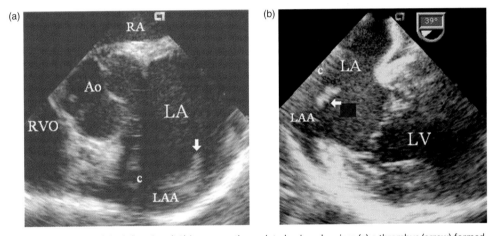

Figure 12.45 ICE image of the left atrium (LA) in an unanticoagulated swine, showing: (a) a thrombus (arrow) formed following catheter/sheath (c) placement in the LA appendage (LAA); and (b) the thrombus (arrow) also imaged comparable by transesophageal echocardiography. Ao: aortic root; LV: left ventricle; RA: right atrium; RVO: right ventricular outflow.

at end-systole and end-diastole/wall thickness at end-diastole) × 100. In the swine model of anteroseptal myocardial infarction, ICE imaging guided linear radiofrequency lesions in the left ventricle cause increased wall thickness (Table 12.7) [23] and immediately decreased regional wall fractional shortening at the ablated site and the normal myocardium adjacent (1 cm) to the ablated site as detected by ICE imaging (Figure 12.42a–d). The time course for functional recovery is short, with fractional shortening returning to pre-ablation values within 30 min (Figure 12.42e,f) (Table 12.8) [17]. The fractional shortening in the opposite or distal wall region can increase as a functional compensation.

Alcohol left ventricular ablation

Limitations in lesion volume and in particular lesion depth may reduce the efficacy of catheter ablation using radiofrequency energy. Absolute ethanol has

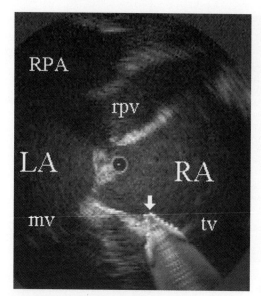

Figure 12.46 Mechanical radial ICE image of the right atrium (RA) in a swine, showing the echocardiographic transponder arrowhead (arrow) indicating the ablation electrode positioning at the tricuspid annulus (the radius of the image = 4 cm). LA: left atrium; mv: mitral valve; RPA and rpv: right pulmonary artery and vein; tv: tricuspid valve.

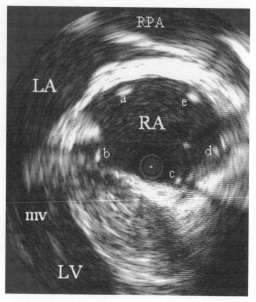

Figure 12.48 Mechanical radial ICE image of the right atrium (RA) in a swine, showing the five poles (marked as "a, b, c, d, and e") of a ventricular mapping basket catheter (50-pole. Cordis Webster, Baldwin Park, CA) positioned in the RA, in which the pole "b" locates at the coronary sinus orifice and the "e" at the crista terminalis (the radius of the image = 3 cm). mv: mitral valve; LA: left atrium; LV: left ventricle; RPA: right pulmonary artery.

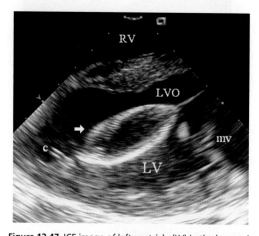

Figure 12.47 ICE image of left ventricle (LV) in the long-axis view with the transducer placed in the right ventricle (RV) in a swine, showing a mapping array (arrow, EnSite system, Endocardial Solutions, St. Paul, MN) positioned near the LV outflow (LVO) in the LV. c: catheter; mv: mitral valve.

proven useful for nonsurgical ablation of myocardial tissue, both for treatment of arrhythmias [24–28] and hypertrophic obstructive cardiomyopathy [29–31]. Real-time ICE-guided direct intramural injection of

ethanol (0.5 ml) into the left ventricular myocardium with a novel injection catheter system that includes an 8 Fr deflectable catheter equipped with a 27-gauge extendable/retractable needle (MyoStar™, Biosense-Webster, Diamond Bar, CA) was performed to evaluate the safety and efficacy of myocardial ablation in nine swine (36–40 kg) [32]. ICE imaging is used to guide catheter positioning, to ensure optimal catheter contact prior to and following needle deployment, and to assess the intramural lesion morphology and to quantify the lesion size. Alcohol injection induces myocardial "targeted" intramural lesions ($n = 86$), all directly adjacent to the needle and is characterized by increased echogenicity and wall thickness (Figure 12.43a,b). Thrombus formation at lesions, and myocardial perforation or ventricular arrhythmias were not observed with needle deployment or lesion creation, whereas single ventricular premature beats were observed with needle deployment and were used to identify satisfactory position within the myocardium. Lesions created with a single port needle are significantly larger in volume and have a greater depth than those created with the multiport needle which has a series of four laser etched holes for terminal exit (Table 12.9) [32]. The findings in the swine model indicates that ethanol injection may prove helpful in selected catheter ablation procedures where deeper lesions are essential for procedural success.

Swine model of thrombus in the left atrial appendage

To evaluate the capability of ICE for diagnosing thrombus in the left atrial appendage a swine model of thrombus is established. A standard coronary catheter (AL1) is advanced into the left atrial appendage through an 8 Fr introducer sheath via transseptal catheterization guided by ICE imaging. Thrombin (250–500 IU) is injected into the left atrial appendage to create thrombus (Figure 12.44a,b) in four swine anticoagulated with heparin and another two thrombi are formed spontaneously on the introducer sheath tip in the appendage (Figure 12.45a,b) in two unanticoagulated swine. The area of the thrombus in the left atrial appendage is 0.7 ± 0.9 cm^2 (0.2–2.6) detected by ICE and 0.8 ± 1.2 cm^2 (0.2–3.2) by transesophageal echocardiography [11]. In this swine model, ICE is comparable to transesophageal echocardiography for the detection of the thrombus in the left atrial appendage. ICE can be considered to be used for detection of the thrombus in the left atrial appendage in patients unable to undergo transesophageal echocardiography or those in sinus rhythm for atrial fibrillation ablation.

Application of catheter-based devices

Echocardiographic transponder

Commercial ablation catheters fitted with an echocardiographic transponder have been studied to improve localization of the electrode during radiofrequency ablation procedure in healthy swine ($n = 15$) and the swine model of anteroseptal myocardial infarction ($n = 5$) [33]. The signal is presented on the ICE image in the shape of an arrowhead (Figure 12.46), with the tip of the arrowhead representing the center on the ablation electrode. The findings demonstrate that echocardiographic transponder-guided catheter ablation is feasible and accurate, especially for normal endocardial targets.

Basket catheter

ICE has been used to test and guide positioning of a variety of basket catheters at endocardial targets in different cardiac chambers (Figure 12.47). Real-time ICE imaging provides an important tool for identification of the pole/electrode contact with endocardial tissue and actual localization of each basket poles (Figure 12.48).

References

1 Ren JF, Schwartzman D, Lighty GW, *et al.* Multiplane transesophageal and intracardiac echocardiography in large swine: imaging technique, normal values, and research applications. *Echocardiography* 1997; **14**: 135–147.
2 Seward JB, Khandheria BK, McGregor CGA, Locke TJ, Tajik AJ. Transvascular and intracardiac two-dimensional echocardiography. *Echocardiography* 1990; **7**: 457–464.
3 Valdes-Cruz LM, Sideris E, Sahn DJ, *et al.* Transvascular intracardiac applications of a miniaturized phased-array ultrasonic endoscope: initial experience with intracardiac imaging in piglets. *Circulation* 1991; **83**: 1023–1027.
4 Schwartz SL, Pandian NG, Kumar R, *et al.* Intracardiac echocardiography during simulated aortic and mitral balloon valvuloplasty: *in vivo* experimental studies. *Am Heart J* 1992; **123**: 665–674.
5 Seward JB, Packer DL, Chan RC, Curley M, Tajik AJ. Ultrasound cardioscopy: embarking on a new journey. *Mayo Clin Proc* 1996; **71**: 629–635.
6 Ren JF, Schwarttzman D, Michele JJ, *et al.* Lower frequency (5 MHz) intracardiac echocardiography in a large swine model: imaging views and research applications. *Ultrasound in Med & Biol* 1997; **23**: 871–877.
7 Chu E, Kalman JM, Kwasman MA, *et al.* Intracardiac echocardiography during radiofrequency catheter ablation of cardiac arrhythmias in humans. *J Am Coll Cardiol* 1994; **24**: 1351–1357.
8 Ren JF, Schwartzman D, Callans D, Marchlinski FE, Gottlieb CD, Chaudhry FA. Imaging technique and clinical utility for electrophysiologic procedures of lower frequency (9 MHz) intracardiac echocardiography. *Am J Cardiol* 1998; **82**: 1557–1560.
9 Packer DL, Stevens CL, Curley MG, *et al.* Intracardiac phased-array imaging: methods and initial clinical experience with high resolution, under blood visualization–initial experience with intracardiac phased-array ultrasound. *J Am Coll Cardiol* 2002; **39**: 509–516.
10 Ren JF, Marchlinski FE, Callans DJ, Herrmann HC. Clinical use of AcuNav diagnostic ultrasound catheter imaging during left heart radiofrequency ablation and

transcatheter closure procedures. *J Am Soc Echocardiogr* 2002; **15**: 1301–1308.

11 Jacobson JT, Ren JF, Michele JJ, Lazar S, Callans DJ. Intracardiac echocardiography for detection of left atrial appendage thrombus.(abstr) *Heart Rhythm* 2005; 2: 5312.

12 Schwartzman D, Ren JF, Devine WA, Callans DJ. Cardiac swelling associated with linear radiofrequency ablation in the atrium. *J Interventional Cardiac Electrophysiol* 2001; **5**: 159–166.

13 Eldar M, Ohad D, Bor A, Varda-Bloom N, Swanson DK, Battler A. A closed-chest pig model of sustained ventricular tachycardia. *Pacing Clin Electrophysiol* 1994; **17**: 1603–1609.

14 Callans DJ, Ren JF, Michele J, Marchlinski FE, Dillon SM. Electroanatomic left ventricular mapping in the porcine model of healed anterior myocardial infarction: correlation with intracardiac echocardiography and pathological analysis. *Circulation* 1999; **100**: 1744–2750.

15 Ren JF, Callans DJ, Schwartzman D, Michele JJ, Marchlinski FE. Changes in local wall thickness correlate with pathologic lesion size following radiofrequency catheter ablation: an intracardiac echocardiographic imaging study. *Echocardiography* 2001; **18**: 503–507.

16 Ren JF, Callans DJ, Michele JJ, Dillon SM, Marchlinski FE. Intracardiac echocardiographic evaluation of ventricular mural swelling from radiofrequency ablation in chronic myocardial infarction: irrigated-tip versus standard catheter. *J Interventional Cardiac Electrophysiol* 2001; **5**: 27–32.

17 Callans DJ, Ren JF, Narula N, Michele J, Marchlinski FE, Dillon SM. Effects of linear, irrigated-tip radiofrequency ablation in porcine healed anterior infarction. *J Cardiovasc Electrophysiol* 2001; **12**: 1037–1042.

18 Ren JF, Schwartzman D, Brode SE, *et al.* Intracardiac echocardiographic monitoring for morphologic changes in radiofrequency ablation atrial lesions: *in vivo* validation and initial clinical observations. *Circulation* 1997; **96**: 1–22.

19 Ren JF, Schwartzman D, Michele JJ, *et al.* Intracardiac echocardiographic quantification of atrial wall thickness changes associated with radiofrequency ablation. *J Am Coll Cardiol* 1998; **31**: 259A.

20 Schwartzman D, Michele JJ, Trankiem CT, Ren JF. Electrogram-guided radiofrequency catheter ablation of atrial tissue: comparison with thermometry-guide ablation. *J Interventional Cardiac Electrophysiol* 2001; **5**: 253–266.

21 Ren JF, Schwartzman D, Brode SE, Callans DJ, Chaudhry FA, Marchlinski FE. Right atrial mural swelling and its effect on adjacent great vessels from linear radiofrequency ablation for atrial fibrillation (abstr). *J Am Coll Cardiol* 1999; **33**: 137A.

22 Ren JF, Schwartzman D, Brode SE. Evolution of right pulmonary vein lumen narrowing after right atrial linear radiofrequency ablation (abstr). *J Am Coll Cardiol* 1999; **33**: 137A–138A.

23 Ren JF, Callans DJ, Michele J, Marchlinski FE. Intracardiac echocardiographic quantification of changes in wall thickness and ventricular function associated with radiofrequency ablation in chronic myocardial infarction (abstr). *J Am Coll Cardiol* 1999; **33**: 140A.

24 Inoue H, Waller BF, Zipes DP. Intracoronary ethylalcohol or phenol injection ablates acontine-induced ventricular tachycardia in dogs. *J Am Coll Cardiol* 1987; **10**: 1342–1349.

25 Brugada P, deSwart H, Smeets JL, Wellens HJ. Transcoronary chemical ablation of ventricular tachycardia. *Circulation* 1989; **79**: 475–482.

26 Kay GN, Bubien RS, Dailey SM, Epstein AE, Plumb VJ. A prospective evaluation of intracoronary ethanol ablation of the atrioventricular conduction system. *J Am Coll Cardiol* 1991; **17**: 1634–1640.

27 Sneddon JF, Ward DE, Simpson IA, Linker NJ, Wainwright RJ, Camm AJ. Alcohol ablation of atrioventricular conduction. *Br Heart J* 1991; **65**: 143–147.

28 Qi XQ, Sun RL, Tang CJ, *et al.* Transcoronary ethanol ablation of experimental ventricular tachycardia after epicardial ice mapping and localizing. *Chinese Med J* 1991; **104**: 639–644.

29 Knight C, Kurbaan AS, Seggewiss H,, *et al.* Nonsurgical septal reduction therapy for hypertrophic obstructive cardiomyopathy: outcome in the first series of patients. *Circulation* 1997; **95**: 2075–2081.

30 Seggewiss H, Gleichmann U, Faber L, Fassbender D, Schmidt HK, Strick S. Percutaneous transluminal septal myocardial ablation in hypertrophic obstructive cardiomyopathy: acute results and 3 month follow-up in 25 patients. *J Am Coll Cardiol* 1998; **31**: 252–258.

31 Lakkis NM, Nagueh SF, Kleiman NS, *et al.* Echocardiography-guided ethanol septal reduction for hypertrophic obstructive cardiomyopathy. *Circulation* 1998; **98**: 1750–1755.

32 Callans DJ, Ren JF, Narula N, *et al.* Left ventricular catheter ablation using direct, intramural ethanol injection in swine. *J Interventional Cardiac Electrophysiol* 2002; **6**: 225–231.

33 Menz V, Vilkomerson D, Ren JF, Michele JJ, Schwartzman D. Echocardiographic transponder-guided catheter ablation feasibility and accuracy. *J Interventional Cardiac Electrophysiol* 2001; **5**: 203–209.

Index

NOTE: Page numbers in italics refer to figures, and tables